ONCOLOGY CERTIFIED NURSE (OCN®) REVIEW

Denise Menonna-Quinn, DNP, RN, NPD-BC, AOCNS, BMTCN, earned her master's degree in clinical nursing from Seton Hall University, South Orange, New Jersey, and DNP degree at William Paterson University, Wayne, New Jersey. Dr. Menonna-Quinn is a classroom and clinical instructor at several colleges and universities in northern New Jersey; however, she has made her greatest contribution to nursing in the clinical arena. She has dedicated her more than 30-year clinical career to the care of oncology patients, holding a variety of roles including staff nurse, clinical nurse specialist, breast cancer nurse coordinator, education specialist, insurance nurse navigator for melanoma patients seeking bone marrow transplants, and ambulatory chemotherapy administration nurse. She brings deep passion and compassion to the care of complex oncology patients, resulting in trusting and meaningful nurse–patient relationships. Dr. Menonna-Quinn also has extensive experience developing and leading review courses for the OCN and Advanced Oncology Certified Clinical Nurse Specialist exams.

Oncology Certified Nurse (OCN®) Review

Denise Menonna-Quinn DNP, RN, NPD-BC, AOCNS, BMTCN

Education Specialist, Oncology Division

Hackensack Meridian Healthcare System

Hackensack, New Jersey

Nursing Faculty Professor, Ameritech
College of Healthcare

Draper, Utah

Adjunct Clinical Professor, Felician University

Rutherford, New Jersey

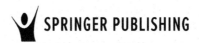
SPRINGER PUBLISHING

Springer Publishing Company, LLC
11 West 42nd Street, New York, NY 10036
www.springerpub.com
connect.springerpub.com/

Acquisitions Editor: Adrianne Brigido
Compositor: Integra

ISBN: 9780826138835
ebook ISBN: 9780826138842
DOI: 10.1891/9780826138842

23 24 25 / 6 5 4 3 2

ONCC® and OCN® are registered trademarks of the Oncology Nursing Certification Corporation. The Oncology Nursing Certification Corporation does not sponsor or endorse this resource, nor does it have a proprietary relationship or other affiliation with Springer Publishing Company.

The author and the publisher of this Work have made every effort to use sources believed to be reliable to provide information that is accurate and compatible with the standards generally accepted at the time of publication. Because medical science is continually advancing, our knowledge base continues to expand. Therefore, as new information becomes available, changes in procedures become necessary. We recommend that the reader always consult current research and specific institutional policies before performing any clinical procedure or delivering any medication. The author and publisher shall not be liable for any special, consequential, or exemplary damages resulting, in whole or in part, from the readers' use of, or reliance on, the information contained in this book. The publisher has no responsibility for the persistence or accuracy of URLs for external or third-party Internet websites referred to in this publication and does not guarantee that any content on such websites is, or will remain, accurate or appropriate.

LCCN: 2021920541

Contact sales@springerpub.com to receive discount rates on bulk purchases.

Publisher's Note: **New and used products purchased from third-party sellers are not guaranteed for quality, authenticity, or access to any included digital components**.

Printed in the United States of America by Hatteras Inc.

For Adrianne Brigido, with genuine gratitude and warm regard. This book would not have come to fruition without her unwavering support, spirited encouragement, and confidence in my abilities. In a time of unprecedented and seemingly insurmountable challenges, Adrianne's kindness, compassion, and inspiration were the driving forces that led me to accomplish my goal of writing an OCN® review book. It was her "voice" that gave me the strength and fortitude to continue to research, write, and edit. I am forever grateful that our paths have crossed. Thank you for being you!

Contents

PART IV. SYMPTOM MANAGEMENT AND ONCOLOGIC EMERGENCIES   247

Contributors

Kathleen D. Clark DNP, RN, RN-BC
Assistant Director of Nursing Faculty
Ameritech College of Healthcare
Draper, Utah
Chapter 33. Practice Test
Chapter 34. Practice Test: Answers With Rationales

Carmela Cuccurullo, AGPCNP-BC
Nurse Practitioner, Multiple Myeloma Division
Tisch Cancer Center
Mount Sinai Hospital
New York, New York
Chapter 19. Multiple Myeloma

Mai-Fung Ho-Law, MSN, RN, OCN
Clinical Level 4 Oncology Nurse, Multiple Myeloma Division
John Theurer Cancer Center
Hackensack Meridian Healthcare System
Hackensack, New Jersey
Chapter 21. Hematologic Side Effects
Chapter 22. Pulmonary Side Effects
Chapter 23. Cardiovascular Side Effects

Jenna M. Forsythe MSN, RN, AOCNS, OCN
Nurse Specialist, Oncology Division
Hackensack University Medical Center
Hackensack Meridan Healthcare System
Hackensack, New Jersey
Chapter 28. Cancer Survivorship
Chapter 33. Practice Test
Chapter 34. Practice Test: Answers With Rationales

Jolanta Jakubowska, MSN, NP-C
Nurse Practitioner
Gastrointestinal Division, Mount Sinai Cancer Center
Mount Sinai Hospital
New York, New York
Chapter 13. Gastrointestinal Cancers

Mary Leban, MEd, MSN, APN, FNP-BC, ONC, PMGT-BC, CNE
Assistant Professor
Phillips School of Nursing
Mount Sinai Beth Israel
New York, New York
Chapter 27. Oncologic Emergencies

Laura Linse MS, BSN, RN
Primary RN The Moffitt Center
Malignant Hematology
Tampa, Florida
Chapter 6. Treatment Modalities for Malignancies
Chapter 29. End-of-Life Care

Gina Lione, BSN, RN
Oncology Nurse, Lymphoma and Leukemia Division
John Theurer Cancer Center
Hackensack Meridian Healthcare System
Hackensack, New Jersey
Chapter 31. Cancer and Sexual Health

Gabriella Gadaleta Magarelli RN, ACNP-BC
Nurse Practitioner, Lymphoma Division
Regional Cancer Care Associates
Hackensack, New Jersey
Chapter 18. Lymphoma

Phyllis McKiernan, MSN, RN, APN, OCN
Nurse Practitioner, Bone Marrow Transplant Division
John Theurer Cancer
Hackensack Meridian Healthcare
Hackensack, New Jersey
Chapter 7. Hematopoietic Stem Cell Transplantation

Patricia V. Newton, DNP, MSN, BBA, RN, CMSRN
Adjunct Professor, RN-BSN Program
Ameritech College of Healthcare
Draper, Utah
Chapter 16. Head and Neck and Thyroid Cancers

Joanne Pasinski, MSN, RN, CCRN, CNL
Clinical Level 4 Nurse
Hackensack Meridian Healthcare System
Hackensack, New Jersey
Chapter 30. Psychosocial Issues Related to Oncology Patients

Kaitlin Pasinski, MS
Vocational Counselor
The Arc of Bergen and Passaic Counties
Hackensack, New Jersey
Chapter 30. Psychosocial Issues Related to Oncology Patients

Kimberly Rivera DNP, RN-BC, OCN, NPD-BC
Specialty Clinician
Baptist Health South Florida
Boca Raton Regional Hospital
Boca Raton, Florida
Chapter 33. Practice Test
Chapter 34. Practice Test: Answers With Rationales

Jayshree Shah, MSN, RN, FPN-C, AOCNP, BSN, BS
Oncology Nurse Educator
AstraZeneca
Hackensack, New Jersey
Chapter 24. Gastrointestinal Side Effects

Anne Marie Shaftic DNP, AOCNP, OCN
Nurse Practitioner
New Jersey Cancer and Blood Associates
Haskell, New Jersey
Chapter 26. Neurological Side Effects

Rebecca Testi MSN, RN, APN, OCN
Nurse Practitioner, Leukemia Division
John Theurer Cancer Center
Hackensack Meridian Healthcare System
Hackensack, New Jersey
Chapter 17. Leukemia

Kristin Wilks, DNP, RN, OCN
Nurse Manager
Regional Cancer Care Associates
North Bergen, New Jersey
Chapter 6. Treatment Modalities for Malignancies
Chapter 32. Standards of Professional Performance
Chapter 33. Practice Test
Chapter 34. Practice Test: Answers With Rationales

Kara Yannotti MSN, MMH, BSN, OCN, CCPR
Oncology Educator
Holy Name Medical Center
Teaneck, New Jersey
Chapter 8. Research and Clinical Trials
Chapter 33. Practice Test
Chapter 34. Practice Test: Answers With Rationales

Preface

Welcome to *Oncology Certified Nurse (OCN®) Review*. This comprehensive print + digital resource is designed to help you study effectively and efficiently for the oncology nursing certification exam developed by the Oncology Nursing Certification Corporation. Each chapter, authored by expert oncology nurses and nurse practitioners, addresses topics on the OCN® exam blueprint with Exam Tips, Key Facts, quick-reference tables, useful illustrations, and end-of-chapter questions to assess knowledge retention. The review concludes with a full 165-question practice test. With more than 300 exam-style practice questions in total, detailed review content and answer rationales, and a convenient print + digital package, *Oncology Certified Nurse (OCN®) Review* gives you the tools you need to study your way and the confidence to pass the first time, guaranteed!

Readers receive 6 months' free digital access to the interactive digital version on ExamPrepConnect (see access details on inside front cover). Features include:

- All of the high-quality content from the book, including the full reference lists and bibliographies
- Personalized study plan based on exam date
- Ability to study by topic area to identify strengths and weaknesses
- Full timed practice tests that simulate the test-taking environment
- Discussion board to connect with your exam-prep community
- Games to make studying fun

It is my hope that this book proves to be a valuable resource as you prepare for success on your certification exam.

Denise Menonna-Quinn

Pass Guarantee

If you use this resource to prepare for your exam and you do not pass, you may return it for a refund of your full purchase price. To receive a refund, you must return your product along with a copy of your original receipt and exam score report. Product must be returned and received within 180 days of the original purchase date. This excludes tax, shipping, and handling. One offer per person and address. Refunds will be issued within 8 weeks from acceptance and approval. This offer is valid for U.S. residents only. Void where prohibited. To initiate a refund, please contact customer service at CS@springerpub.com.

Part I
Certification and Exam Information

Oncology Nursing Certification

INTRODUCTION

Congratulations on making the decision to pursue your certification in oncology nursing. Oncology nursing practice encompasses numerous nursing arenas, including medical, surgical, and critical care. Choosing to pursue certification requires commitment, determination, time, patience, and strategic planning, and the benefits to both oncology nurses and their employers are significant. While certification is an individual decision, healthcare organizations support and highly encourage nurses to pursue specialty certification, particularly hospitals and healthcare networks that hold Magnet® status. Nurse managers and educators often help oncology nurses pursue their oncology certification. In some cases, organizations will provide a financial reward for successfully completing the certification process. Please consult with your current employer and review their certification policies and procedures.

There are many benefits and reasons for obtaining certification in oncology nursing, including:

- Personal growth
- Professional growth
- Increased compensation and career mobility
- Commitment to the specialty and oncology patients
- Validation of competencies and skills
- Organizational requirements: clinical ladder requirements, Magnet, and individual unit

ONCOLOGY NURSING CERTIFICATION

The Oncology Nursing Certification Corporation (ONCC®) is a nonprofit organization that develops and administers the Oncology Certified Nurse (OCN®) certification examination and other related certifications. The OCN® credential symbolizes advanced knowledge of oncology practice, focus on the provision of the highest quality and safe care, and the nurse's ability to:

- Provide direct patient care, including the administration of chemotherapy and biotherapy agents
- Counsel and provide emotional support to the patient and family
- Identify and manage side effects and provide effective patient education
- Act as a clinical resource and advocate for the patient and family

---

The bibliography and references for this chapter are available on ExamPrepConnect; see inside front cover for access instructions.

► ELIGIBILITY REQUIREMENTS

To qualify to take the OCN® exam, the nurse must meet all of the following eligibility requirements:

1. A current, unrestricted RN license in the United States and its territories or Canada at the time of application and examination

2. A minimum of 2 years of experience as an RN within the 4 years prior to application

3. A minimum of 2,000 hours of adult oncology nursing practice within the 4 years prior to application (practice can include clinical practice, nursing administration, education, research, or consultation)

4. A minimum of 10 contact hours of nursing continuing education in oncology within the 3 years prior to application (a maximum of 5 of the 10 required contact hours may be continuing medical education (CME) in oncology)

► APPLICATION PROCESS

Applicants may submit an online application. Approved applicants will receive an Authorization to Test (ATT) notification within 2 weeks of applying, which will include a 90-day testing window. The ATT notification will include information on how to schedule an exam appointment at a PSI Testing Center. The exam fee is $296 for members of the Oncology Nursing Society (ONS) or Association of Pediatric Hematology/Oncology Nurses (APHON), and $416 for nonmembers. Complete application process and fee details are available on the ONCC website.

► ABOUT THE EXAMINATION

The OCN® exam is 3 hours and consists of 165 multiple-choice questions with four answer options. You must select the single best answer. Only 145 questions are scored, and the remaining 20 questions are used as pre-test items. It is impossible to know which questions are scored, so be sure to answer all questions to the best of your ability.

The exam is based upon the OCN® content outline, which outlines the exam domain areas and topics that will be covered on the exam. This should serve as a guide for the oncology nurse to develop a study plan. Each domain is given a percentage to indicate the total number of related questions the nurse can expect to encounter on the exam. The higher the percentage, the greater the number of questions on that topic. For example, the exam will have more questions related to the Symptom Management and Palliative Care domain than the Psychosocial Dimensions of Care domain. See Table 1.1 for OCN® exam domains and question distribution. For the full list of exam subject areas, refer to the test content outline on the ONCC website.

Table 1.1 OCN® Exam Domains and Question Distribution

Exam Domain	Percentage of Questions
Care Continuum	19%
Oncology Nursing Practice	17%
Treatment Modalities	19%
Symptom Management and Palliative Care	23%
Oncologic Emergencies	12%
Psychosocial Dimensions of Care	10%

Source: Data from Oncology Nursing Certification Corporation. Oncology Certified Nurse (OCN®) Test Content Outline. 2018. https://www.oncc.org/files/2018OCNTestContentOutline.pdf

▶ **EXAM TIP**

Review the OCN® Test Content Outline prior to developing a study plan.

SCORING OF OCN® EXAMINATION

The OCN® exam is calculated based on a scaled score. A scaled score is the transformation of a raw score, which represents the number of correct items into a different unit of measurement. For example, two common standardized tests that utilize a scaled score system are the ACT and SAT examinations. The required passing scaled score of the OCN® examination is 55.

▶ MAINTENANCE AND RENEWAL OF CERTIFICATION

The OCN® certification is valid for 4 years. To qualify for renewal, the nurse must have a current, active, and unencumbered RN license. There are three different renewal options:

1. Practice Hours and Professional Development (Points)
2. Practice Hours and Successful Testing
3. Points and Successful Testing

The majority of nurses review with practice hours and professional development (points), which does not require them to retake the certification exam. The point system is based on the initial learning assessment that is completed after successfully passing the first exam. The learning assessment will be sent by ONCC to the oncology nurse will all the details of the process. It is important to pay special attention to all the details to ensure the ability to collect the necessary data and paperwork to renew. Regardless of the method, necessary information should be sent to ONCC according to renewal deadlines to ensure that there is no lapse in certification. In the event that the renewal deadline is missed, the nurse can apply to be reinstated (fee required). To reinstate via the points system, the points must be earned and provided by December 31 of the year of expiration.

The bibliography and references for this chapter are available on ExamPrepConnect; see inside front cover for access instructions.

Exam Preparation

● DEVELOPING A STUDY PLAN

▶ STEP 1: DETERMINE LEARNING STYLE

Nurses preparing for the OCN® examination should create a solid study plan and foundation of information. The first step is to explore and understand individual learning styles to determine how knowledge can best be learned and retained. Most learners use a combination of the learning styles, including:

- Visual/spatial: The learner needs to see the information presented via written material and in images. Reading is a form of visual learning.
- Auditory/verbal: The learner needs to hear the information presented by another person or repeat the information themselves. Auditory learners often read aloud the study questions.
- Psychomotor: The learner needs to use their body, hands, and sense of touch. This is a style that can be used when learning a new task or physical procedure in nursing.
- Logical/mathematical learning style: The learner needs to use logic and reasoning techniques to identify patterns and connections between information. A logical learner is more concerned with understanding the information and process than memorizing the information.
- Social/interpersonal: The learner needs to study with partners or in groups.
- Solitary/intrapersonal learning style: The learner needs to study alone without distraction.

▶ STEP 2: DEFINE STUDY TIMELINE

The second step is to develop a clear, concise study timeline based on the extent of oncology experience and overall confidence taking standardized tests. For an experienced oncology nurse who feels comfortable with the material and taking standardized tests, 3 months of study prior to the examination should be sufficient. For a new oncology nurse, a study timeline of up to 6 months is recommended. It is better to take more time to study than rush to take the examination and not be successful.

▶ STEP 3: IDENTIFY STUDY TOPICS

Once the general study timeline has been established, the next step is to develop the study plan. This begins by thoroughly reviewing the OCN® exam content outline available on the Oncology Nursing Certification Corporation website. The learner should then engage in a detailed self-assessment to determine difficult topic areas and areas of strength and weakness. This is essential because the most difficult areas should be studied first, as it ensures that there is plenty of time to master those areas, which will help to build confidence.

Estimate the number of days it will take to adequately review study for each of the domains and key topic areas on the exam. This time estimate (hours or days) should be enough time to completely digest and understand the study materials. For example, a reader may set aside 3 to 5 days to review oncologic emergencies and 1 to 2 days to review information related to prevention. Set a goal for when you hope to finish studying each domain are on the exam. Deadlines help to maintain motivation and keep the learner on track.

Another technique that is helpful in studying is journaling with positive self-talk. Journaling is a great stress reliever and can provide mental and physical health benefits. A journaling method that is recommended for individuals studying for examination is bullet journaling or personal planning. Personal planning journaling helps to maintain the study schedule, as well as to provide an environment for positive self-talk and affirmations such as, "I will pass the OCN exam." Also, practice writing your full name with OCN credentials. These techniques are motivating and provide confidence during the studying process.

▶ STEP 4: MASTER ANSWERING PRACTICE QUESTIONS

QUESTION LOG

First, it is important to manage the practice-question process as well as progress. A strategy that has been successful with previous students is to use a notebook or computer-based log to keep track of difficult questions during the study process. Note question number (if relevant), the topic, and why it was challenging. This will help identify review content that needs to be further studied. When you encounter a difficult practice question, before trying to answer it or guess, STOP and research the topic. Then return to the question, determine the correct answer, and then write the information in the tracking log. This is a more efficient means of study and knowledge retention and will help to prevent frustrations that can arise when answering questions incorrectly.

At the end of studying the practice questions, the log will serve as an individual personal study guide to the questions that were difficult and act as an individual review specific to the weakest areas that should be studied prior to the examination.

QUESTION ANALYSIS

Exams with multiple-choice questions require the learner to recognize exactly what the question is asking. Closely review the stem of the question (the scenario or information presented in the question) and the lead-in (the actual question or statement). Identify whether the question is a simple recall or "fact" question. For example: "Which of the following medications is used to decrease nausea and vomiting?" All that is required is for the learner to understand anti-nausea medications available.

Some questions will require critical thinking and application of knowledge. For example: "A new nurse is assigned to a bone marrow transplant patient who is experiencing shaking chills after the infusion of stem cells. What measures will the nurse anticipate performing?" This question requires the nurse to be prepared for the next step, which is based upon the knowledge of stem-cell infusion reactions.

The learner must then decipher whether the question is looking for the correct or incorrect response. These types of questions can be difficult and require a close reading of the stem and lead-in. Pay attention to the use of "EXCEPT" or "NOT," which indicates that the incorrect response is required. For example, "The nurse is teaching the patient and family members home care instructions regarding post care of chemotherapy administration. The patient received their first cycle of doxorubicin and cyclophosphamide for the treatment of breast cancer. The nurse will include all of the following in the teaching, EXCEPT:"

The question is asking for what not to do. This question requires the nurse to know the side-effect profile of the chemotherapy agents and how to relay the information in the form of patient teaching. Then, the nurse needs to identify what statement would not be included in the teaching.

ANSWER SELECTION

To choose the correct multiple-choice response, first narrow down the choices to two options. Choices with qualifiers such as "commonly" and "possibly" are more likely correct. Choices with absolutes such as "always," "none, or "never" are typically distractors. The rationale for not selecting an absolute is that in nursing no situation is an always, none, or never, especially when dealing with patients and healthcare. Look for common elements within the question and choices to identify clues. If a choice does not align with the facts presented in the stem, then it is probably wrong. Most importantly, read each answer choice before jumping to select an answer.

● PREPARING FOR THE EXAM

▶ THE NIGHT BEFORE THE EXAM

All of the studying should be done by this point—no cramming! The most you should do is read over any notes regarding difficult topics. Gather all necessary supplies for the examination, but do not bring any study materials. Most importantly, eat a healthy balanced meal and get a good night's sleep.

▶ THE MORNING OF THE EXAM

Wake early to ensure you have enough time to prepare for the day without rushing or stress. Eat a balanced breakfast of protein and carbohydrate. Avoid sugar-filled cereals and/or breakfast bars. Drink the same amount of caffeine that you would normally have in the morning—no more, no less. Excessive caffeine can cause jitteriness and the need to urinate, and a reduction in caffeine may cause withdrawal and a headache. Wear comfortable clothing and dress in layers to maintain a comfortable temperature during the examination.

Additional tips on what to expect:

1. Plan to arrive at least 30 minutes prior to the testing time. Late arrivals will not be accepted.
2. Prepare to be scanned with a metal detector wand. Pants will be raised above the ankles, and sleeves will be raised above the wrist. Pockets will be pulled inside out for inspection.
3. Only a wedding band and/or engagement rings are acceptable; no other jewelry is allowed. Eyeglasses may be worn, but they will be inspected.
4. Bring two forms of current, valid ID: one primary form and one secondary form or two primary forms (Table 2.1).
5. Only soft earplugs are allowed in the testing center.
6. Scratch paper will be provided; however, it will be collected before leaving the testing area.
7. The following items are prohibited:
   - Weapons of any type
   - Cold weather clothing (e.g., hats, gloves)
   - Purses, briefcases, cell phones, recording devices, and cameras
   - Food, drinks, or gum
   - Study guides, educational, or written material

Table 2.1 Appropriate Forms of Identification

Primary ID (must include photo and signature)	Secondary ID (must include signature)
■ Passport or Passport Card ■ Government-issued driver's license or learner's permit ■ National/state/country or government-issued local language ID ■ Military ID (including spouse/dependent) ■ Alien Registration Card (Green Card, Permanent Resident Visa) ■ Employee or school ID	■ U.S. Social Security Card ■ Debit/ATM card ■ Credit card ■ RN license

Source: Data from https://www.oncc.org/find-test-center

Key Facts

- There are no scheduled breaks during the examination. If you need to leave the room, the clock will not be stopped.
- If you do leave the room, no cells phones or electronic devices are allowed during the break.
- All security procedures need to be re-addressed before returning to the testing room.
- Excessive breaks during the examination will be reported to ONCC.

TEST-TAKING TIPS

1. Carefully read the directions and pay attention to any information provided by the testing center. Once settled at the computer terminal, read the directions on how to navigate through the test and be sure to understand how to review the answers before submitting the final test.
2. It is imperative to watch the time and keep track of the clock on the screen that displays the amount of time remaining.
3. Choose your answers carefully, but do not waste too much time on one question. If you are unsure about the answer, leave it blank and return to it before the end of the test.
4. Use your best judgment and follow your intuition. Your first instinct is often the correct answer; however, ensure that you understand EXACTLY what the test question is asking before selecting a response.
5. Do not change an answer unless you are close to 100% sure that it is not the correct response. In some circumstances, it can be counterproductive to change an answer, especially if you are struggling with the test.
6. Do not answer questions based on your personal individual practice. Each organization has different policies and procedures, as well as study protocols, different clinical settings, and provider preferences in caring for oncology patients. Therefore, it is vital that you use the academic information that you used to study to answer questions. In practice, you will be exposed to many chemotherapy and biotherapy agents, procedures and techniques that are current, and cutting-edge treatments that have not yet been added to the exam blueprint and test bank. Practice is usually ahead of testing.

Becoming certified requires self-confidence and dedication. The most effective way to build self-confidence is to study thoroughly and be prepared. The following chapters will provide you with review content and practice questions necessary to understand the exam topics and apply your knowledge to the exam. Develop your plan, know your strengths and weaknesses, STUDY, and PRACTICE, PRACTICE and PRACTICE.

Part II
Foundations of Oncology Practice

Health Promotion and Disease Prevention Concepts

INTRODUCTION

Epidemiology is the method used to find the causes of health outcomes and diseases in populations. Essentially, it is the study of how often a disease is present in specific groups of individuals, as well as the reason why the disease occurs. The information obtained from epidemiology allows healthcare professionals to develop plans and strategies to prevent diseases and manage the disease in those individuals who have been affected. There are two terms related to cancer epidemiology that are important to understand: prevalence and incidence. *Prevalence* refers to the proportion of diagnosis of cancer within a population at a given time (i.e., how widespread the disease is). *Incidence* is the rate of individuals who develop cancer during a particular time period and the risks of developing the disease.

The American Cancer Society (ACS) is a leader in researching and studying epidemiology. Each year the ACS publishes the *Cancer Facts & Figures*, which provides the most current information related to cancer developments within the year. Race, age, and gender all play a vital role in the development of cancer and the risks related to cancers.

Epidemiology also addresses *death rates*. The ACS *Cancer Facts & Figures 2021* estimated that there was an estimated 1.9 million new cancer cases diagnosed and 608,570 cancer deaths in the United States in 2021. Each disease has specific death rates.

> ### ▶ EXAM TIP
>
> Take time to review the ACS *Cancer Facts & Figures* for the current year and prior year before taking the certification exam.

CANCER-RELATED STATISTICS

Heart disease still remains the leading cause of death in the United States, and cancer is the second leading cause of death in the United States. According to the ACS (2019), more than 15.5 million Americans have had a history of some form of cancer. Many of these Americans have no evidence of the disease. Approximately 80% of the cancers in the United States will be diagnosed in individuals over the age of 55 years. It is important to be aware that the growing elderly population (individuals over the age of 85) is at increased risk of numerous types of cancers. However, screening is not recommended for this patient population since the risk of harm from treatments outweighs the benefits after the age of 75 years. ACS (2019) projected that by the year 2030, the average remaining life expectancy at the age of 65 will be 20 years for men and 22 years for women. Table 3.1 describes the top four newly diagnosed cancers in men and women.

The bibliography and references for this chapter are available on ExamPrepConnect; see inside front cover for access instructions.

Table 3.1 The Top Four Newly Diagnosed Cancers for Men and Women (2021)

Male		Female	
Disease Site	**Percentage of Cases**	**Disease Site**	**Percentage of Cases**
Prostate	26%	Breast	30%
Lung and bronchus	12%	Lung and bronchus	13%
Colon and rectum	8%	Colon and rectum	8%
Urinary/bladder	7%	Uterine corpus	7%

Source: Adapted from ACS. (2021). *Cancer Facts and Figures.* https://www.cancer.org/content/dam/cancer-org/research/cancer-facts-and-statistics/annual-cancer-facts-and-figures/2021/cancer-facts-and-figures-2021.pdf

▶ SURVIVAL RATES

Survival rates have dramatically changed since the early 1960s from 39% to 70% among the white population and 27% to 63% among the Black population. These increased rates of survival can be directly related to early-detection practices, early diagnosis, and vast improvements in oncology treatments, including biotherapy, targeted therapy, and new diagnostic markers. Actual survival rates differ according to the specific oncology disease, stage of disease, age of the patient, and other comorbidities of the patient. See the ACS *Cancer Facts & Figures* for additional information.

● HEALTH PROMOTION

Health promotion is the process of enabling people to increase control over, and to improve, their own health and is an important factor for all individuals. In addition, it moves beyond a focus on individual behavior toward a wide range of social and environmental interventions for populations. Health promotion does not focus on individuals who are at risk for specific diseases.

It is imperative to understand that health promotion is not the sole responsibility of healthcare professionals. Health promotion concepts have also been adopted by the government as an important issue to be addressed, monitored, and reinforced. Health promotion encompasses a holistic approach that includes physical, mental, and social well-being. Health is viewed as a requirement for everyday living and not a goal of living. The following resources must be available to have a solid foundation of health: peace, basic living requirements (e.g., housing, food, water), education, social balances, and financial resources.

▶ OTTAWA CONFERENCE FOR HEALTH PROMOTION

In 1986, the first Ottawa Conference on the Assessment of Competence in Medicine and the Healthcare Professions was held in Ottawa, Canada. It presented a charter to create action to achieve health for all individuals by the year 2000 and beyond. The international conference was established as a direct result of the growing need for a public health movement around the globe. At the conference, the participants made a pledge of commitment to health. The following elements are included in the pledge:

1. Develop healthy public policy and concise political commitment to health.
2. Avoid pressure to use harmful products.
3. Decrease unhealthy living conditions.
4. Promote proper nutrition.

5. Focus on addressing pollution and occupational hazards.
6. Address the inequities of heath within societies.
7. Recognize that people are the main health resource and support them in their endeavor to remain healthy and offer the appropriate resources.
8. Educate the public, healthcare professionals, and other disciplines on the importance of health promotion.
9. Acknowledge the importance of health and health maintenance as a social challenge as well as vital investment.

Since the inception of the conference, there have been many more conferences over the past two decades. It is important to understand that the health promotion plans and strategies identified in the pledge are continually being addressed and evaluated. See Box 3.1 for examples of health promotion programs.

Box 3.1 Examples of Heath Promotion Programs

- Urban and rural health programs
- Health literacy programs
- Breastfeeding for newborns
- Proper nutritional programs (decrease obesity)
- Sudden infant death syndrome prevention and education
- Injury prevention (e.g., use of seatbelts, car seats, and helmets)
- Promoting physical activity
- Smoking cessation programs

▶ HEALTHY PEOPLE 2030

To combat the risk of cancer and promote health for all Americans, the U.S. government developed *Healthy People 2020*, which was a 10-year plan of complete national objectives and health goals for all Americans. *Healthy People 2020* encompassed 42 topics with more than 1,200 objectives. *Healthy People 2030* includes a smaller set of objectives that are divided into 355 core objectives, 114 developmental objectives, and 40 research objectives.

In addition, *Healthy People* includes a subset of leading health indicators (LHIs) that focus on high-priority health issues. The LHIs are divided into the following categories: access to health services; clinical preventive services; environmental quality; injury and violence; maternal, infant, and child health; mental health; and nutrition, physical activity, and obesity. These health indicators are monitored and tracked on a regular basis to determine if improvement and/or detectable changes have been met. The Office of Disease Prevention and Health Promotion (2014) noted that progress had been made with indicators that are directly related to cancer, namely that:

- Fewer adults are smoking cigarettes.
- Fewer children are exposed to secondhand smoke.
- Adults are more physically active.
- Fewer adolescents are engaging in alcohol and drug use.

However, in some cases, the indicators for health promotion are worsening, and new strategies are being discussed to potentially meet the goals (*Healthy People 2020*).

There have been tremendous improvements within the past decade in relation to increased birth rates and death rates from heart disease and strokes. Although great strides have been made, health promotion remains a challenge and is a constant process for all healthcare professionals and policy makers.

PREVENTION

Prevention is a term that addresses a large range of techniques aimed at reducing the threats and risks to an individual's health. The goal of prevention is to avoid a disease before it begins. According to the ACS (2019), approximately 42% of new diagnoses of cancer (approximately 740,000 cases) are potentially preventable. The CDC (2019) developed a prevention framework that includes the following:

1. **Local prevention:** An example is the development of safe bike paths for cyclists.
2. **State prevention:** Examples include the regulations and inspections of food services and community swimming pools, as well as the disposal of hazardous wastes materials in work environments.
3. **National prevention:** There are numerous programs and initiatives that are developed by various governmental agencies and have a direct and powerful impact on health prevention for Americans. Programs such as Clean Water Act and the National Asthma Control and Tobacco Control Program have been instrumental in addressing national prevention. The government agencies that develop these programs include the U.S. Department of Health and Human Services (HHS), the U.S. Centers for Disease Control and Prevention (CDC), and the U.S. Food and Drug Administration (FDA).

Over the past decade, public health has improved. Improvements include a decrease in lead poisoning cases in children, a reduction in air pollution, and an increase in mandate smoke-free environments, such as work environments, hospitals, restaurants, and bars. The government and associated laws have been instrumental in promoting these improvements to all Americans (CDC, Picture of America).

▶ CANCER PREVENTION

Cancer prevention is characterized by the actions that are taken to reduce the chance of being affected by a cancer diagnosis. Prevention is divided into three categories:

1. **Primary prevention**: Prevention of disease or injury before it occurs (e.g., asbestos ban, use of seatbelts and bike helmets, immunizations against specific diseases)
2. **Secondary prevention**: Early detection of disease or injury and measures to prevent it from worsening (e.g., screening tests and early-detection measures)
3. **Tertiary prevention**: Lessening the impact of existing disease to reduce long-term effects (e.g., rehabilitation, diabetic foot care)

> ▶ **EXAM TIP**
>
> Understand the differences between primary, secondary, and tertiary prevention and memorize several examples of each.

RISK

Another element that is important to understand in relationship to prevention is the analysis of risk. *Risk* can be explained as the likelihood that malignancy will develop after exposure to specific factors that may cause cancer. The following terms are different types of risk related to health promotion.

- **Relative Risk (RR)**: Also known as the *risk ratio*, it is the risk of cancer between groups—one group exposed to a particular factor and the other unexposed to that factor. For example, when investigating the risk of lung cancer among factory workers, individuals would be divided into smoking and nonsmoking groups. The ACS (2019, p. 2) identified that "men and women who smoke are approximately 25 times likely to develop lung cancer than non-smokers." The relative risk for smokers is a 25 times increase in the likelihood of developing lung cancer.
- **Attributable Risk**: The number of diseases that could have been avoided by reducing or avoiding the risk factors of the disease. Attributable risk is a better indicator to measure the success of prevention strategies/techniques. For example, if all the factory workers did not smoke, then the rate of lung cancer would have been significantly reduced.
- **Absolute Risk**: The actual numeric value of probability that cancer will develop during a specific time frame. For example, men have a 17% chance of developing prostate cancer by the age of 70.

▶ RISK FACTORS FOR CANCER

Risk factors for cancer are divided into two groups: modifiable and nonmodifiable risk factors. Modifiable risks can be controlled and/or eliminated. For example, smoking and drinking are considered modifiable risk factors. An individual can choose not to smoke and not to drink, thereby "modifying the risk." Nonmodifiable risk factors are ones that cannot be changed or eliminated—for example, sex, age, race, genetic background, and family history. The most common modifiable risk factors for cancer include tobacco use, alcohol consumption, exposure to sunlight, excess body weight, sedentary lifestyle, and poor diet/nutrition. Environmental risk factors for cancer such as radiation, infectious agents, and workplace exposures may be nonmodifiable or modifiable. For example, exposure to the pollution resulting from the 9/11 terrorist attack is a nonmodifiable risk factor versus occupational exposure to chemotherapy, which is a modifiable risk factor. Each of these risk factors can be associated with different types of cancers. Table 3.2 summarizes common risk factors for cancer based on site/type.

Table 3.2 Common Risk Factors for Cancer

Cancer Type	Non-Modifiable Risk Factors	Modifiable Risk Factors
Brain cancer	Family history, gene mutations	Ionizing radiation
Bladder cancer	Age, family/personal history race/ethnicity, sex	Arsenic in drinking water, certain drugs, exposure to workplace chemicals (e.g., hairdressers), radiation therapy, smoking
Breast cancer (women)	Age, family/personal history, gene mutations, race/ethnicity	Alcohol, hormone replacement therapy, ionizing radiation, lack of physical activity, night-shift work, obesity
Cervical cancer (women)	Age, race/ethnicity	HPV infection, oral contraceptive use, smoking
Colorectal cancer	Age, family/personal history, race/ethnicity	Alcohol, obesity, poor diet, smoking

(continued)

Table 3.2 Common Risk Factors for Cancer (*continued*)

Cancer Type	Non-Modifiable Risk Factors	Modifiable Risk Factors
Endometrial cancer	Age, family/personal history	Contraceptive use, lack of physical activity, obesity, poor diet, tamoxifen use
Esophageal cancer	Age, history of other forms of cancer (e.g., lung, oral), sex	Alcohol, obesity, GERD/Barrett's esophagus, lack of physical activity, obesity, poor diet, tobacco use (e.g., smoking, chewing tobacco)
Larynx cancer	Age, race, sex	Alcohol, occupational exposures, smoking
Leukemia	Age, family history, genetics, race, sex	Benzene exposure, certain chemotherapy drugs, HTLV-1 infection, ionizing radiation
Liver cancer	Race/ethnicity	Alcohol, anabolic steroids, HBV or HCV infection, obesity
Lung and bronchus cancer	Age, sex, family/personal history, race/ethnicity	Arsenic in drinking water, exposure to asbestos/radon/other chemicals, smoking/secondhand smoke
Lymphoma (Hodgkin's/ Non-Hodgkin's)	Age, family history, race, sex	Benzene exposure, infections (EBV, HCV, *Helicobacter pylori*, HIV, HTLV-1)
Melanoma	Age, fair skin, family/personal history, immunosuppression, race, sex	Sun exposure and history of sunburns
Oropharynx cancer	Age, history, sex	Alcohol, HPV infection, obesity, sun exposure, tobacco use (e.g., smoking, chewing tobacco)
Ovarian cancer	Age, gene mutations	Obesity, oral contraceptive use, reproductive history
Pancreatic cancer	Diabetes, family history	Obesity, smoking
Prostate cancer	Age, family history, gene mutations, race/ethnicity	Increased consumption of dairy and calcium, obesity, smoking
Renal cancer	Family history, genetics	Hypertension, obesity, occupational exposures, smoking
Skin cancer	Age, fair skin, family/personal history, immunosuppression, race, sex	Sun exposure and history of sunburns, ultraviolet radiation
Stomach cancer	Family history	Obesity, *Helicobacter pylori* infection, lack of physical activity, poor diet, tobacco use
Testicular cancer	Age, family/personal history, race	Ionizing radiation
Thyroid cancer	Age, family history, sex	Ionizing radiation

GERD, gastroesophageal reflux disease; HBV, hepatitis B virus; HCV, hepatitis C virus; HIV, human immunodeficiency virus; HPV, human papillomavirus; HTLV-1, human T-cell leukemia virus type 1.

▶   **EXAM TIP**

Know the difference between the modifiable and non-modifiable risk factors for cancer development.

AGE AND SEX

Non-modifiable risk factors include sex, age, ethnicity, and family history/genetic mutations. The sex of an individual can make individuals predisposed to certain cancers based upon their anatomy. Women are predisposed to breast, cervical, ovarian, uterine, and vaginal cancers. Men are predisposed to prostate and testicular cancers.

Age itself is a risk factor, one that cannot be changed. Many cancers are identified during the aging process, including:

- Breast cancer: 95% diagnosed in women over the age of 40
- Cervical cancer: Diagnosed in women aged 35 to 55
- Colorectal cancer: Diagnosed over the age of 45 in both sexes
- Larynx cancer: Diagnosed after the age of 65
- Lymphomas: Diagnosed in early adulthood (age 15 to 40) and after the age of 55
- Lung cancer: Diagnosed after the age of 65
- Multiple myeloma: Diagnosed before the age of 35 and after the age of 65
- Ovarian and uterine cancer: Diagnosed after the age of 50; usually postmenopausal
- Prostate cancer: Diagnosed after the age of 65

> ### ▶ KEY POINT
>
> Testicular cancer does not develop as a result of the aging process, although it typically occurs between ages of 20 and 34.

RACE/ETHNICITY

Like age, ethnicity and race are factors that cannot be changed. Unfortunately, there are some ethnic groups that are at higher risk for specific cancers, resulting in a potential cancer disparity. The National Cancer Institute (NIH 2020, Cancer Disparities) has described cancer disparities as differences within a specific group in relation to the incidence, prevalence, mortality, morbidity, survivorship, screening, and diagnosis rates.

Cancer disparities involve the interplay among many factors, including social determinants of health, behavior, biology, and genetics. Certain groups in the United States experience cancer disparities because they are more likely to encounter obstacles in obtaining healthcare (NIH 2020, Cancer Disparities). For example, some ethnic groups may not have access to healthcare and appropriate screening due to financial constraints. The limited access to care may result in cancers being diagnosed at later stages, leading to higher mortality rates. Medically underserved populations have increased rates of behavioral risk factors, such as smoking, drinking, obesity, and limited physical activity, which also increase cancer risk. In addition, genetic variants in these groups may play a part in the development of cancer. The following are notable, current cancer disparities (NIH 2020, Cancer Disparities):

- African Americans have elevated death rates for many cancers compared to other groups and are at greater risk for colorectal cancer than Whites.
- African American women have higher death rates from breast cancer than White women and have higher deaths rates from cervical cancer.
- African American men are twice as likely to die of stomach cancer than White men, have higher deaths rates from prostate cancer than white men, and are at greater risk for incidence and death from lung cancer.

■ American Indian and Alaska Native populations are at greater risk for cervical cancer, liver cancer, and biliary duct cancer, and have the highest death rates for renal cancer.

■ Renal cancer death rates are highest in American Indian and Alaska Native populations.

FAMILY HISTORY AND GENETICS

Genes are the basic physical and functional unit of heredity. Genes are made up of DNA, which is in every cell within the body. There are approximately 20,000 to 30,000 genes in each cell. These genes create sex and physical characteristics, such as hair and eye color, as well as other defining characteristics. Genes have essential functions such as promoting the creation of proteins that create the structure and function of cells within the body and acting as messengers that provide cells with vital information.

For multiple reasons (which will be discussed in Chapter 5), genes can develop mutations, which can be genetically inherited and create a pathway for familial links of specific cancers. For example, families that have the BRAC1 and BRAC2 gene mutations have a higher risk of developing breast and ovarian cancer. Cancer research focuses on identifying and examining gene mutations that cause cancer to develop screening and treatment options and potential elimination of the mutation.

ALCOHOL AND TOBACCO USE

Alcohol has a relationship to many cancers. Alcohol causes direct cell damage with the production of a byproduct called acetaldehyde. When alcohol is metabolized, the chemical acetaldehyde damages the DNA of cells and inhibits the body from repairing the damage. Unfortunately, the DNA damage can be the promotor for abnormal cells to multiply and replicate, creating an environment for malignant cells to thrive.

Tobacco use includes the use of cigarettes, chewing tobacco, cigar smoking, and e-cigarettes, also known as "vaping." The Centers for Disease Control and Prevention (CDC) (2019) has identified numerous reports regarding lung diseases related to vaping, especially in the adolescent and young adult population; however, the full effects and long-term risks of vaping have not yet been determined. Recent government banning of certain vaping products may help to reduce the incidence of lung disease related to vaping. Studies suggest that quitting smoking before the age of 40 years significantly decreases the risk of dying early from smoking-related diseases, including lung cancer by 90%, and stopping by 54 reduces the risks by two-thirds (Johns Hopkins, 2020).

Secondhand smoke is a combination of smoke from the burning cigarette as well as the smoke being eliminated from the lungs of the smoker. According to the CDC (2018), secondhand smoke exposure is responsible for approximately 20% to 30% of lung cancers in nonsmokers. Secondhand smoke for infants and adolescents is a major health risk factor. Sudden infant death syndrome (SIDS) has a direct effect with secondhand smoke, and infant death has been noted when mothers smoke during pregnancy.

INFECTIONS

Several million cancer diagnoses each year can be linked to an infectious process. Both viruses and bacteria are known to be precursors to cancers. There are several infections (e.g., HIV, HPV) that are considered modifiable risk factors due to their relationship to high-risk behaviors such as multiple sex partners and unprotected sex with either sex. Otherwise, they are considered modifiable risk factors since the virus and bacteria are insidious, and the exact cause may be unknown. Common bacteria and viruses and bacteria that increase the risk for cancer include:

- *Helicobacter pylori* (bacterium): *H. pylori* is a gram-negative bacterium that is usually found in the stomach. It is estimated that approximately two in three adults worldwide have *H. pylori* (ACS). It is spread via the fecal-oral route, contaminated food and water, and mouth-to-mouth contact.
- **Hepatitis B and C viruses:** They cause acute inflammation and damage to the liver and are the most common chronic viruses linked to liver cancer. According to the Hepatitis B Foundation, individuals infected with hepatitis B have a 25% to 40% lifetime risk of developing liver cancer. Hepatitis B and C can be spread via blood, semen, and other body fluids infected. It can also be passed from infected mother to child. Common forms of transmission include engaging in sexual relations with an infected person; sharing needles and syringes; sharing toothbrushes, razors, or medical equipment; coming into contact with blood or open wounds; and engaging in homosexual activity. High-risk groups for contracting the virus include healthcare professionals (e.g., needlestick exposure) and patients receiving hemodialysis.
- **Epstein-Barr virus (EBV):** The virus that causes mononucleosis. The primary route of transmission is through saliva; however, it can also be transmitted by sharing personal items such as toothbrushes and eating utensils. EBV is related to lymphoma (e.g., Burkitt's, Hodgkin's, non-Hodgkin's) and gastric cancer.
- **HIV:** The virus that causes AIDS. It grossly affects the immune system and alters the body's response to defend against oncovirus, which increases the risk of cancer. It is transmitted via bodily fluids such as semen, vaginal fluids, blood, and breast milk.
- **HPV:** HPV is transmitted via sexual contact and occurs rather quickly after a sexual experience. There are over 100 types of HPV. Fourteen of the HPV strains are linked to cervical cancer; however, most diagnoses are related to types 16 to 18.
- **Human T-cell leukemia virus (HTLV-1):** HTLV-1 is a retrovirus that can lie dormant for decades and, in many individuals, will not cause any harm. However, it can cause leukemia in a small percentage of infected individuals. Approximately 1 in 20 of infected individuals can develop leukemia. The most common forms of transmission are unprotected sex, sharing IV needles and syringes, breastfeeding, and blood and organ transplantation.

RADIATION EXPOSURE

There are two types of radiation exposure that increase the risk for cancer: ultraviolet light, which is derived mainly from the sun and/or tanning beds, and ionizing radiation, which is derived from radiation therapy and medical diagnostic testing (e.g., x-rays, CT scans). Ultraviolet light can cause skin cancer, including basal cell, squamous cell, and melanoma.

Exposure to ionizing radiation is seen with radiation therapy and medical diagnostic testing such as x-rays, CT scans, and nuclear medicine scans. Risk is increased in young women, as studies have demonstrated that young women treated with radiation therapy for lymphoma above the diaphragm had a higher incidence of developing breast cancer later in life, which is known as a secondary malignancy. It is important for healthcare professionals to pay attention to the amount of radiation exposure related to the diagnostic tests ordered, especially in the younger population. Risk for benefits measures need to be addressed before proceeding with potentially unnecessary imaging.

OBESITY

Obesity is a risk factor for several cancers and is strongly linked to breast cancer. Obesity increases the risk for cancer due to the following factors:

- Obesity can cause a chronic low-level inflammatory response in the body, damaging cell DNA.
- Fat cells can develop increased amounts of estrogen, which has been correlated with breast, ovarian, and other female reproductive cancers.
- Fat cells can release hormones and other chemicals that inhibit cell growth, as well as other regulating factors of cell development.
- Obesity can increase insulin blood levels, leading to hyperinsulinemia. The elevated amounts of insulin can promote the development of colon, kidney, prostate, and endometrial cancers.

Women who are obese and have a sedentary lifestyle are significantly at risk. Weight loss and associated programs help to decrease the risk of cancers that have been associated with obesity.

DIET

Poor diets, including high-fat, high-protein, and heavily processed foods, can increase the risk for several cancers, include gastric and colorectal cancer. Red meats that increase the risk for cancer include beef, pork, veal, and lamb. Charred meat (e.g., barbecue) increases the risk for gastric cancer further. Processed and cured meats increase risk due to the use of the preservative nitrates. Processed meats include bacon, smoked meats, deli meats, beef/turkey jerky, hot dogs, salami, and other cured meat products. The quantity of red meat consumed also impacts risk. Eating more than 18 oz of meat per week is associated with an increased risk of cancer, especially gastric and colon/rectal cancers.

According to the National Cancer Institute, artificial sweeteners can pose a potential risk for cancer; however, the studies are not conclusive. There have not been definitive studies that prove that artificial sweeteners cause cancer in humans, but saccharine is known to cause bladder cancer in animals. It is important for oncology nurses to be aware of the potential, especially when educating patients.

Cancer Preventive Diets

There are many foods that can help reduce the risk of cancer; however, there is conflicting information regarding the exact benefits. An antioxidant is a chemical connection that neutralizes free radicals and stops them from causing damage to the cell. Antioxidants are found in fruits and vegetables and some grains:

- Beta carotene (vitamin A): Acts as antioxidant and immunostimulant.
- Lycopene: A red carotenoid that has anti-inflammatory and chemopreventive properties.
- Selenium-containing proteins: Selenium was involved in a large chemoprevention trial named SELECT (discussed further in Chapter 4). Note that it can reduce the absorption of vitamin C supplements when taken together.

High-fiber diets may help to reduce the incidence of colorectal cancers. The recommended daily amount of fiber is 25 to 30 g/day, obtained from food and not supplements. There are two types of fiber: soluble and insoluble. Soluble fiber is responsible for bulking the stool by absorbing water during the digestion process. Common sources of soluble fiber include apples, oranges, grapefruit, lentils, peas, and barley. Insoluble fiber is responsible for motility within the colon and does not change during the digestion process. Common sources of insoluble fiber include fruits and vegetables with seeds and peel, brown rice, pasta, whole-wheat products, cornmeal, and rolled oats.

> ### ▶ CLINICAL PEARL

High-fiber diets should not be promoted for patients with Crohn's or irritable bowel syndrome, as it can aggravate their symptoms.

OCCUPATIONAL EXPOSURES

There are many occupations that can place an individual at risk for health issues such as cancer due to related hazardous exposures on the job. Hazardous agents that are correlated with cancer include asbestos, benzene, chemotherapy and biotherapy, and other chemicals. Occupations at high risk for cancer include steel, rubber, and chemical workers (e.g., hairdressers, printers, painters, truck drivers); mechanics; and healthcare professionals.

MEDICATIONS

While medications are a tremendous asset to the healthcare profession, they can cause complications such as malignancies. Medications that are known to be promotors of cancer include hormones; immunosuppressants; and chemotherapeutic, biotherapy, and immunotherapy agents.

Diethylstilbestrol (DES) is a synthetic estrogen that was prescribed from 1940 to 1980s for women who were experiencing fertility issues. Incidence of reproductive system issues, breast cancer, and clear cell adenocarcinoma were increased in individuals whose mothers took DES during pregnancy.

⬤ CONCLUSION

This chapter reviewed the health promotion concepts, health disparities, risk factors, and related cancers. It also provided an overview of modifiable and nonmodifiable risk factors for specific cancers. The next chapter discusses the screening and preventive measures currently available.

The bibliography and references for this chapter are available on ExamPrepConnect; see inside front cover for access instructions.

1. Which of the following is the BEST example of a health promotion strategy that has a direct effect on cancer prevention?

    A. *Healthy People 2030*
    B. Health literacy program
    C. Smoking cessation program
    D. SIDS awareness program

2. An example of a secondary health prevention intervention is:

    A. Use of seatbelts
    B. Immunization
    C. Screening tests
    D. Stroke rehabilitation program

3. Which of the following are considered nonmodifiable risk factors for cancer?

    A. Gender, safe sex practices, diet
    B. Genetics, race, alcohol use
    C. Age, gender, genetics
    D. Obesity, ethnicity, tobacco use

4. HTLV-1 is defined as:

    A. Bacteria that cause liver cancer
    B. Bacteria that cause renal cancer
    C. Virus that causes cervical cancer
    D. Virus that causes leukemias

5. A 30-year-old female tells the nurse that her mother took DES (diethylstilbestrol) while she was pregnant and she is concerned about the long-term effects of being exposed to the drug in the womb. The nurse's BEST response is:

    A. "I understand your concern. Are you practicing breast self-examinations?"
    B. "I understand your concern. Let's talk to the doctor and order a mammogram."
    C. "Don't worry about that. You are too young for any diagnostic tests."
    D. "Don't worry about that. It was so long ago; there are no lasting effects of the drug."

1. C) Smoking cessation program
A smoking cessation program is the best example of a health promotion strategy because the reduction in smoking has a direct effect on decreasing the risk of cancers related to smoking. *Healthy People* (2020 and 2030) is a program of a nationwide health-promotion and disease-prevention goals set by the U.S. Department of Health and Human Services. Health literacy programs are designed to help individuals better comprehend and use the information to make informed decisions about their health. A SIDS (sudden death infant syndrome) awareness program increases awareness of risk factors and interventions to prevent SIDS.

2. C) Screening tests
Secondary prevention interventions aim to reduce the impact of a disease or injury that has already occurred. This can be done by detecting and treating a disease as soon as possible, such as with screening tests. Primary prevention is aimed at preventing a disease or injury before it occurs, such as with the use of seatbelts or smoking cessation programs. Tertiary prevention is aimed at lessening the impact of an ongoing illness or injury to increase the quality of life and long-term health outcomes, such as with rehabilitation programs.

3. C) Age, gender, genetics
Age, gender, genetics, race, and ethnicity are nonmodifiable risk factors. Diet, safe sex practices, alcohol and tobacco use, and obesity are modifiable risk factors.

4. D) Virus that causes leukemias
HTLV-1 (Human T-cell leukemia virus) is a retrovirus that causes leukemias. Liver cancer can be caused by the hepatitis B or C virus, and cervical cancer can be caused by the human papillomavirus (HPV). Renal cancer is not commonly caused by bacteria or viruses.

5. A) "I understand your concern. Are you practicing breast self-examinations?"
DES (diethylstilbestrol) exposure has been linked to breast cancer; however, due to the patient's age, breast self-examination (BSE) is the most appropriate preventive measure. Option A is the best response because it uses therapeutic communication skills, first validating the patient's concern and then opening a dialogue about practicing BSE. If the patient does not currently practice BSE, the nurse can provide teaching about the benefits and proper techniques. The patient is too young to begin screening with mammography; baseline mammogram begins at age 40.

Screening and Early Detection

4

INTRODUCTION

Screening and early detection practices are vital for the identification of cancer development before any signs or symptoms of the disease exist, leading to better prognostic outcomes. Screening techniques include physical examinations, blood tests, and imaging. Research demonstrates that cancer screenings have decreased the death rates of certain cancers, including cervical, colorectal, and lung (National Cancer Institute [NCI], 2019). However, not all screening methods are proven to decrease cancer mortality rates, and results can vary depending on the patient's overall health status and access to the healthcare system.

While screening can be beneficial to the patient and the healthcare team, it can also cause potential risks. Healthcare providers need to review statistical data and evidence-based screening guidelines to determine the most appropriate screening tools for their patients. Risks related to cancer screening include:

- **Overdiagnosis:** Screening identifies a potentially slow-growing, nonaggressive cancer that would likely not cause any harm to the patient. Instead, the patient may be subjected to invasive, expensive, painful, and unnecessary treatments.
- **Overutilization of Medical Tests**: The initial screening process can be inconclusive and additional tests may be suggested and required. Again, this potentially subjects the patient to invasive, expensive, stressful, and unnecessary diagnostic tests, including exposure to radiation due to unnecessary imaging.
- **False Positives**: Screening erroneously identifies cancer, which is discovered after further testing and potential treatment.
- **False Reassurance**: Screening does not detect an existing malignancy.

> ▶ **EXAM TIP**
>
> Review screening recommendations for each cancer site and the appropriate age groups.

SCREENING AND EARLY DETECTION

Although there are risks concerning screening and preventions strategies, these measures have been successful in recognizing cancers for many patients. Table 4.1 summarizes the *American Cancer Society (ACS) Guidelines for the Early Detection of Cancer.*

The bibliography and references for this chapter are available on ExamPrepConnect; see inside front cover for access instructions.

Table 4.1 American Cancer Society Guidelines for the Early Detection of Cancer

Cancer	Population	Recommendation
Breast cancer	All women High risk: Family history of breast cancer; genetic predisposition	Age 20–74: Monthly breast-self exams, annual clinical breast exam Age 30: Annual breast MRI and mammography (high-risk individuals) Age 40–44: Option to start annual mammography Age 45–74: Annual mammography
Cervical cancer	All women High risk: History of serious cervical precancer	Age 25–65: A primary HPV test every 5 years. If a primary HPV test is not available, a Pap test every 3 years or an HPV test with a Pap test every 5 years Age 65+: Do not test if normal results for past 10 years History of serious cervical precancer: Test for 25 years after diagnosis, even if testing goes past age 65
Colorectal cancer	All adults High risk: Family history of colon cancer and genetic predispositions (screening age may be earlier than 45); history of inflammatory bowel disease	Age 45–75: Annual physical examination and fecal occult blood test; colonoscopy every 3–5 years
Lung cancer	Adults who are current smokers and former smokers who quit in the past 15 years with at least a 20 pack-year smoking history	50–80 years: Annual low-dose helical CT
Ovarian cancer	Women High risk: Strong family history of breast or ovarian cancer, or genetic predisposition to ovarian cancer (e.g., Lynch syndrome, BRCA gene mutations)	Average risk: no recommendations High risk: Transvaginal ultrasound plus CA-125 Test
Prostate cancer screening	Men aged 50 years High risk: Men aged 40–45 years with $\geq$1 first-degree family history diagnosed at <65 years of age; African Americans aged $\geq$45 years	Age 45 years: If high risk, discuss pros and cons of PSA blood test with/without DRE with healthcare provider Age 50 years: Discuss pros and cons of PSA blood test with/without DRE with healthcare provider

Source: From the American Cancer Society. 2021. *American Cancer Society Guidelines for the Early Detection of Cancer.* https://www.cancer.org/healthy/find-cancer-early/american-cancer-society-guidelines-for-the-early-detection-of-cancer.html

▶ **KEY FACT**

There are no specific screening tests available for testicular cancer; however, it is highly recommended that men practice self-testicular examination as well as have an annual physical exam.

▶ BREAST CANCER SCREENING

There are several modifiable and nonmodifiable factors risk factors for breast cancer. Gender is a primary risk factor; female patients are at higher risk, particularly those over the age of 50. Individuals with previous breast cancer are at increased risk. For example, if a patient had a left-sided mastectomy, then the right breast is at risk for breast cancer and needs to be followed closely. Other high-risk groups include individuals with a family history of breast cancer and positive testing for *BRAC1* and *BRAC2* genes (MRI of the breast for patients that are positive for *BRAC1* and *BRAC2*).

Screening for breast cancer is an essential component to identify the disease at the earliest stage possible, which can yield the best prognostic indicator for cure. Screening and early-detection methods include:

- Annual complete breast health history
- Monthly breast self-examination (BSE): Although most organizations do not recommend BSE as a viable screening technique, many healthcare providers encourage female patients to be familiar with the changes within their breasts, which can be an early alert to potential breast issues.
- Mammogram: Mammography is breast imaging using 3D techniques to visualize the breast tissue and compare changes from year to year. ACS recommends that women aged 40 to 44 start annual screening with mammograms if they wish to do so. Women aged 45 to 54 should get mammograms every year (ACS, 2021). Women 55 and older should switch to mammograms every 2 years or can continue yearly screening. Screening should continue as long as a woman is in good health and is expected to live 10 more years or longer. Women with a family history of breast cancer should start mammograms 10 years before their first-degree relative is diagnosed. For example, if a patient's mother was diagnosed at 40, the patient should have her first mammogram at age 30. MRI of the breast is recommended if strong family history and/or genetic link to breast cancer is identified. Prophylactic bilateral mastectomies for patients diagnosed with positive BRAC1 and BRAC2 genes have also been recommended in specific cases.

NURSING CARE CONSIDERATIONS

1. Teach how to perform monthly breast self-examination.
2. Encourage annual physical examination by healthcare provider and/or breast surgeon.
3. Encourage and recommend annual mammography at the age of 50 or earlier depending on age of the patient.
4. Encourage genetic testing when appropriate.

▶ CERVICAL CANCER SCREENING

High-risk individuals for cervical cancer include females younger than age 30 and females with multiple sex partners, immunocompromised status (e.g., HIV), history of organ transplant, and those exposed to DES in utero.

Screening and prevention strategies for cervical cancer are based on age:

- Age 25–65: A primary HPV test every 5 years. If a primary HPV test is not available, a Pap test every 3 years or an HPV test with a Pap test every 5 years.
- Age 65+: Do not test if normal results for past 10 years.
- History of serious cervical precancer: Test for 25 years after diagnosis, even if testing goes past age 65.

In addition, HPV is recommended for both boys and girls between the ages of 9 and 11 before they become sexually active. HPV is responsible for genital warts and can be transmitted via skin-to-skin contact during sexual activity. The virus is most common in men and women in their late teens, and many have been exposed to the virus at one point during a lifetime. The HPV virus most often presents with no symptoms and will disappear naturally due to the body's properly functioning immune system. HPV strains 16 to 18 are most closely linked to cervical, rectal, anus, penile, vaginal, vulva, and oropharynx malignancies.

NURSING CARE CONSIDERATIONS

1. Encourage and recommend annual screening testing.
2. Educate patients regarding safe sex practices.
3. Encourage and recommend HPV vaccines.

▶ COLORECTAL CANCER SCREENING

Colorectal cancers are strongly linked with diet, weight, and exercise. High-risk group includes patients over the age of 50 and those with a family history of colon polyps (adenomatous polyps; precancerous lesions) and/or colon cancer. Individuals with a first-degree relative with colorectal cancer are at a higher risk, especially if the relative was affected before the age of 45. For the full list of risk factors, see Chapter 3.

Screening and prevention strategies for colorectal cancer include an annual physical examination by healthcare provider and:

- **Fecal Occult Blood Test (FOBT):** Determines if blood is present in the stool due to colon polyps (sometimes hemorrhoids may be the cause of the bleeding).
- **Colonoscopy**: An invasive screening and diagnostic test to examine the colon for polyps and abnormal cells. Colonoscopies should begin at the age of 50 or earlier if family and genetic history is present, then every 3 to 5 years, depending on the results and healthcare provider's recommendations.
- **Genetic Testing** (if appropriate)

NURSING CARE CONSIDERATIONS

1. Assess family history related to colorectal cancer.
2. Encourage appropriate screening measures.
3. Educate patients regarding healthy diet and nutritional programs, as well as the importance of exercise programs.
4. Educate patients regarding the risks of alcohol and tobacco use and its potential relationship to colorectal cancers.

▶ LUNG CANCER SCREENING

Lung cancer is a leading cause of death for both sexes. Lung cancer screenings are recommended for those at high risk of developing lung cancer. Smoking, secondhand smoke, and radon are the primary causative factors of lung cancer. It is imperative to screen high-risk patients to identify lung cancer at the earliest possible stage. High-risk populations for lung cancer include current smokers, heavy smokers (≥20 pack-year history), and smokers who have quit within the past 15 years; individuals who use tobacco plus alcohol; and individuals whose occupations have exposed them to asbestos and other known carcinogens.

> ▶ **KEY FACT**

Pack year = the average of one pack of cigarettes per day for one year. A patient who smokes a pack a day for 20 years has a 20 pack-year history.

Prevention options for patients who are at high risk for lung cancer include smoking cessation programs to help individuals quit smoking. Annual low-dose helical computer tomography (LDCT) is recommended for adults aged 50 to 80 who are current smokers or former smokers who quit in the past 15 years with at least a 20 pack-year smoking history.

NURSING CARE CONSIDERATIONS

1. Complete a detailed lung and family history assessment.
2. Educate individuals about the harmful effects of smoking and alcohol use.
3. Recommend and assist with smoking cessation programs.

▶ OVARIAN CANCER SCREENING

Ovarian cancer screening for ovarian cancer has provided the least amount of success. Currently, there are no recommended screening tests for ovarian cancer for women who do not have any evidence of disease or signs or symptoms of ovarian cancer. According to the ACS (2018), ovarian cancer is discovered in the earliest stage only 20% of the time, which yields poorer prognoses. Screening works best in the high-risk population, including women with a family history of ovarian or breast cancer and women who are *BRAC1* and *BRAC2* positive.

Screening and prevention strategies for ovarian cancer include an annual GYN examination.

■ Annual transvaginal ultrasound (TVUS) which uses sound waves to examine the uterus, fallopian tubes, and ovaries. The ultrasound can discover abnormalities within the ovaries before symptoms occur.
■ CA-125 is a laboratory blood test that measures the protein CA-125 within the blood. The blood test can be drawn on high risk patients such as genetically predisposed to ovarian cancer. The CA-125 is most often used as a tumor marker to determine how an ovarian cancer patient is responding to cancer treatment. However, an elevation of CA-125 in a patient that does not have presence of ovarian cancer can be a precursor to the disease. The concern for using the CA-125 as a screening measure is that the elevated CA-125 blood levels may not always indicate ovarian cancer. Endometriosis and pelvic inflammatory disease can also cause an increase in CA-125 levels. Therefore transvaginal ultrasound and CA-125 blood tests are used in high risk populations.
■ Prophylactic totally hysterectomy for *BRAC1* and *BRAC2* positive patients may also be a recommendation to prevent ovarian cancer.

NURSING CARE CONSIDERATIONS

1. Encourage annual GYN examination.
2. Assess family history for ovarian cancer.
3. Recommend genetic testing when appropriate.
4. Teach the signs and symptoms of ovarian cancer.

▶ PROSTATE CANCER SCREENING

Prostate cancer is a slow-growing malignancy that, in many cases, may not cause a man to experience significant issues. Therefore, the decision to screen is a decision that should be made with the healthcare provider to minimize the risk of potential treatment options that cause unnecessary long-term side effects, such as urinary incontinence and/or sexual dysfunction (ACS, 2018). ACS (2018) suggests that men be informed of the following statistics:

1. Men aged 50 who are at average risk can be expected to live 10 years or more after diagnosis.
2. Men aged 45 are at the highest risk if a first-degree relative such as father and/or brother have been diagnosed with prostate cancer before the age of 65. This also includes the African American population.
3. Men aged 40 are at the greatest risk of prostate cancer if one first-degree relative has been diagnosed with prostate cancer at an early age.

Screening and prevention strategies for prostate cancer include annual physical examination, including a digital rectal examination (DRE), which allows the healthcare provider to assess and palpate the prostate gland to determine if it is enlarged or irregular in shape. Prostate-specific antigen (PSA) is a laboratory test that identifies protein produced by normal and cancer cells of the prostate. The PSA is obtained via a blood sample. The PSA was first created as a tumor marker to manage prostate cancer treatments. The PSA test can be elevated with prostate cancer, prostatitis, and benign prostatic hyperplasia (BPH). Recommendations based on PSA results:

- PSA <2.5 ng/mL: Repeat test every 2 years.
- PSA >2.5 ng/mL: Repeat test annually.

NURSING CARE CONSIDERATIONS

1. Provide accurate information regarding prostate screening measures.
2. Encourage annual DRE and PSA testing in high-risk patients.

▶ SKIN CANCER SCREENING

High-risk groups for skin cancer include individuals who are fair-skinned with light hair and eyes; work primarily outdoors, especially those who live in warmer climates; have a history of multiple sunburns or more than one blistering sunburn; have a family history of skin cancers (e.g., melanoma); have more than 50 moles; and regularly visit tanning salons.

Screening and prevention are key factors in finding a potential malignancy at the earliest stage. Skin cancer prevention methods include:

- **Regular Self Skin Assessment**: It is important for a person to know their body and identify any changes in their moles and skin. Oncology nurses play a vital role in educating patients on how to perform self-skin assessments as well as how to identify changes at the onset of discovery.
- **Regular Use of Sunscreen**: The number of sun protection factor (SPF) determines how long the sun's UVB rays will take to penetrate and cause redness to the skin. In other words, if a patient uses SPF 50 product correctly, it will take 50 times longer to burn the skin than using no sunscreen.

■ Avoid sunlight from 12 noon to 3 p.m. and wear sun-protective clothing when outdoors for extended periods of time, especially during the summer months.

NURSING CARE CONSIDERATIONS

1. Complete a detailed skin assessment.
2. Teach self-skin assessment.
3. Teach the identification of any skin and mole changes.
4. Teach the ramifications of overexposure to ultraviolet light and tanning beds.
5. Encourage sunscreen usage, especially in the summer months.

● CONCLUSION

This chapter provides the foundation of the prevention methods for specific malignancies, including breast, cervical, lung, ovarian, prostate, and skin cancers. However, it is important to understand that not all cancers have recommended screening measures.

The bibliography and references for this chapter are available on ExamPrepConnect; see inside front cover for access instructions.

1. A Pap smear test is used to screen for:

   A. Vulva cancer
   B. Uterine cancer
   C. Cervical cancer
   D. Ovarian cancer

2. A 62-year-old male patient visits the clinic with the chief complaint of difficulty with urinary flow. The nurse anticipates that the provider will order:

   A. CBC, chem screen, and CA-125
   B. Chem screen, CEA, and CA-125
   C. CBC, chem screen, and PSA
   D. Chem screen, hemoglobin A1C, and PSA

3. Which of the following patient populations is at the highest risk for colorectal cancer?

   A. African American males
   B. Hispanic females
   C. Asian females
   D. Non-Hispanic males

4. Which of the following is the MOST accurate statement regarding breast cancer screening?

   A. It is recommended to have a mammogram every 3 years after the age of 50
   B. It is recommended to have a mammogram every year after the age of 50
   C. It is recommended to perform breast self-examination every month after the age of 20
   D. It is recommended to perform breast self-examination every other month after the age of 20

5. Which of the following factors identified in a patient's medical history should the nurse recognize as causing the highest risk for cancer development?

   A. Family history of colorectal cancer
   B. Positive for *BRAC1* and *BRAC2* genes
   C. Working in the healthcare field
   D. Patient has limited physical activity and is moderately overweight

1. C) Cervical cancer
The Pap test is used for the screening and prevention of cervical cancer. There are no screening tools for vulva, uterine, and ovarian cancers.

2. C) CBC, chem screen, and PSA
Complete blood count (CBC) is used to measure elevated or decreased white blood cells (WBC), hemoglobin (HGB), and hematocrit (HCT). The chem screen is used to monitor liver, kidney, and electrolytes. An elevated prostate-specific antigen (PSA) level can be related to benign prostatic hyperplasia (BPH), prostatitis, and/or prostate cancer. CEA levels are used as tumor markers for colon cancer, and CA-125 is used in ovarian cancer.

3. A) African American males
African American males have the highest risk for colorectal cancers, which may be associated with high-fat, high-calorie, red-meat-heavy diets.

4. B) It is recommended to have a mammogram every year after the age of 50
The American Cancer Society (ACS) recommends that women start screening mammograms at the age of 45 and then annually after the age of 50. Breast self-examinations are not used as screening measures.

5. B) Positive for *BRAC1* and *BRAC2* genes
A known genetic malfunction such as *BRAC1* and *BRAC2* poses the greatest risk for developing breast and ovarian cancer. Family history is also a concern; however, identified genes carry a higher risk. Working in healthcare can be a potential risk, but further information would be required. Limited physical activity and extra weight are also risks but not as strong as gene identification.

Carcinogenesis and the Role of Genes

● INTRODUCTION

Carcinogenesis is the ever-evolving process of the development of cancer cells. Researchers have acknowledged that cancer development is not related to one process or theory. Cancer development is an advanced multilayered process caused by several mechanisms and multiple carcinogens that threaten the hosts/human life.

● CANCER CELLS

Cancer cells are normal cells that have a genetic mutation, abnormal proliferation, and innate ability to spread throughout the body. In other words, cancer cells are normal cells that have gone awry. A malignant cell has unregulated cell division, the inability to stop replicating, and the ability to travel via the lymphatic and circulatory systems. Most importantly, cancer cells lose the function to die.

There are distinct differences between a healthy normal cell and a cancer cell. Healthy cells appear normal in shape and size, with smooth round edges. A healthy cell will present in a uniform manner and possess a fixed cell membrane, which enables the proper function of the cell. In contrast, a malignant cell will present with an abnormal shape and size, irregular borders, and edges and will have a permeable or nonfixed cell membrane (Figure 5.1).

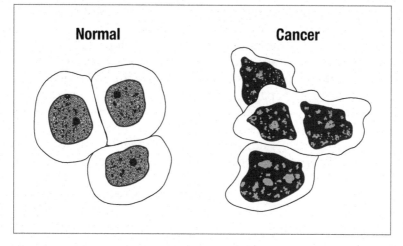

Figure 5.1 Normal cells versus cancer cells.

THE CELL CYCLE

The cell cycle includes several important tasks that every cell within the body will perform. For a cell to successfully divide and produce two new daughter cells, the cells must move through the resting phase, interphase, and mitotic phase:

The bibliography and references for this chapter are available on ExamPrepConnect; see inside front cover for access instructions.

- **Resting phase—Gap 0 (G0):** The cell rests and, in some cases, waits for the signal to start the division process. Some cells can permanently remain in the resting phase (e.g., heart and nerve cells). Most cancer cells do not engage in the GO phase as they tend to divide rapidly.
- **Interphase:**
  - Gap 1 (G1): The cell grows and gathers nutrients to prepare for DNA replication and cell division. G1 phase is responsible for RNA and protein synthesis.
  - Synthesis (S): The cell continues to grow and replicates DNA.
  - Gap 2 (G2): The cell continues to grow and obtains the necessary proteins for cell division. This is also called the premitotic phase.
- **Mitotic (M):** Cell division occurs in four phases: prophase, metaphase, anaphase, and telophase. These four phases describe the separation of the chromosomes within the cell, the creation of mitotic spindles, the signals to start cell division, and the creation of two new daughter cells. Cytokinesis, the process of division of cytoplasm within the cell, ensures the separation of chromosomes at the right time and the right place to create each daughter cell appropriately.

> ▶ **EXAM TIP**
>
> It is important to understand the cell cycle. This information will help you answer questions related to carcinogenesis and the mechanisms of action of chemotherapy agents.

● ROLE OF GENES IN CANCER DEVELOPMENT

Genes are messengers within the cell that make proteins with the information necessary to perform the vital tasks such as cell growth and division. When a gene has a missing protein (a genetic mutation), the cell does not replicate properly, creating an abnormal cell that divides rapidly and leads to malignancy. Genetic mutations interfere with the replication of the DNA in a single cell or multiple cells. A single mutation is not likely to cause cancer as the body can often self-correct the mutation. Cancer development usually occurs in the older adult population due to the accumulation of mutations over the lifespan. Acquired and germline are two common types of genetic mutations. Acquired mutations occur during an individual's lifetime and are not passed from mother or father to child. They are isolated to a specific cell and caused by extrinsic factors such as exposure to carcinogens such as tobacco smoke, alcohol, viruses, and chemicals.

Germline, or heredity, mutations are passed from mother/father to child, resulting in inherited cancers. Up to 20% of cancers are caused by inherited cancers (e.g., breast and colon cancer). The genetic mutation or malformation is found in the sperm and/or the egg of the parent and starts at conception. Germline mutations are permanent and affect every cell within the body. When a mutation is present, the cells grow and divide with the DNA malformation. Lynch syndrome is an example of an inherited gene and is associated with colon cancer.

▶ MUTATIONS OF NORMAL GENES

There are several genes that act as the gatekeepers and regulatory agents to promote the proper functions of the cells. A disturbance in gene function is a gene mutation of which there are several types:

- Missense mutation: A change in one DNA pair
- Nonsense mutation: A reduction in protein production

- Insertion mutation: An addition of DNA within the gene
- Deletion mutation: A removal of DNA within the gene
- Duplication mutation: Improper copying of the gene
- Frameshift mutation: A coding defect within the gene
- Repeat expansion: The DNA is shortened and repeated in several sequences, causing the gene to malfunction

▶ TUMOR SUPPRESSOR GENES

Tumor suppressor genes are ordinary genes within cells that act as protectors to decrease cell division activity, correct DNA mistakes, and promote apoptosis (programmed cell death). When tumor suppressor genes are not functioning appropriately, the gene is inactivated, which fosters an environment for cells to rapidly replicate with the DNA mistakes and the inability to perform programmed cell death. This leads to the development of a cancer cell and/or tumor. Most tumor suppressor genes mutations are acquired and not inherited. An example of a tumor suppressor gene is *TP53* (or *p53*), which is found in approximately half of all cancers.

▶ EXAM TIP

Understand the concept of *apoptosis*, its role in cancer cell development, and how it contributes to the mechanisms of oncologic treatments.

▶ PROTO-ONCOGENES

Proto-oncogenes are part of the normal process of cell division. When they mutate or produce too many copies, they can become an unhealthy gene, known as an oncogene. During this change process, they become activated and replicate without regard for the malformation and contribute to cancer development. This form of mutation is acquired, not inherited. Examples of oncogenes are as follows:

- *HER2*: More than a quarter of breast cancer cells will overexpress *HER2*, which is a protein that monitors and controls cancer growth and metastases. *HER2* is also found in ovarian cancers.
- *RAS* genes: Found in approximately a third of pancreatic, lung, and colorectal cancers. A mutated RAS gene causes uncontrolled cellular growth and impaired cell death signals, potentially causing resistance to chemotherapy and other anti-cancer agents.

▶ DNA REPAIR GENES

DNA repair genes correct the DNA replication mistakes. Many of the DNA repair genes function as tumor suppressor genes. If the mutated gene continues to replicate and the DNA repair genes are unsuccessful, the cancer cell has the chance to develop. Examples of DNA repair genes are *BRAC1* and *BRAC2* and *p53*.

▶ EPIGENETIC CHANGES

Epigenetics describes how DNA modifications interfere with the activity of the gene rather than not changing the sequence of DNA. The most common type of epigenetic modification is methylation. An excess or reduction in methylation directly impacts the function of the gene, either turning it on or silencing it. Epigenetics has been associated with cancers and other diseases such as degenerative and metabolic disorders and can be influenced by environmental carcinogens.

▶ CHROMOSOMAL TRANSLOCATION

Chromosome translocations occur when one chromosome is split and then fuses to a different chromosome. An example of chromosomal translocation is the Philadelphia chromosome, in which the short chromosome on chromosome 22 translocates to chromosome 9. This translocation is indicative of chronic lymphocytic leukemia, which is presented with the *BCR* gene on one chromosome and *ABL* gene on the other chromosome, thus creating the *BCR-ABL* connection.

▶ GENOMIC INSTABILITY

As previously discussed, tumor suppressor genes are abnormal cells that are disorganized and unstable compared to healthy cells. Genomic instability is a defining characteristic of many cancer cells and is a defect in the regulation mechanisms such as immune surveillance, DNA damage checkpoint, DNA repair, and self-correction. When one or all these mechanisms fail, the genomic integrity is comprised and creates the potential for abnormal, malignant growth. The hereditary gene *HNPCC* is an example of genomic instability. The DNA damage is found on the germline and is caused by microsatellites (MSI) which are an abnormal accumulation of DNA pairs that are repeated between 5 and 50 times.

▶ HIT THEORY

The two-hit theory was discovered by Alfred Knudson in 1971 and is recognized as part of the carcinogenesis process. The hit theory is based upon a finding that tumor suppressor genes have two mutations and was discovered when studying retinoblastoma in children. While one gene mutation may not necessarily develop cancer, damage to the same gene on the second chromosome can produce cancer. For example, individuals with hereditary or familial cancers have an inherited damaged gene that occurs during conception; this is considered the first hit. The second hit or damage can occur after birth and/or later in life, thus creating cancer. The second mutation can be caused by an immune surveillance failure, environmental exposures, inability to perform programmed cell death, and gene malfunctions.

CAUSATIVE FACTORS FOR CANCER DEVELOPMENT

As discussed in Chapter 3, there are countless factors that can cause a malignant cell to originate. Intrinsic factors include age, sex, genetic predisposition, immune system, hormone levels, metabolism, and nutritional status. Extrinsic factors include exposure to chemicals, smoking, drinking, environmental pollution such as air, water and soil, radiation exposure, sexual behaviors, and cultural traits. Both intrinsic and extrinsic factors impact the development of cancer and act as a vehicle for promoting cancer at the cellular level, thus the foundation of carcinogenesis.

Inflammation is another component related to cancer development. The inflammatory process has been directly related to the exposure of viruses and bacteria. For example, *Helicobacter pylori*, a bacterial infection, is linked to gastric cancer, HPV virus is linked to cervical cancer, hepatitis B and C are linked to liver cancer, and inflammatory bowel disorder is linked to colon cancer.

Exposure to environmental carcinogens such as air and water pollutants are also contributing factors that can spark the inflammatory process. For example, asbestos can cause chronic lung irritation that can lead to cancer development.

STAGES OF CARCINOGENESIS

Carcinogenesis is a multi-step process that is continually evolving. It includes four stages: initiation, promotion, transformation, and progression (Figure 5.2).

1. **Initiation Phase:** Development of a permanent genetic mutation (acquired or inherited) within a tumor suppressor gene or an oncogene. Cellular immortalization and uncontrolled cell growth occur during this phase.
2. **Promotion Phase:** The stage between premalignant and invasive cancer development. It can take an extended period to develop a cancer cell, so progression has the potential to be reversible with chemoprevention medications, such as Tamoxifen and Proscar.
3. **Transformation Stage:** The cells are deprived of necessary oxygen and exposed to elevated levels of cellular waste products, which promotes the cells to transform into unhealthy cells. They also signal that would impede uncontrolled proliferation.
4. **Progression Stage:** The rapid proliferation of the mutated unhealthy cell. During this phase, the cancer cell is well developed and has the opportunity for local invasion as well as the potential to cause metastases.

▶ TUMOR DEVELOPMENT

Carcinogenesis describes the changes of genes and cells. As the cancer cells grow, especially in solid tumor malignancy, there are specific stages that a cancer cell will move through to develop into a tumor. The growth of tumor cells is measured in time. Growth fraction is the number of cancer cells proliferating within the tumor compared to the remainder of the cells within the body. Doubling time refers to the amount of time it takes to multiple or double in size. Each cancer cell's doubling time is different depending on the type of cancer cell. The stages of tumor development are:

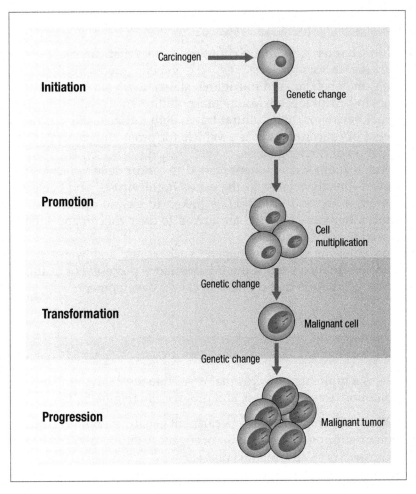

Figure 5.2 The four stages of carcinogenesis.

1. **Stage I—hyperplasia (hyper prefix means "more"):** Healthy cells look and act normal but are overexpressed (too many of them within the organ). An example is endometrial hyperplasia.
2. **Stage II—dysplasia:** Builds upon hyperplasia; cells look disorganized, rather than normal. An example is cervical dysplasia, which can be moderate to severe.
3. **Stage III—carcinoma in situ:** Cells have grown and spread within the organ; isolated to the organ of origin with no spread. It does not resemble the cell of origin and is abnormal, which is referred to as *anaplasia*.
4. **Stage IV—cancer:** Tumors have the ability to invade surrounding tissues and/or metastasize to areas outside the local tissue.

NOMENCLATURE AND CLASSIFICATIONS OF CANCERS

Terminology is a key component to determining the cancer cell origin. Table 5.1 presents the body's cells and corresponding prefixes. In addition to the cancer prefixes, cancer classifications are determined by the histology type of the tissue. The six categories classify over hundreds of cancers, include carcinomas, sarcomas, myeloma, leukemia, lymphoma, and mixed types (Table 5.2).

Table 5.1 Prefixes of Human Cancers

Pre-Fix for Cancers	Tissue and Organ Origin
Adeno	Glandular tissue cells
Chondro	Cartilage cells
Erythro	Red blood cells
Fib	Fibrous tissue cells
Hemangio	Blood vessels
Hepato	Liver cells
Leiomyo	Smooth muscle cells
Lipo	Fat cells
Lympho	Lymphocyte cells
Melano	Pigment cells
Myelo	Bone marrow cells
Myo	Muscle cells
Oseto	Bone cells
Rhabdomyo	Striated muscle cells

Table 5.2 Cancer Categories

Category	Cell Type	Organs
Carcinomas: Adenocarcinomas (glandular tumors) and squamous carcinomas (solid nest of cells with specific borders)	Epithelial tissues	Biliary tissue, breast, colon, gastrointestinal tract, lungs, pancreas, urogenital tract, skin
Sarcomas (e.g., osteosarcomas, leiomyosarcomas)	Connective tissues	Bone, cartilage, fat, muscle, tendons
Leukemia (acute or chronic)	Precursor	Cells/blood cells
Lymphoma	Lymphatic tissue	Blood vessels, nodes, spleen, thymus, tonsils
Mixed types (e.g., adenosquamous carcinoma, carcinosarcoma, teratocarcinoma)	Tissues from different categories and/or different cell types	Various

⬤ BIOMARKERS

Biomarkers, or tumor markers, are used to determine the number of potential cancer cells that are active within the body and monitor the progress of cancer treatments. They can be tested in the blood, urine, bone marrow, and tumor tissue. Genetic testing can also be viewed as biomarkers, which assists in determining the cancer disease state and aggressiveness of the cancer. There are several different types of biomarkers; some are isolated to specific cancers, and others are related to multiple malignancies.

Although biomarkers are useful, they can sometimes provide inaccurate information or misleading results because certain healthy normal cells can also elevate a tumor marker level. For example, PSA levels, which are used to identify and monitor prostate cancer, can also be increased in benign disorders such as benign prostate hypertrophy, thus showing a false positive. Laboratory scientists spend a tremendous amount of time to ensure that the tumor markers have both specificity and sensitivity. Specificity is the ability of a test to correctly identify patients *without* the disease, while sensitivity is the ability of a test to correctly identify patients *with* the disease. This means that the test is not sensitive enough for cancer, thus resulting in false negative. For the full list of the most common biomarkers in practice, visit https://www.cancer.gov/about-cancer/diagnosis-staging/diagnosis/tumor-markers-list.

▶ EXAM TIP

Review the full list of the most common biomarkers in practice at https://www.cancer.gov/about-cancer/diagnosis-staging/diagnosis/tumor-markers-list

⬤ TUMOR GRADING

Tumor grading is a system that measures how the tumor is growing within the body. Tumor grading is provided by the pathologist, who examines the cancer cells under the microscope to identify cell differentiation. Cell differentiation reveals the morphology and function of the cancer cell. In other words, it determines how much or how different it resembles the cell of origin. The less it resembles the original cell, the higher the grade. The four grades are:

1. Grade I—well-differentiated/low-grade: Resembles the cell of origin.
2. Grade II—moderately differentiated/intermediate grade: Somewhat resembles the cell of origin.
3. Grade III—poorly differentiated/high grade: Does not accurately resemble the cell of origin.
4. Grade IV—undifferentiated/high grade: Does not resemble the cell of origin.

Tumor staging determines the size, location, and extent of cancer. Staging for solid cancers is based upon the TNM staging system: T represents tumor, N represents lymph nodes, and M represents distant metastases. Each solid tumor has specific classifications regarding the size, nodal status, and metastatic sites. For example, breast cancer spreads to the brain, bone, lungs, and liver, whereas colorectal cancer spreads to lungs, liver, and peritoneum. Liquid tumors use different staging systems that will be discussed in related chapters.

ANGIOGENESIS

Angiogenesis, the development of blood vessels from the existing vasculature, is another mechanism cancer cells use to promote growth. Capillaries, which are the primary vehicle for angiogenesis, require oxygen to successfully complete the process. An important component of angiogenesis is the vascular endothelial growth factor (VEGF). VEGF is a powerful angiogenic factor to promote the growth of vascular endothelial cells. VEGF receptors are found on non-endothelial tumor cells, which increases the ability of the cancer cells to create new blood vessels and obtain nutrients for tumor growth and development.

METASTASIS

The final concept of carcinogenesis to review is metastasis. In metastasis, cancer cells can break away from the original tumor and travel through the blood or lymph system to distant locations in the body, where they exit the vessels to form additional tumors. The metastasis process includes direct invasion, seeding, and dissemination. The cancer cells multiply within a specific organ and break through the cell membrane into the surrounding tissue, which leads to seeding. Cancer cells have the innate ability to detach through chemical signals and growth factors from the primary tumor. Once detached, the cancer cells enter the lymph nodes and blood vessels, which promotes the locomotion of the abnormal cells to other organs (Figure 5.3). For example, in prostate cancer, the cancer cells leave the contained prostate and spread via the lymph nodes to the bone.

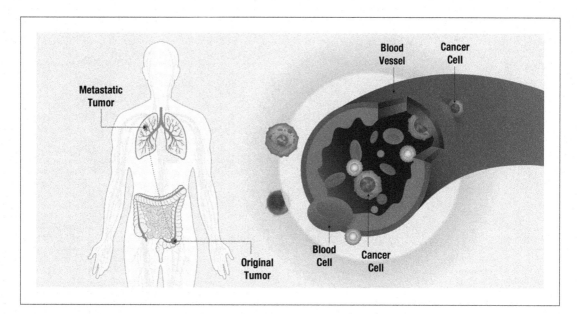

Figure 5.3 Cancer metastasis.
Source: National Cancer Institute.

The bibliography and references for this chapter are available on ExamPrepConnect; see inside front cover for access instructions.

1. Which factors in a patient's history will the nurse recognize as a risk for cancer development?

   A. First cousin diagnosed with colon polyps
   B. Father diagnosed with irritable bowel syndrome
   C. Mother diagnosed with a positive *BRAC2* test
   D. Paternal aunt diagnosed with a positive RAS test

2. Which of the following mechanisms is involved in the carcinogenesis process?

   A. Immune surveillance
   B. Genomic instability
   C. Apoptosis
   D. Chromosomal replication

3. The correct order of the stages of carcinogenesis is:

   A. Initiation, promotion, progression transformation
   B. Initiation, promotion, transformation, progression
   C. Promotion, initiation, progression, transformation
   D. Promotion, initiation, transformation, progression

4. Which of the following biomarkers should be ordered with a diagnosis of stage 2 breast cancer?

   A. CEA
   B. CA-125
   C. *HER2*
   D. AFP

5. A patient is informed that they have cancer of the cartilage of the right knee. Which of the following terms BEST describes this cancer?

   A. Osteosarcoma
   B. Leiomyosarcoma
   C. Liposarcoma
   D. Chondrosarcoma

(See answers next page.)   **47**

1. C) Mother diagnosed with a positive *BRAC2* test
A first-degree relative, such as mother, with a genetic mutation such as *BRAC2* would be most concerning for potential cancer development as *BRAC2* is an inherited tumor suppressor gene. A first cousin with colon polyps is not concerning now. Father with irritable bowel syndrome would not affect the patient unless they had a genetic colon mutation. An aunt with a positive *RAS* gene would be a potential concern, but a mother with an inherited gene would take precedence and further investigation would be required.

2. B) Genomic instability
Genomic instability is a mechanism related to carcinogenesis. Immune surveillance, apoptosis, and chromosomal replication are normal gene functions that help to protect against cancer development.

3. B) Initiation, promotion, transformation, progression
The order of the carcinogenesis stages is initiation, promotion, transformation, and progression.

4. C) *HER2*
HER2 is oncogene related to breast cancer. CEA is a marker for colorectal cancer, CA-125 is a marker for ovarian cancer, and AFP is a marker for testicular cancer.

5. D) Chondrosarcoma
Chondrosarcoma is the malignancy of the cartilage. Osteosarcoma is cancer of the bone. Leiomyosarcoma is a cancer of smooth muscle. Liposarcoma is a cancer of fat.

Treatment Modalities for Malignancies

INTRODUCTION

Oncology treatment does not typically utilize just one modality; instead, it often incorporates multiple treatment modalities, including surgery, radiation, chemotherapy, biotherapy, targeted therapy, and/or hormone therapy. The combination of the modalities depends on a number of factors:

1. Type of cancer: Solid or liquid malignancy, location of tumor, grade of tumor, and stage of tumor
2. Patient information: Age, comorbidities, previous cancers and treatments, family history, and patient consent
3. Goal of treatment:
   a. Cure: Elimination of the cancer
   b. Control: Management to stop the progression
   c. Palliation: Management of side effects of the disease, when cure is not an option
4. Quality of life: Side effects of proposed treatment

This chapter provides an overview of the different types of treatment options available. Individual treatments specific to each cancer will be discussed in their respective chapters.

SURGICAL TREATMENT

Surgical treatment is often the first choice for solid malignancies. Surgery is localized treatment; however, a patient may require more than one surgical procedure. For example, initially, a patient will require a biopsy, which is the removal of cells and/or a small amount of tissue to determine if cancer cells are present. Once a cancer is identified, then the recommended surgery will be discussed and performed. Biopsy options include fine-needle biopsy, core biopsy, incisional biopsy, laparoscopic biopsy, and diagnostic-guided biopsy (ultrasound, MRI, CT).

▶ KEY FACTS

Local excision: Removal of cancer cells and tumor

Wide excision: Removal of the tumor and surrounding tissue

Debulking: Elimination of as much of the bulk of a tumor as possible to aid chemotherapy and radiation

Ablation: Elimination of cancer cells via burning or freezing the cells

---

The bibliography and references for this chapter are available on ExamPrepConnect; see inside front cover for access instructions.

Surgery for cancer can be preventive, curative, palliative, or reconstructive (Table 6.1). While the goal is to cure cancer, not all diagnosed cancers are able to be cured, especially cancers that are identified at later stages.

Table 6.1 Types of Surgery for Cancer

Type of Surgery	Purpose	Examples of Surgical Procedures
Preventive	Used to prevent cancer development before it occurs; common with genetic and familial predispositions (e.g., *BRAC1* and *BRAC2*)	Prophylactic bilateral mastectomy, prophylactic hysterectomy
Curative	Used to remove the tumor and/ or diseased organ to achieve cure (limited disease; first line of defense with solid malignancies	Mastectomy, prostatectomy, colon resection, lung resection, and lobectomy
Palliative	Used to relieve symptoms such as pain and obstruction	Nerve blocks, stents (renal and bladder cancers)
Reconstructive	Used to reconstruct and/or replace the diseased organ	Breast reconstruction (implants or autologous reconstruction), facial reconstruction for head and neck malignancies

There are several methods used to perform surgery, which are highly dependent on the age and overall health of the patient, type of cancer, location of tumor/tumors, and stage of the disease. The different types of surgical approaches are discussed subsequently.

▶ ENDOSCOPIC SURGERY

Endoscopy is used to examine the internal aspects of the body, including the head and neck, cardiac area, thoracic area, digestive tract, bladder, and joints, as well as to obtain biopsies and remove tissue. If a procedure name ends in "oscopy," endoscopy is used. A variety of tools can be used in endoscopy, including flexible and biopsy forceps to remove tissue samples to determine if cancer is present, cytology brushes to take cell samples to determine if cancer cells are present, and suture removal forceps to remove sutures within the body.

There have been several advancements in endoscopy procedures, including virtual and capsule endoscopy. Virtual endoscopy is primarily used for colonoscopy and uses a CT scan to visual polyps. The scope is not inserted into the body. Bowel prep is still required because if polyps are found, a traditional coloscopy is required. Capsule endoscopy requires a patient to swallow a small pill with a camera inside, which takes pictures of the entire GI tract for 8 hours. The healthcare provider then reviews and makes determination based upon the pictures. This procedure is used to find polyps and cancer, as well as for gastric bleeding, Crohn's disease, and celiac disease. Advantages include less trauma to the tissues and decreased blood loss, scarring, and pain.

▶ LAPAROSCOPIC SURGERY

Minimally invasive surgery uses several small incisions within the abdomen for the transmission of multiple tools and a camera to obtain a biopsy or remove the tumor/ cancer. It is commonly used for cervical, ovarian, endometrial, colon, and kidney cancers. Its advantages include less invasive and decreased pain and length of stay.

▶ LASER SURGERY

Laser surgery is the use of narrow, focused light beams to reduce and destroy cancer cells. It is typically used for skin cancers and tumors that obstruct organs such as the stomach, esophagus, and colon. Lasers can also be used to stop localized bleeding and cover nerve endings to decrease or eliminate pain. CO_2 lasers use carbon dioxide to remove the first layer of tissue from an organ site. They are used for skin cancers and gynecologic cancers (e.g., cervix, uterine, vulva) at early stages. Photodynamic therapy (PDT; Argon laser) utilizes light energy to eliminate cancers. Advantages of laser surgery include targeted treatment area and decreased treatment time and damage to surrounding tissue.

▶ ROBOTIC SURGERY

This is the use of a specialized robotic equipment with computers and cameras to provide the surgeon with a 3D view of the surgical site; considered minimally invasive as it only produces small incisions. Advantages include less invasive, increased vision of surgical site; ability to reach difficult locations; decreased blood loss, postop pain, and recovery time.

> ### ▶ KEY FACT
>
> Signed consent must be received prior to any surgical procedure.

▶ ANESTHESIA

There are several categories of anesthesia. The type of anesthesia used depends on the type of surgery, the length of surgery, and the patient's overall health status. General anesthesia uses a combination of inhaled and/or IV anesthetics to cause a loss of unconsciousness and amnesia, decreased sensations and reflexes, and relaxation of muscles including the diaphragm. This method requires that the patient have an endotracheal tube to breathe during the procedure. The most common side effects are drowsiness, which wears off with time, and nausea and vomiting. Patients with a history of motion sickness are at a higher risk for post-anesthesia nausea and vomiting.

Regional anesthesia is used to block the sensation of pain in specific areas of the body. The patient can be awake during the procedure; however, a sedative is typically administered to relax the patient. While the patient's breathing pattern is not altered, regional anesthesia can cause permanent nerve damage, specifically with epidural blocks. These procedures should be performed by highly skilled healthcare providers to reduce the risk of nerve damage. There are several forms of regional anesthesia:

- **Peripheral nerve blocks:** Anesthetic agents are injected into a nerve or nerve bundle to eliminate the sensation of the nerve fiber. The most common types include brachial plexus block, which numbs the shoulder and arm, and femoral nerve block, which numbs the leg and thigh.
- **Epidural/spinal anesthesia:** Anesthetic agents are injected close to the spinal cord, which stops the feeling of the lower positions of the body (e.g., abdomen, hips, and legs). The most common side effect is a headache.

- **Local anesthesia:** Anesthetic agents such as lidocaine are injected into local site to eliminate sensation in that particular area. The patient will feel a numbing sensation. This is used for deep cuts or before a bone marrow biopsy. Local anesthesia can also be used in combination with sedation. Topical medications can also be applied to mucous membranes or the skin to numb the area. For example, Elma Cream can be applied to the skin over an implanted central access device, such as a port a catheter.
- **Sedation (conscious sedation or twilight sleep):** Narcotics and sedatives are administered to induce relaxation and drowsiness. Sedation does not require the patient to have an endotracheal tube; however, respirations will be decreased. Sedation is used for endoscopy and eye procedures.

▶ POSTOPERATIVE NURSING CONSIDERATIONS

1. Assess the patient's level of pain and pain tolerance level.
2. Take measures to reduce the risk of infection in the surgical wound, especially if surgical drains are placed. For example, post-mastectomy patients may have Jackson Pratt drains, which have a higher risk of infection. Nursing care should include proper handwashing, the administration of prophylactic antibiotics, sterile dressing changes, aseptic technique when emptying drains, and monitoring for signs/symptoms of infection (e.g., fever, chills, redness, pain, swelling at insertion site/surgical site, and drainage at the surgical site).
3. Take measures to reduce the risk of deep vein thrombosis (DVT). Surgery is a risk factor for developing a DVT. The nurse should encourage ambulation and the use of compression stockings and a sequential compression device.

● RADIATION THERAPY

Radiation is the use of high-energy waves—x-rays, gamma rays, electron beam, and protons—to eradicate cancer cells. Radiation works at the cellular level by destroying parts of the DNA of the cancer cell and inhibiting the ability of the cancer cell to replicate, divide, and grow. Radiation is a localized treatment effective against many types of cancers. The different forms of radiation particles include:

- **Alpha radiation:** Heavy, short-ranged particles that do not penetrate human skin. Examples are radon, radium, uranium.
- **Beta radiation:** Light, short-ranged particles that can penetrate the first layer of skin. Examples include pure beta emitters: strontium-90, carbon-14, tritium, and sulfur-35.
- **Gamma and X radiation:** Long-range electromagnetic radiation that is able to penetrate skin. Examples include gamma emitters: iodine-131, cesium-137, cobalt-60, radium-226, and technetium-99m.

Radiosensitive cancers are more receptive to radiation therapy and typically include rapidly dividing cancers versus cancer cells that are slower growing. Radiation therapy work bests on cancer cells that are in the active phases of cancer's cell cycle. Tumors that are slower growing have decreased replication time and do not benefit from radiation therapy as much as rapidly dividing cancer cells. The most common highly radiosensitive tumors include leukemia and lymphoma cells. Moderate highly sensitive tumors include squamous cell cancers of the head and neck and oropharyngeal and cervical cancers. Moderately low-sensitive cancers include salivary gland, breast, hepatomas, renal, pancreatic, and osteogenic. Significantly low-sensitive cancers include leiomyosarcoma and rhabdomyosarcoma.

Radio curability is identified as the relationship between normal tissue and tumor. The goal is to obtain a cure by radiating the cancer cells without causing damage to the surrounding healthy tissue. Radio curable tumors may only require radiation as the primary treatment.

Tumor location plays a vital role in the effectiveness of radiation therapy. Tumors that are easily accessible and adjacent to vital organs have the potential to be radiated without severe side effects. For example, breast and testicular cancers are easily accessible to be radiated with limited side effects versus providing radiation to brain cancer at the base of the brain stem.

▶ DOSING OF RADIATION

Dosing of radiation is considerably different from medication dosing. The dose of radiation is described as a gray (Gy) and is known as the international system of units for radiation. One gray is equal to 1 joule/kilogram, which is equal to 100 rads. Radiation therapy can continue to make changes at the cellular level, up to 6 weeks from the last dose of radiation. Radiation is similar to the dose of sunlight in the sense of intensity, duration of exposure, and sensitivity from the skin. Dosing concepts include:

1. **Absorbed dose:** The amount of radiation absorbed into the tissue to create a change at the cellular level.
2. **Equivalent dose:** The estimated dose of radiation that will produce a cellular change from the absorbed dose of radiation.
3. **Effective dose:** The calculated dose of radiation that can provide long-term effects of radiation.
4. **Fractionated dosing:** The dose of radiation is divided over days and weeks. Hyper fractionated is the delivery of smaller doses that are administered more than once per day. Hypo fractionated is the delivery of higher doses that are administered once a day or less often. The goal is to reduce the number of treatments provided.

▶ TYPES OF RADIATION THERAPY

There are two primary delivery methods of radiation therapy: internal radiation and external radiation. In internal radiation, or brachytherapy, radioactive material is placed inside a cavity of the body (e.g., prostate gland, vaginal vault, rectum) for a specific amount of time. Radiation implants include pellets, seeds, ribbons, wires, or tubes. Internal radiation can be delivered in low doses (LDR) or high doses (HDR).

External (XRT), or teletherapy, is sent from outside of the body and delivered daily over the course of several weeks, depending on the type and location of the tumor. Table 6.2 describes the different types of external radiation.

Table 6.2 Types of External Radiation Therapy

Type of Radiation Therapy	Description
Three-dimensional conformal radiation therapy (3D-CRT)	Provides radiation beams in several different directions to match the shape of the tumor; decreases radiation damage to normal tissues and maximizes cancer cell death
Image-guided radiation therapy (IGRT)	CT scans are performed prior to the radiation to direct the position of the radiation beam to the exact spot of the tumor and decrease exposure to normal tissues
Intensity-modulated radiation therapy (IMRT)	Radiation is delivered in 3D-CT, which allows for the strength of the radiation beam to be altered in specific areas to deliver a higher dose to eradicate cancer and preserve healthy tissues
Helical-tomotherapy (another form of IMRT)	Small beams of radiation are delivered in several different angles around the tumor to provide a more precise amount to the cancer
Photon beam radiation	Photons are delivered by a linear accelerator machine; increases the risk of destroying healthy tissue
Stereotactic radiosurgery (SBRT)	CT scans are used to determine the exact location of the tumor; a large dose of radiation to a small tumor from different angles during one session (CT scans determine location); used to treat primary brain tumors and lung, liver, and spinal cancers
Intraoperative radiation therapy (IORT)	Radiation delivered directly into a tumor or organ with tumors (e.g., hepatic cancers)

▶ RADIATION SAFETY PRACTICES

Radiation is a hazardous agent and requires safety precautions for the healthcare provider, patient, and family members post internal radiation, system radiation, or radioactive isotopes. Radiation dosing badges should be worn by healthcare providers. A dosimeter badge calculates how much radiation the provider is exposed to during their shift. The goal is to limit time and exposure to the source of the radiation, which can be remembered with the mnemonic ALARA:

A—As
L—Low
A—As
R—Reasonably
A—Achievable

The best method to achieve ALARA is via time, distance, and shielding. The nurse should reduce the time with the radiation source. Avoid being close to the source of radiation. For example, if a patient has cervical implanted radiation, the nurse should stand at the head of the bed and not at the foot of the bed. Shielding is the barrier protection from radiation, including lead aprons, portable lead shields, and drapes. These are tools that block the radiation field.

Sealed Versus Unsealed Sources

Radiation can be a sealed or unsealed source. A sealed source is a radioactive material that is encapsulated, fixed, and/or bonded to prevent the release of the radiation during handling, transportation, and change in temperatures. An example of a sealed source of radiation is radiation pellets used in brachytherapy to treat prostate cancer.

Unsealed sources included liquids, powders, and potential gases that are radioactive material and can cause exposure if not secured within containers. Examples include IV radioisotopes, which can be injected into a patient. Shielding is imperative for both sealed and unsealed sources during the transportation process prior to the delivery of either source.

Patient Education

Patient education for internal/systematic radiation therapy includes:

1. Practice proper hand hygiene.
2. Wash linens, towels, and personal laundry separate from other family members.
3. Sit while urinating to avoid splashing of urine (both men and women) and double flush the toilet.
4. Increase fluid intake to flush the radioactive material.
5. Do not share utensils.
6. Avoid sexual and intimate contact for at least a week after systemic radiation.
7. Keep a distance of 6 feet apart and avoid extensive visits by other family members.
8. Avoid contact with children, pregnant women, pets, and public areas for a designated time as instructed by a healthcare provider.

▶ SIDE EFFECTS

Radiation side effects tend to be localized and less systematic than chemotherapy and biotherapy. Skin discoloration and irritation of the area being irradiated are common with external beam radiation. To minimize, instruct the patient to avoid using creams or lotions on the area during radiation therapy. Mucositis typically occurs with head/neck malignancies. In some cases, it can be so severe that it impairs the ability to maintain adequate nutrition, necessitating a feeding tube for a short period of time. Patients typically experience fatigue toward the latter portion of the radiation treatment. They should be instructed to rest and exercise as able. Bone marrow suppression may occur when bones are being radiated and in stem cell transplant patients.

● CHEMOTHERAPY

Chemotherapy, antineoplastic agents, and cytotoxic drugs are interchangeable terminology to describe the chemical agents that are used to treat countless types of oncologic disorders. There are several specific terms that are associated with chemotherapy ordering and administering parameters. Chemotherapy agents are categorized as either cell-cycle specific or cell-cycle non-specific. Cell-cycle specific means that the chemotherapy agent will affect/destroy the cancer cell within a specific phase of the cell cycle. Cell-cycle non-specific means that the chemotherapy agent will affect/destroy the cancer cell in any phase, including the resting phase (when the cancer cell is least active). Understanding if the chemotherapy agent is cell-cycle specific or non-specific is important because most chemotherapy treatment regimens use a combination of chemotherapy agents to promote maximum cell death. Single agents are typically used in some maintenance regimens, advanced treatment, and treatment for palliation.

Dose-dependent refers to the amount of drug administered and the related amount of side effects. Therefore, if a lower dose is administered, there are fewer potential side effects. Dose limiting refers to increased side effects with a standard dose. With dose-limiting side effects, the drug dose needs to be decreased or eliminated altogether.

> ▶ **EXAM TIP**
>
> Know and understand chemotherapy terminology.

▶ CHEMOTHERAPY DRUG CLASSIFICATIONS

Table 6.3 describes the chemotherapy drug classifications. Although these medications are highly effective in treating oncology patients, these agents are considered hazardous material and can be a health threat to nurses and other healthcare providers. According to NIOSH (2014) and ONS (2018), hazardous drug (HD) criteria, an HD is any drug that meets at least one, if not more, of the following complications: carcinogenic, teratogenic, and/or causing developmental toxicity, reproductive toxicity, organ toxicity, and genotoxicity.

Table 6.3 Chemotherapy Drug Classifications

Chemotherapy Drug Classifications	Examples of Chemotherapy Agents	Cell-Cycle Specific or Non-Specific
Alkylating agents	Mustard gas derivatives: Cyclophosphamide, Ifosfamide Alkylsulfonates: Busulfan Hydrazines and triazines: Procarbazine, dacarbazine, temozolomide Nitrosoureas (only chemotherapy that can cross the blood–brain barrier): Carmustine, lomustine Metal salts: carboplatin, cisplatin, oxaliplatin	Cell Cycle Non-Specific
Plant alkaloids	Taxanes: Taxol, taxotere Vinca alkaloids: Vincristine, vinorelbine, vinblastine Podophyllotoxins: Etoposide Campthothecas: Irinotecan, topotecan	Cell Cycle Specific (tend to be more active in the S- and M-phases)
Antitumor antibiotics	Anthracyclines: Doxorubicin, daunorubicin, epirubicin, mitoxantrone Chromomycins: Dactinomycin Miscellaneous: Mitomycin, bleomycin	Cell Cycle Specific Non-Specific
Antimetabolites	Folic acid antagonists: Methotrexate. Pyrimidine antagonists: 5-Fluorouracil, cytarabine, capecitabine, gemcitabine. Purine antagonists: 6-Mercaptopurine Adenosine deaminase inhibitors: Fludarabine, nelarabine	Cell Cycle Specific
Topoisomerase inhibitors	Topoisomerase I inhibitors: Topotecan Topoisomerase II inhibitors: Amsacrine, teniposide	Cell Cycle Specific

ROUTES OF CHEMOTHERAPY ADMINISTRATION

Chemotherapy agents can be classified as irritants, non-vesicants, and vesicants. Irritants are medications that can cause moderate to severe irritation to the vein. For example, dacarbazine (DTIC) is known to cause severe pain if administered peripherally. Non-vesicants are medications that would not cause any harm to the surrounding tissue if they were to leak out of the vein. Vesicants are medications that are highly caustic to the veins, and, if leaked from the vein, can cause severe damage to the surrounding tissue.

Most vesicants must be administered via direct IVP to control the risk of extravasation. Adriamycin and Vinca alkaloids are well-known vesicants.

Chemotherapy agents can be administered via several different pathways depending on the treatment regimen and disease. The most common routes include:

- Oral: There are many more oral agents available to date than in the past years. The primary barriers to the oral route of chemotherapy are patient compliance and the potential for high costs. It is especially important to teach the patient that these agents should not be crushed, and any family member should wear gloves if assisting the patient in taking pills.
- Intravenous (IV): Agents can be administered via IVP or IVSS. IVP can be administered in less than 15 minutes and is directly administered into the vein or central venous device. Vesicants should be administered via IVP, with the exception of Vincristine, which should be administered via IVSS. IVSS is a short-term IV infusion that takes 15 minutes to 2 hours. With continuous IV, chemotherapy agents are infused over for 24 hours or more.
- Intramuscular (IM): Agents administered into the muscles. Barrier to administering via the IM route is the ability to maintain an adequate platelet count.
- Subcutaneous: Agents administered into the subcutaneous tissue.
- Intrathecal: Agents administered into the cerebrospinal column. This is used when cancer has spread to the central nervous system, which is common with lymphoma, leukemia, and metastatic breast cancer. The chemotherapy can be administered via the lumbar puncture or through an Ommaya reservoir, which is a surgically implanted device place in the head.
- Intrapleural: Agents administered into the pleura cavity.
- Intra-artery: Agents administered into an artery. This route is commonly used to treat hepatocellular cancer. A device is surgically implanted to deliver the medication via the artery directly to the liver. A primary barrier to this method is the risk of infection.
- Intraperitoneal: Agents administered into the abdominal cavity. This is common practice for ovarian and omental cancers. This also requires a surgically implanted device such as a Tenckhoff catheter or an abdominal port.

▶ SIDE EFFECTS

Chemotherapy agents do not have the ability to differentiate between a malignant cell versus a healthy cell. Thus, these agents have a large acute systematic side effect profile, which includes alopecia, skin/nail reactions, mucositis/stomatitis, nausea/vomiting, myelosuppression (neutropenia [infection], anemia, thrombocytopenia), constipation/ diarrhea, peripheral neuropathy, infusion/hypersensitivity reactions, and extravasations with vesicants.

▶ SAFETY MEASURES

Chemotherapy safety measures are essential. Organizations not only have the responsibility to take care of patients but the staff as well. The safety measures start with ensuring that appropriate education regarding HDs is well instituted. Safety guidelines and standards involving chemotherapy and all HD handling are created based upon the standards set by:

- Occupational Safety and Health Administration (OSHA)
- National Institute for Occupational Safety and Health (NIOSH)
- American Society of Health-System Pharmacists (ASHP)
- Oncology Nursing Society (ONS)
- American Society of Clinical Oncology (ASCO)
- United States Pharmacopeia (USP) Chapter 800 (ONS, 2018) requires all organizations to create and maintain an updated list of practice-specific HDs adapted from the comprehensive NIOSH list, as well as maintain and regularly update policies and procedures.

Hazardous Drug Education and Training

HD education and training should be based upon regulatory body standards and organization-specific training requirements. Two phases of education include orientation and annual competency assessments utilizing skills checklists and knowledge assessments. All oncology nurses who administer chemotherapy and/or immunotherapy at least once per month or less should further their knowledge by taking appropriate online courses provided by the Oncology Nursing Society.

Chemotherapy Orders

Chemotherapy orders must be standardized; no handwritten or telephone orders are acceptable. A completed and appropriate chemotherapy must include the following requirements:

- Patient's name
- Second patient identifier
- Order date
- Accurate height and weight
- Regimen name or protocol number and cycle number
- All medications are listed using general names, no abbreviations.
- Appropriate sequencing of drugs, if necessary
- Drug dosages are written following organizational standards.
- Dosage calculation and method
- Date of administration
- Rate and route of administration
- Allergies
- Laboratory parameters for withholding the chemotherapy
- Supportive care treatments: Pre-medications, pre- and post-hydration, if applicable, and growth factors, if applicable

Preparation of Hazardous Drugs

All HDs need to be prepared in a biological safety cabinet in a specifically designated pharmacy area. In addition, HDs need to be mixed, prepared, and drug calculation checked by a licensed pharmacist, a pharmacy technician, physician, or a registered nurse with sufficient education, training, and documented validation of competencies before administration of HDs.

Safe administration of HD requires a qualified physician, physician assistant, APN, and/or oncology registered nurse. Prior to each administration of HDs, two approved practitioners need to verify and document the following parameters are correct and appropriate:

- Drug name and dose
- Infusion or syringe volume
- Rate and route of administration
- Expiration dates/times
- Physical integrity of the drugs and bag or syringe—no visible particulate and color is appropriate
- Rate of the infusion pump, when appropriate
- Appropriate access site assessed and documented
- Maintaining positive blood return from either PIV or CVC obtained before, during, and after infusions.
- Completed documentation of administration of HDs
- Documented patient education
- Proper use of personal protective equipment (PPE).

Personal Protective Equipment

Personal protective equipment (PPE) is required for healthcare providers who are handling HDs, especially pharmacy and nursing staff. PPE includes the use of chemotherapy-designated gloves and gowns. Eye protection and respiratory protection need to be worn when appropriate. Two pairs of HD-tested and approved gloves should be worn for any activity involving HDs, including receiving and unpacking; preparing; administering and discarding; and disposing of, cleaning, and handling of patient excreta within 48 hours of receiving HDs. Only one pair of HD-approved gloves is necessary when dispensing intact oral chemotherapy pills (ONS, 2016b).

Gowns that are HD-tested and approved should be worn for any handling of HDs, including disconnecting HDs (ONS, 2016b). Gowns are for single use only and should be discarded in appropriate waste receptacles once removed. Goggles and/or face shields should be worn during any contact with HD that will be at risk for splashing or exposure. Respiratory protection (e.g., use of N95 mask) should be used when there is a risk of aerosolization and during spill cleanup (ONS, 2016b). Spill kits need to be readily available on the unit in case of a large spill. Finally, closed system transfer devices (CSTDs) should be used to prime HD without exposure to the environment and healthcare providers.

BIOTHERAPY AND IMMUNOTHERAPY

Biotherapy/immunotherapy is a broad term that includes monoclonal antibodies, gene therapy, and targeted therapy for solid and liquid cancers. To understand how biotherapy agents work, it is important to review basic immune system functions. The immune system promotes hemostasis by protecting and identifying pathogens. There are two forms of immunity:

1. Innate immunity: Refers to the genetic makeup, what is encoded on the DNA. It is the body's innate ability to create an inflammatory response (e.g., fever) once a pathogen is introduced to the immune system.
2. Adaptive immunity: Immunity that is acquired via active or passive means (Figure 6.1).

Biotherapy/immunotherapy agents work by changing and manipulating the environment in which the cancer cell lives within the body. In addition, certain biotherapy agents can directly connect with a specific receptor on the cancer cell to ultimately cause cell death.

They can also target, signal, turn on, and in some cases, suppress the immune system. See Table 6.4 for common biotherapy/immunotherapy classifications, their mechanisms of action, and side effects.

Table 6.4 Common Biotherapy/Immunotherapy Classifications

Classification/Mechanism of Action	Examples	Side Effects
Antiangiogenetic agents: Impair the ability of cancer cells to create a new blood supply to obtain nutrients to grow	Bevacizumab, sorafenib	Bleeding, peripheral neuropathy, nausea/vomiting
Cancer vaccines: Trigger the immune system to attack and kill the cancer cells	Sipuleucel-T, talimogene, laherparepvec	Flu-like symptoms, joint and back pain, nausea/anorexia, myalgia, neuralgia
Chimeric antigen receptor (CAR) T-cell therapy: Attach laboratory-altered T-cells to cancer cells to initiate cell death. Patient T-cells are extracted via pheresis, processed, and then infused back into the patient	Axicabtagene ciloleucel, brexucabtagene autoleucel, tisagenlecleucel	Cytokine storm syndrome (life-threatening), high fever, redness and swelling, severe fatigue, confusion
Cytokine therapy: Stimulate the growth of T-cells and natural killer cells	Interleukins, interferon	Severe allergic reaction, myelosuppression, thrombosis, skin rashes, depression (Interferon)
Immune checkpoint modulators: impair immunosuppression mechanism, preventing cancer cells from escaping immune surveillance	Thalidomide, lenalidomide, pomalidomide	Severe birth defects, somnolence, peripheral neuropathy, thrombosis formation, flu-like symptoms
Monoclonal antibodies: Target specific antigens to cause cell destruction or block the antigen protein to prevent cell growth	Alemtuzumab, rituxamaub	Infusion reactions/hyersensisity, skin rashes, flu-like symptoms
Targeted agents: Target the signaling, blocking, and/or turning off of the mutated genes of the cancer cell to stop cell growth	Cetuximab, trastuzumab, dasatinib	Skin reactions, rash, thrombosis formation, hypertension, GI perforation in rare cases with some targeted therapies

▶ TREATMENT ACCESS DEVICES

If the patient is receiving chemotherapy or biotherapy/immunotherapy, venous access is required. The two primary routes of administration are either peripheral venous access (PVC) or central venous (CVC) catheters. The route is determined based upon the diagnosis, age of the patient, lifestyle, and most importantly, the chemotherapy/biotherapy regimen. For example, some chemotherapy agents can only be administered via central venous (CVC) catheters, such as continuous 5FU infusion. CVC are devices that may require a surgical procedure and are inserted or implanted into the internal jugular vein and/or the subclavian vein. Oncology nurses should be aware of which vein is accessed because the subclavian approach is associated with an increased risk of pneumothorax. If a patient is receiving multiple agents and requires hydration and other supportive medications, two peripheral IVs may be required. The second option is to obtain central venous access. There are several central venous access devices that can be used, including implanted port A catheter (PAC), peripherally inserted central venous catheter (PICC), triple lumen catheter (short-time use only), and apheresis catheter (used for stem cell transplantation).

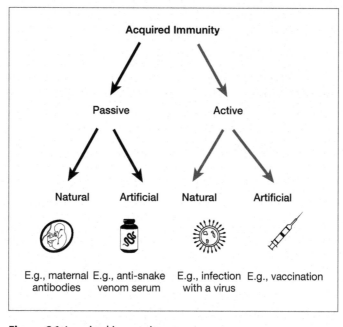

Figure 6.1 Acquired immunity.

Source: Reprinted from Gawlik, KS, Melnyk, BM, and Teal, AM. *Evidence-Based Physical Examination: Best Practices for Health and Well-Being Assessment (2021).* Springer Publishing Company.

Although CVCs are convenient for patients and providers, they can cause acute complications such as vascular perforation, hemothorax, pneumothorax, hematoma, and device malposition. They can also cause late complications such as infection, thrombosis, and occlusions.

▶ NURSING CARE CONSIDERATIONS

CVC requires specific care to maintain the catheters. When working with CVCs, the oncology nurse must adhere to organization-specific policies and procedures and:

1. Assess for blood return before administering any HD.
2. Perform sterile dressing and cap changes when appropriate.
3. Flush with saline and heparin as policy.
4. Scrub all ports with chlorhexidine before use of CVC.
5. Monitor for signs and symptoms of infection.
6. Ensure appropriate patient education is completed and document on how to successfully care for CVC.

COMPLEMENTARY AND ALTERNATIVE CANCER THERAPIES

Complementary and alternative medicine (CAM) is the term for medical products and practices that are not part of standard medical care. CAMs can be beneficial to oncology patients because they enhance the ability to cope with the side effects of cancer treatments, such as nausea, pain, and fatigue; increase the patient's ability to comfort themselves and decrease stress; and enable patients to participate in the cancer recovery process more actively. There are four different categories of CAM used for cancer treatment:

- **Mind–Body Therapies:** These therapies combine thinking, breathing, and body movements to help relax the body and mind.
  - Meditation: Focused breathing or repetition of words or phrases to quiet the mind.
  - Biofeedback: Using simple machines, the patient learns how to affect certain body functions that are normally out of one's awareness, such as heart rate and respirations.
  - Hypnosis: A state of relaxed and focused attention in which a person concentrates on a certain feeling, idea, or suggestion to enhance the healing process.
  - Yoga: Ancient practice developed in India, which uses the body to stretch and maintain numerous different poses. The primary focus is to pay attention to the breathing patterns during each pose. Yoga supports the mind, the body, and the spiritual aspect.
  - Tai Chi: Involves slow, gentle movements with a focus on the breath and concentration.
- **Biological-Based Practices**
  - Vitamins and supplements: such as high levels of antioxidants like vitamin C
  - Botanicals/herbal medicine: Herbs like turmeric are used frequently for its anti-inflammatory and anti-carcinogenic properties. Medical cannabis is another example of botanical medicine for oncology patients that helps to increase appetite and decrease insomnia and nausea and vomiting.
- **Body-Based Practices**
  - Chiropractic care: Alignment of bones and joints.
  - Massage: Rubbing and kneading of muscles and joints of the body to relieve tension and/or pain.
  - Reflexology: Type of massage used to relieve tension and treat illness, based on the theory that there are reflex points located within the head, hands, and feet. The points are linked to support other parts of the body.
- **Biofield Therapy (or energy medicine):** Biotherapy involves the belief that the body is based on energy fields that can be aligned to promote healing and wellness. Therapists use their hands to move the energy in a positive and natural flowing direction to restore balance and wellbeing. Techniques include Reiki and therapeutic touch.
- **Aromatherapy:** The use of essential oils to alter mood or improve wellbeing. Interventional use of aromatherapy in cancer patients suggests a short-term benefit to reduce anxiety and depression, improve sleep and increase overall wellbeing lasting up to 2 weeks (Boehm et al., 2012). Oils can be applied topically in diluted forms, used in massage therapy, inhaled by adding a few drops to steaming water and using an atomizer or humidifier, or added bathwater or placed on linens. The oils also can cause local skin irritation, especially with prolonged skin contact, allergic contact dermatitis, and phototoxicity from reaction to sunlight. Repeated topical administration of lavender and tea tree oil was associated with reversible prepubertal gynecomastia (*"Aromatherapy,"* 2009). These oils can mimic estrogenic and antiandrogenic activities and, therefore, are not recommended for patients with estrogen-dependent tumors, such as breast cancer. Common oils used in aromatherapy include:
  - Lavender: Used to modify mood, decrease anxiety, and improve sleep.
  - Eucalyptus oil: Used for antimicrobial and anti-inflammatory effects.
  - Roman chamomile: Used to reduce anxiety and stress.

The bibliography and references for this chapter are available on ExamPrepConnect; see inside front cover for access instructions.

1. Which of these education points should be addressed when a patient is being discharged from receiving internal cervical radiation therapy?

    A. Tell the patient they have no restrictions

    B. Tell the patient to avoid direct contact with small children

    C. Explain to the patient that their blood counts will be affected within the next 10–14 days

    D. Explain to the patient that they will need to wear a radiation badge for the next week

2. A patient is receiving rituximab for the treatment of lymphoma. Which of the following nursing interventions should be included in the patient's care plan?

    A. Monitor for neutropenia

    B. Monitor for anemia

    C. Monitor for extravasation

    D. Monitor for infusion reaction

3. A 49-year-old patient who is 48 hours post right-sided implanted PAC for large-cell B lymphoma and is starting Hyper C Vad A is complaining of right-sided arm pain. The patient's BP is 120/70 mmHg, pulse is 100 bpm, respiration is 18 breaths/min, and temperature is 99.8°F. The nurse suspects that the patient is experiencing:

    A. Hemothorax

    B. Pneumothorax

    C. Device malfunction

    D. Infection

4. The correct order of a properly completed chemotherapy order is:

    A. Patient ID, cycle, pre-medications, drug, dose, route, and rate

    B. Patient ID, pre-medications, drug, dose route, and time

    C. Patient ID, regimen, drug, dose, route, rate, and time

    D. Patient ID, cycle, regimen, drug, dose, route, and rate

5. The nurse is preparing to administer cisplatin to a lung cancer patient. All of the following measures are required before administration of this agent, EXCEPT:

    A. Obtain accurate height and weight

    B. Review allergies

    C. Calculate drug dose

    D. Plan for infusion reaction

1. B) Tell the patient to avoid direct contact with small children

Patients who receive internal radiation need to avoid children and pregnant women for a specific time frame. Internal radiation therapy does have restrictions. Blood counts are typically affected with chemotherapy, not radiation therapy. Radiation badges are used only by healthcare providers.

2. D) Monitor for infusion reaction

Monoclonal antibodies such as rituximab pose the greatest risk for infusion reactions. Neutropenia, anemia, and extravasation are side effects related to chemotherapy agents.

3. D) Infection

Infection is a potential complication from PAC insertion. The nurse should suspect an infection due to the patient's pain and low-grade temperature of 99.8°F, which are early signs of in fection. The patient would have pain and an altered respiratory rate with hemothorax or pneumothorax. If there were a device malfunction, the nurse would not be able to access, flush, or infuse.

4. A) Patient ID, cycle, pre-medications, drug, dose, route, and rate

The correct order of a properly completed chemotherapy order is patient id, cycle, pre-medications, drug, dose, route, and rate.

5. D) Plan for infusion reaction

Cisplatin is a chemotherapy agent. Before administration of this agent, the nurse should obtain accurate height and weight, review allergies, calculate drug dose, and don personal protective equipment (PPE). The nurse does not need to plan for infusion reactions that are typically associated with biotherapy agents.

Hematopoietic Stem Cell Transplantation

INTRODUCTION

Hematopoietic stem cell transplantation (HCT) is a potentially curative treatment modality used to treat a variety of hematological malignancies, solid tumors, and nonmalignant conditions. Over the past several decades, advances in the scientific and clinical management of patients have led to improved outcomes and made the therapy available to a wider range of patients.

Historically, HCT centered around using high-dose chemotherapy to eradicate tumor cells, followed by infusion of stem cells to "rescue" the bone marrow and reestablish hematopoiesis. Although this principle remains, capitalizing on the immunologic effects of donor T cells leading to a graft versus tumor effect has become a focus of study and continues to evolve in the field.

TYPES OF HEMATOPOIETIC STEM CELL TRANSPLANTATION

The disease process, stage of diagnosis, age and comorbidities of the patient, and potential availability of donors will help determine which HCT treatment is best for the patient. Although HCT therapy is effective for various solid and liquid tumor malignancies, it has also been shown to be effective in autoimmune disorders due to the immune effect created by this treatment. There are three types of HCT:

1. Autologous (Auto): Uses the patient's own stem cells collected prior to the conditioning regimen.
2. Allogeneic (Allo): Uses donor cells that are harvested from another person, related or unrelated to the patient.
3. Syngeneic: Uses stem cells that are harvested from an identical twin sibling. This is comparable to an autologous HCT without the possibility of tumor contamination.

There is no graft versus tumor effect due to identical immune cells of patient and donor.

Boxes 7.1 and 7.2 list the malignant and nonmalignant indications for autologous and allogeneic HCT therapy.

The bibliography and references for this chapter are available on ExamPrepConnect; see inside front cover for access instructions.

Box 7.1 Malignant and Nonmalignant Indications for Autologous Stem Cell Transplantation

Malignant Indications

- Acute myeloid leukemia
- Acute promyelocytic leukemia
- Ewing sarcoma
- Germ cell tumors
- Hepatoblastoma
- Hodgkin's lymphoma
- Medulloblastoma
- Multiple myeloma and other plasma cell disorders
- Neuroblastoma
- Non-Hodgkin's lymphoma
- Osteosarcoma

Nonmalignant Indications

- Amyloidosis
- Autoimmune diseases
- Chronic inflammatory demyelinating polyradiculoneuropathy (CIDP)
- Multiple sclerosis
- Systemic lupus erythematosus (SLE)
- Systemic sclerosis

Box 7.2 Malignant and Nonmalignant Indications for Allogeneic Stem Cell Transplantation

Malignant Indications

- Acute lymphoblastic leukemia
- Acute myeloid leukemia
- Chronic lymphocytic leukemia
- Chronic myelogenous leukemia
- Hodgkin's lymphoma
- Myelodysplastic syndrome
- Myeloproliferative disorders
- Multiple myeloma
- Non-Hodgkin's lymphoma

Nonmalignant Indications

- Aplastic anemia (severe)
- Diamond-Blackfan syndrome
- Combined immunodeficiency (severe)
- Dyskeratosis congenita
- Fanconi anemia
- Hemoglobinopathies
- Inborn errors of metabolism
- Inherited bone marrow failure syndromes
- Osteopetrosis
- Paroxysmal nocturnal hemoglobinuria
- Sickle cell disease
- Thalassemia major
- Wiskott-Aldrich syndrome

SOURCES OF TRANSPLANT CELLS

There are three sources of cells that can be collected or harvested to perform a hematopoietic transplant: peripheral stem cells, bone marrow cells, and umbilical cells. See Table 7.1 for the advantages and disadvantages of each source.

Table 7.1 HCT Cell Types: Advantages and Disadvantages

Cell Type	Advantages	Disadvantages
Bone marrow cells	■ Short collection time ■ Low T-cell count—less chronic GVHD (allo) ■ No need for growth factors or apheresis catheter ■ Minimal risk to donor	■ Slower engraftment of neutrophils/platelets ■ Surgical procedure with an anesthesia risk
Peripheral stem cells	■ No need for anesthesia ■ Rapid hematologic recovery ■ Low risk of contaminated tumor cells (auto)	■ May require a central venous catheter ■ Requires growth factors; side effect bone pain ■ May require multiple sessions ■ Higher risk for chronic GVHD (allo)
Umbilical cell	■ Prompt availability and decreased cost ■ Noninvasive to donor ■ Increased pool of donors ■ Requires less stringent HLA match ■ Lower risk of infection	■ Cell size limits ■ Donor not available for future cell collections ■ Increased risk of graft failure/delayed engraftment ■ Less graft versus tumor effect ■ Possible maternal T-cell contamination ■ Possible transmission of unknown genetic anomaly

GVHD, graft versus host disease; HLA, human leukocyte antigen.

Bone marrow cells are harvested directly from the bone marrow. This is a surgical procedure that requires multiple injection sites in the bilateral posterior iliac crests to collect as many cells as possible. This procedure can be done for both auto and allo transplants. Bone marrow cells are known as "immature cells" and can take longer to engraft.

Peripheral stem cells are collected from peripheral blood, with a procedure known as "apheresis." Apheresis uses a special machine to remove the blood from the body to remove the stem cells, then the rest of the blood is placed back into the patient's body. This is performed via an outpatient procedure, usually requiring several days to collect enough cells. Cells can be collected for auto and allo transplants.

Umbilical cells are collected from the umbilical cord after the birth of a baby. Individuals can choose to donate the cells or store them after delivery in a stem cell laboratory in the event they would be needed for their child or other family members.

> ▶ **EXAM TIP**
>
> Know the terms related to the HCT process, as well as the steps and timeline.

⬤ OVERVIEW OF THE TRANSPLANT PROCESS

See Figures 7.1 and 7.2 for an overview of the autologous and allogeneic transplant process.

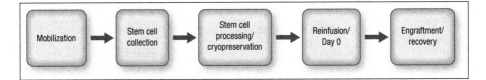

Figure 7.1 Autologous Stem Cell Transplantation Process.

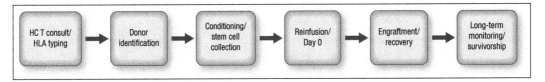

Figure 7.2 Allogeneic Stem Cell Transplantation Process.

▶ STEP I: IDENTIFICATION OF DONOR

The first step is to identify an appropriate donor for transplant. If the patient is proceeding with an auto stem cell there is no donor selection process. However, if an allogeneic transplant is the recommendation, then a donor needs to be identified. The process can be cumbersome depending on the culture and genetic makeup of the patient.

For an allogeneic transplant, the HLA typing of the patient and donor needs to be addressed. The key is to have the closest HLA match as possible between the patient and donor. The human leukocyte antigen (HLA) complex determines an individual's ability to recognize "self" versus "non-self." This function protects the body from foreign pathogens and other invaders. Histocompatibility testing is performed to determine if a donor and recipient have compatible genetic complexes. **The degree of histocompatibility between the donor and recipient can greatly influence the risks of complications and the success of the transplant**.

The major histocompatibility complex (MHC) is encoded by genes received from each parent, located on chromosome 6. There are five loci of primary importance when determining a match for an allogeneic HCT: HLA-A, B, C, DRB1, and DQB1. Each locus has a pair of antigens (one from each parent), resulting in a total of 10 antigens used to determine compatibility. Of note, for umbilical cord blood, only HLA-A, B, and DRB1 are tested for a total of six antigens.

In most cases, family members are assessed first to find a related donor. However, there is a 25% chance for two siblings to be a full HLA match. Therefore, when family members are not a match, or the patient does not have siblings, an unrelated donor is researched. According to the National Marrow Donor Program, a national bone marrow registry, there is an approximately 60%–70% chance of finding a histocompatibility donor through the registry. This percentage decreases for patients of mixed ancestry, race, and for minority populations.

Another option is to use haploidentical donor, which can be siblings, parents, or extended family. Haplo identical donors have been used more frequently in recent years. Donors who match with one haplotype (inherited from one parent) can be used safely with newer techniques, such as administration of post-transplant cyclophosphamide. This has greatly expanded the donor pool and allowed more patients to have the option of transplantation. There are additional molecular testing techniques being developed and researched to improve tissue typing and matching for patients and donors, such as killer cell immunoglobulin-type receptor (KIR) typing. Preliminary work is promising and may predict future outcomes.

▶ STEP II: PATIENT EVALUATION

After the type of transplant is determined and a donor is identified, the patient will begin the transplant process. To determine suitability for HCT, the patient undergoes a comprehensive evaluation that includes the following:

1. Physical examinations
   a. Dental and gynecologic examinations
   b. Comorbidity index
   c. Psychosocial assessment to determine available support systems for the patient during the transplant and recovery
2. Laboratory testing
   a. CBC
   b. Full chemistry panel
   c. PT/INR
   d. ABO typing, high-resolution HLA typing
   e. Pregnancy testing for women
3. Diagnostic testing
   a. Cardiac evaluation—EKG, echocardiogram, or MUGA scan
   b. Pulmonary evaluation including pulmonary function test (PFT) and CXR
   c. Kidney and liver function tests
   d. Infectious disease testing
   e. Full disease staging depends on the patient's diagnosis may include an MRI, CT, or PET scan
      i. Bone marrow biopsy and aspirate
      ii. Serum or urine disease biomarkers
4. Financial, spiritual, cultural, and emotional factors should be explored to address concerns and issues that could affect the patient's ability to have access to post-transplant therapies and symptom management.
   a. Written and verbal education should be provided to the patient and family and reinforced throughout the transplant process.

Donor Testing

The donor for an allogeneic transplant undergoes an evaluation to determine eligibility and suitability for donation. Donor assessment includes:

1. Comprehensive history and physical exam
2. CBC, full chemistry panel, PT/INR, infectious disease testing, ABO typing, high-resolution HLA typing, kidney and liver function testing, and pregnancy testing for women
3. EKG and CXR prior to anesthesia; some may require an anesthesia consultation

▶ STEP III: STEM CELL COLLECTION

Stem cell sources include bone marrow, peripheral blood, or umbilical cord. Bone marrow procurement is usually performed in the operating room under general anesthesia, and multiple aspirations from the bilateral posterior iliac crest yield the marrow. The product is filtered for blood and fat, then infused fresh or cryopreserved for later use.

Peripheral blood stem cells (PBSC) are collected via apheresis using peripheral venous access or a central venous apheresis catheter. Stem cells are mobilized out of the bone marrow into the peripheral blood using hematopoietic growth factor, most commonly filgrastim either alone or in combination with chemotherapy. Plerixafor, a CXCR4 antagonist, may be added to facilitate mobilization in patients with multiple myeloma or non-Hodgkin's lymphoma. Target collection dose is a minimum of 2.5×10^6 CD34+ cells for successful engraftment.

Umbilical cord blood (UCB) is cryopreserved after birth and stored in a registry bank. Due to the limited number of stem cells in a cord blood unit, two units can be infused into the recipient to facilitate engraftment. In addition, due to the immaturity of the T-cells, stringent HLA typing is not required for a UCB transplant, allowing for easier procurement.

Stem cells or bone marrow may be processed to reduce tumor contamination or T-cell population. Manipulation of the stem cells can potentially cause damage with delayed engraftment or rejection and is performed on a limited basis. T-cell depletion can decrease the risk of GVHD but may increase the risk of relapse due to reduced graft versus tumor effect, although the data is conflicting.

Bone marrow products from donors with a different blood type than the recipient will be processed to remove red cells to prevent hemolytic infusion reaction. Peripheral blood stem cells can be cryopreserved in specific aliquots for potential future use, either for a second transplant or for donor lymphocyte infusion for maintenance or in the event of relapse. Cryopreservation is done with dimethylsulfoxide (DMSO) to protect the cells during freezing and prevent lysis on thawing.

▶ STEP IV: CONDITIONING

The conditioning or preparative regimen can include any combination of chemotherapy, radiation, or monoclonal antibodies. The purpose is to eliminate as much tumor as possible, to suppress the immune system of the donor to prevent rejection (allo), and to create space in the bone marrow for the donor stem cells. Conditioning regimens can be myeloablative or non-myeloablative, depending on the patient, comorbidities, and disease.

1. **Non-myeloablative or reduced-intensity** regimens refer to agents that do not cause nonreversible cytopenia and are used to reduce the toxicities normally associated with high-dose chemotherapy. Patients who are older or who have comorbidities could be candidates for HCT using these lower intensity regimens.

2. **Myeloablative regimens** refer to the ability to cause nonreversible cytopenia and are associated with a higher risk of toxicities. These regimens are used to treat aggressive diseases in patients with fewer risk factors for toxic effects. Table 7.2 lists the common chemotherapy and biotherapy agents used in transplant therapy. Please note many of these chemotherapy agents are used in combination; they are rarely administered as a single agent.

Table 7.2 Common Chemotherapy and Biotherapy Agents Used in Transplant Therapy*

Agents Used in Transplant Therapies	Monitoring Considerations
Cyclophosphamide (Cytoxan)[†]	Hemorrhagic cytosis; nausea/vomiting; severe myelosuppression
Busulfan (Myleran)[†]	Hepatic toxicity; pneumonitis
Etoposide (VP-16)[†]	Hypotension; severe myelosuppression
Fludarabine (Fludara)[†]	Neurotoxicity; pulmonary toxicity; severe myelosuppression
Thiotepa (Tepadina)[†]	Severe myelosuppression
Carmustine (BCNU, BICNU)[†]	Pulmonary toxicity; renal toxicity; severe myelosuppression
Bortezomib (Velcade)	Peripheral neuropathy
Melphalan (Alkeran)	Gastrointestinal toxicity; severe myelosuppression
Rituximab (Rituxan)	Infusion-related reactions

*Many of these agents are used in combination; they are rarely administered as a single agent.

[†]These agents are administered in high/elevated doses.

Radiation as a Conditioning Regimen

Total body irradiation (TBI) can be used as a single conditioning agent typically used in a non-myeloablative regimen or in combination with chemotherapy in myeloablative regimens. TBI is given in fractions depending on the dose, 12–15 Gy for myeloablative and 2–8 Gy in non-myeloablative regimens.

Nurses are responsible for patient education, providing premedications prior to the radiation session, and managing side effects. The most common side effects of TBI include nausea and vomiting, enteritis, and mucositis. Administering anti-emetics, anti-diarrheal medications, pain medications, and IV fluids, in addition to meticulous oral and skincare, are some interventions for prevention and management of radiation effects. Radiation can increase the risk of gastrointestinal, pulmonary, and hepatic complications.

Oncology and transplant nurses should be familiar with the side effects of each chemotherapy and biotherapy agent in the conditioning regimen and routinely monitor patients for adverse effects. All organ systems are susceptible to adverse effects, including the hematopoietic, gastrointestinal, integumentary, pulmonary, hepatic, renal, urologic, cardiac, and neurologic systems.

Monitoring of vital signs, weight, blood counts, chemistry, and organ function should be performed regularly and documented as per institution guidelines. Preventative measures to reduce the risk of infection, mucositis, nausea and vomiting, and tumor lysis are standard of care for transplant recipients. Nutritional services and physical therapy should be provided to prevent malnutrition and muscle weakness. Intravenous fluids, pain medications, antimicrobial medications, anti-emetics, and anti-diarrheal medications are some of the pharmacologic interventions to support the patient after conditioning. In addition, nonpharmacologic interventions including ambulation, hygiene, oral care, and toileting, will promote comfort and well being. Providing emotional support and encouragement fosters patient involvement in their care and recovery.

▶ DAY 0

The day of stem cell reinfusion is identified as Day 0, and the post-transplant days are numbered sequentially going forward. The stem cell product is brought to the bedside and identified, and cryopreserved cells are thawed gently in a water bath.

Fresh or thawed cells are infused into the patient via central venous catheter either by direct slow push or by gravity drip. The patient is monitored for infusion reaction to the product or DMSO. Common HCT reactions include nausea, vomiting, and hypotension (vagal response to the cold infusion).

Rarely, more severe reactions including hypertension, arrhythmias, tachycardia, respiratory arrest, or diffuse alveolar hemorrhage may occur. The patient should be carefully monitored during and after the infusion for an adverse reaction.

▶ ENGRAFTMENT

Engraftment occurs when stem cells in the marrow start hematopoiesis, as evidenced by improvement of peripheral blood counts. The definition of engraftment can vary, but typically it occurs with:

1. Absolute neutrophil count (ANC) $\geq 0.5 \times 10^8$ on the first of 3 consecutive days
2. Platelet counts of $>20 \times 10^9$ with platelet transfusion independence for 7 days

Timing of engraftment depends on the source of stem cells, conditioning, prior disease, and infections. Peripheral blood stem cells will engraft more quickly than bone marrow or UCB.

The percentage of donor cells can be measured in the peripheral blood or bone marrow and is known as donor chimerism. Once the patient has successfully engrafted, donor chimerism should reach 100% and is monitored after HCT.

▶ ACUTE COMPLICATIONS POST HCT

PANCYTOPENIA

An expected side effect of the conditioning regimen, pancytopenia is managed with growth factors and supportive care. Common growth factors include:

1. Granulocyte colony-stimulating factor (G-CSF): stimulate neutrophils
2. Granulocyte-macrophage colony-stimulating factor (GM-CSF): stimulate neutrophils
3. Erythropoietin (EPO): stimulate red blood cell

Transfusion support is provided, with threshold parameters dependent on institutional guidelines, clinical symptoms, and comorbidities. Blood products should be irradiated to prevent transfusion-related graft versus host disease and alloimmunization. Leukocyte-reduced products will decrease the risk of viral transmission and exposure to cytomegalovirus (CMV).

INFECTION

Patients can develop bacterial, viral, parasitic, or fungal infections because of the immunosuppression of conditioning regimen and neutropenia, and their previous infection history. A comprehension history of previous infections should be done prior to HCT to allow for appropriate prevention and monitoring strategies. The most common organisms, types of infections, and occurrences in the transplant timeline are noted in Figure 7.3.

Treatment for Infections

Prophylactic antibiotics, antivirals, and antifungals start during the conditioning regimen and continue for 1 year after transplant or until the patient is off immunosuppressive medications. Fever is the hallmark of infection, and the patient should be pan-cultured and started on broad-spectrum antibiotics in the event of a temperature >100.4°F. Additional testing such as CT scans, MRIs, or biopsy can be done for persistent fever to identify the source. The patient should be monitored for viral infections during the early post-transplant phase and while receiving immunosuppression. Most common viral infections include:

- Herpes simplex
- CMV
- Epstein Barr
- BK human polyoma virus
- Respiratory syncytial virus
- Enteric viruses

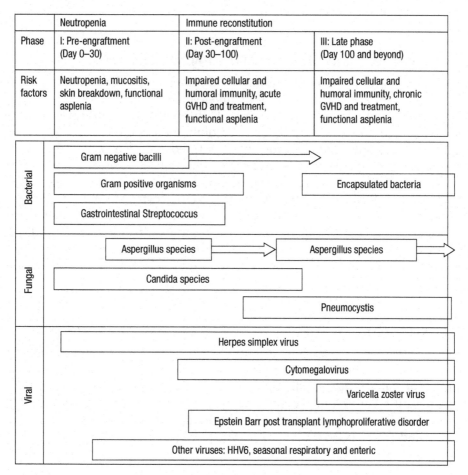

Figure 7.3 Common Infections That Occur in Transplant Patients

Source: From figure 2 of Tomblyn, M., et al. (2009). Guidelines for preventing infectious complications among hematopoietic cell transplantation recipients: A global perspective. *Biology of Blood and Marrow Transplantation*, 15, 1143–1238, with permission from Elsevier.

Patients and families should be educated on recognizing symptoms of infection and how to notify the HCT team. Education should include prevention strategies such as handwashing, oral care, skincare, and personal hygiene. Methods to mitigate environmental risks such as restricting visitors, avoiding crowds, avoiding dust or mold, and consuming a low microbial diet should be discussed.

HEPATIC SINUSOIDAL OBSTRUCTIVE SYNDROME

Hepatic sinusoidal obstructive syndrome (SOS) can occur in up to 50% of patients undergoing HCT, with the highest risk in matched unrelated donor transplants and patient who receive TBI. The conditioning regimen causes damage to the sinusoids of the liver, leading to obstruction of the sinusoidal flow. Additionally, cytokine release activates the coagulation and fibrinolytic pathways, precipitating coagulopathy. Diagnostic criteria include at least two of the following: weight gain, elevated bilirubin, and right upper quadrant pain.

Treatment For SOS includes pharmacologic interventions such as defibrotide, ursodiol, diuretics, and heparin, while fluid management, pain control, and liver function monitoring are nonpharmacologic adjuvants. Severe SOS can be up to 80% fatal in transplant recipients, therefore careful screening and monitoring of patients with higher risk and prompt diagnosis and treatment are critical to reducing mortality.

IDIOPATHIC PULMONARY INTERSTITIAL PNEUMONITIS

Idiopathic pulmonary interstitial pneumonitis (IPIP) can be caused by infectious pathogens or be noninfectious, and the risk increases with myeloablative regimens and TBI. Symptoms include dyspnea, cough, fever, and hypoxia. Diffuse alveolar infiltrates, fibrosis and inflammation are seen, likely a result of the conditioning regimen.

Treatment includes antimicrobials for any identified pathogens, corticosteroids, and oxygen support. Other pulmonary complications include diffuse alveolar hemorrhage (DAH), infectious pneumonia, and peri-engraftment respiratory distress syndrome (PERDS). DAH and PERDs are mainly treated with corticosteroids and respiratory support. Pulmonary infections can be bacterial, viral, or fungal and are treated with the appropriate antimicrobial agent once the organism is identified, and possibly corticosteroids. Opportunistic infections should be considered, especially in patients who have been or who are currently being treated for GVHD with immunosuppressive therapy.

GRAFT VERSUS HOST DISEASE

Graft versus host disease (GVHD) is an immune response where immunocompetent donor T-cells attack recipient host tissues leading to varying degrees of end-organ damage. It is the most frequent complication of allogeneic HCT and is a leading cause of morbidity and nonrelapse mortality. The risk of GVHD increases with disparate HLA histocompatibility, unrelated donors, age, and myeloablative conditioning. Table 7.3 describes the differences between acute and chronic GVHD.

Table 7.3 Differences Between Acute and Chronic Graft Versus Host Disease

Characteristics	Acute GVHD	Chronic GVHD
Timing	Within the first 100 days after allogeneic transplant	Occurs after day 100 of transplant
Presentation	Occurs in 30%–60% of patients	Risk factors for cGVHD include prior aGVHD, age, PBSC transplant, HLA disparity, and unrelated donor transplant
Organ involvement	Skin, liver, gastrointestinal tract	Skin, gastrointestinal tract, oral cavity, eyes, lung, liver, and joints
Symptoms	Rash, nausea, vomiting, diarrhea, jaundice, and weight loss	Related to the inflammatory and fibrotic changes in organs, similar to autoimmune disorders
Treatment	Prophylaxis: Calcineurin inhibitors, low-dose methotrexate, reduced-intensity conditioning regimens First-line therapy: Corticosteroids, typically 1–2 mg/kg of body weight daily, tapered off over several weeks once symptoms resolve Second-line therapy: Ruxolitinib	First-line therapy: Topical medications, corticosteroids, calcineurin inhibitors Second-line therapy: Mycophenolate mofetil, monoclonal antibodies, sirolimus, extracorporeal photopheresis (ECP), clinical trials

GVHD, graft versus host disease; HLA, human leukocyte antigen; PBSC, peripheral blood stem cell.

Nurse Role in Graft Versus Host Disease

Nurses can provide education to patients and families regarding signs and symptoms of GVHD. Immunosuppressant-related side effects should be managed to promote comfort and adherence to the regimen, and levels of calcineurin inhibitors monitored. Interventions to preserve integrity of skin and mucous membranes should be employed, and good personal hygiene and nutrition should be maintained. Due to profound immunosuppression, infection is the most common cause of mortality for patients with GVHD. Patients should be monitored for infection and prompt treatment initiated. Psychosocial support is critical to promote coping strategies and provide support to families.

▶ RECOVERY

Recovery is dependent on the type of transplant (auto versus allo), GVHD, complications post-HCT, and other patient factors including age, comorbidities, and psychosocial issues.

● FOLLOW-UP CARE

A multidisciplinary team is essential to address the variety of post-HCT effects and the impact on the patient's quality of life. Monitoring post-HCT includes regular follow-up evaluations with the transplant team to identify complications, management of therapeutic drugs, levels, and interactions, and to monitor for disease persistence or recurrence. In the unfortunate event of relapse, donor lymphocyte infusions (DLI) can be used as part of reinduction or maintenance. Patient and family education continues throughout the recovery phase, and psychosocial support should be available. Partnering with the patient's medical team outside of HCT can ensure prompt recognition of complications and promote good preventative healthcare maintenance. Patients will require regular vaccinations to prevent pneumococcal pneumonia, meningitis, hepatitis, polio, tetanus-diphtheria, influenza, and measles, mumps, and rubella, among others. Good dental care and skin surveillance, as well as recommended health screenings such as mammography, colonoscopy, and endocrine monitoring, should be part of the post-HCT survivor plan.

As the field of HCT continues to evolve, and outcomes improve, more HCT survivors are in the community and will continue to require long-term monitoring and support. Survivorship programs are increasing in numbers, and nurses will play a critical role in managing and facilitating these programs. Nurses need to stay current with knowledge of the latest scientific and technological advances in the field to provide patients and families with ongoing education and assistance to achieve a high quality of life as a cancer and HCT survivor.

The bibliography and references for this chapter are available on ExamPrepConnect; see inside front cover for access instructions.

1. Which type of donor cells are used for an allogeneic HSCT?

   A. Patient's own stem cells
   B. Patient's twin stem cells
   C. HLA-matched donor stem cells
   D. Non-HLA-matched donor stem cells

2. A 60-year-old patient who is 30 days post allogeneic stem-cell transplant presents with a red rash all over the body. The nurse recognizes that the patient is experiencing which complication?

   A. Chemotherapy-induced rash
   B. Acute skin GVHD
   C. Chronic skin GVHD
   D. Acute liver GVHD

3. Which of the following BEST describes bone marrow transplant procurement?

   A. Bone marrow transplant harvest and peripheral stem cell collection
   B. Bone marrow biopsy and bone marrow harvest
   C. Bone marrow biopsy and peripheral stem cell collection
   D. Donor harvest and bone marrow biopsy

4. Umbilical cord transplants have a high risk for engravement failure because the:

   A. Cells are immature
   B. Cells have been treated with chemotherapy
   C. Cells have been irradiated
   D. Cell count is low

5. What preservative is used to protect the stem cell during the freezing process?

   A. Custodiol
   B. Dimethylsulfoxide (DMSO)
   C. Viaspan
   D. IGL-1

1. C) HLA-matched donor stem cells

Allogeneic HSCT uses HLA-matched donor stem cells, not non-HLA-matched donors. Autologous HSCT uses a patient's own stem cells. A patient's twin stem cells are used in a twin syngeneic transplant.

2. B) Acute skin GVHD

Acute GVHD occurs within the first 100 days of transplant and manifests with rash and redness on the skin. Chronic GVHD occurs post 100 days, and GVHD of the liver presents with jaundice and abnormal liver functions.

3. A) Bone marrow transplant harvest and peripheral stem cell collection

In bone marrow transplant procurement, bone marrow is harvested, and peripheral blood stem cells are collected. Bone marrow biopsy is used to determine if cancer is in the bone marrow and as a tool to stage disease.

4. D) Cell count is low

Umbilical cords tend to have fewer cells infused and typically require more than one donor. Bone marrow cells are immature. Transplant cells are not irradiated or treated with chemotherapy.

5. B) Dimethylsulfoxide (DMSO)

DMSO is used to protect the cells during freezing. Custodiol, Viaspan, and IGL-1 are used in kidney transplantation.

Research and Clinical Trials

INTRODUCTION

The definition of research as it relates to human subjects comes from the Code of Federal Regulations (CFR) Part 46 Protection of Human Subjects (2009): "Research means a systematic investigation, including research development, testing, and evaluation, designed to develop or contribute to generalized knowledge." Each study is designed to answer a question with the intent to formulate or reinforce new knowledge that intends to benefit a specific population. Clinical trials are designed to generate data for prevention, screening, device implantation, investigational new drugs or products, and quality of life.

CLINICAL RESEARCH

Types of clinical research include experimental/interventional studies and observational studies. In an *experimental study*, an intervention is introduced to participants for the purpose of studying the effects of that intervention. They are typically randomized controlled trials (RCTs) in which participants are randomly assigned to a group. One group receives the intervention and the other group—the control group—receives a placebo or no intervention. In an *observational study*, an area of interest is simply observed (e.g., condition, risk factor, treatment) without the introduction of an intervention.

▶ THE REVIEW PROCESS

The U.S. Food and Drug Administration (FDA) constructed four types of review processes for clinical trials to accelerate the process and bring important drugs to market more rapidly. This is especially important for first-available treatments or if a drug is showing advantages over existing therapies. The processes are (i) priority review, (ii) breakthrough therapy, (iii) accelerated approval, and (iv) fast track.

1. **Priority Review:** The FDA's commitment to review an application within 6 months as opposed to a 10-month standard review process. Priority review highlights the trial as paramount and suggests the products would give patients options for life-saving medical treatment compared to the available standard of care. Priority review can be requested if the treatment shows evidence of increased effectiveness in the treatment, prevention, or diagnosis of a condition; elimination or substantial reduction of a treatment-limiting drug interaction; documented enhancement of patient compliance that is expected to lead to an improvement of serious outcomes; or evidence of safety and effectiveness in a new subpopulation (*The FDA's Drug Review Process: Ensuring Drugs Are Safe and Effective*, 2020). Priority review will not affect the overall length of the clinical trial period. The applicant will be made aware within 60 days of the receipt of the original application if the product is approved for priority review.

The bibliography and references for this chapter are available on ExamPrepConnect; see inside front cover for access instructions.

2. **Breakthrough Therapy:** Intended to expedite the development and review of drugs for serious conditions based on preclinical evidence that the product is superior to standard of care therapy (FDA, 2018). Breakthrough therapy utilizes morbidity and mortality data and is requested by the applicant or pharmaceutical company, but the FDA may also recommend that the product qualifies for breakthrough therapy based on preclinical and clinical data review. The request for breakthrough therapy should be received by the FDA by the end of phase II meetings. The intent of breakthrough therapy is to gather data to support product approval as quickly and safely as possible.

3. **Accelerated Approval:** Incorporates surrogate end points into data review to save precious time during the drug approval process. Patients diagnosed with cancer may not have years to wait to ascertain if a drug extends meaningful survival; the FDA can approve a drug if the target (e.g., tumor) shrinks, and this is extrapolated to demonstrate a clinical benefit. The drug can be approved as accelerated and then also move into phase IV trials to continue to collect long-term data and the drug becomes approved. If phase IV trials do not confirm the projected benefits, a drug can be pulled from the market, or the labeling can be amended to incorporate the information from the phase IV trial.

4. **Fast Track:** Expedites review of new drugs that treat serious medical conditions or conditions that classify as unmet medical needs. A drug that is in development to provide treatment for a diagnosis without any currently available treatment classifies as an unmet need. Fast track is also available to drug therapies that show an advantage over available treatments. Fast-track designation must be requested by the pharmaceutical company and can be done at any time during the drug development process (*The FDA's Drug Review Process: Ensuring Drugs Are Safe and Effective*, 2020). The FDA will review the application and notify the applicant within 60 days with their determination.

TYPES OF CLINICAL TRIALS

Clinical trials are not only for investigational agent approvals, but these also answer questions regarding cancer prevention, cancer screening, and quality of life concerns. These trials are associated with lower risk to participants because no early phase investigational products are being tested (*Types of Clinical Trials*, NIH, 2020). Types of trials are as follows.

1. **Prevention trials** are conducted in healthy individuals who are at high risk for developing cancer. Prevention trials are designed to reduce the risk of developing cancer. Prevention trials are further sub classified as action trials or agent studies. Action trials are focused on the actions patients can take to reduce their risk of developing cancer, such as exercise and diet. Agent trials, also known as chemoprevention studies, focus on whether taking certain vitamins or supplements can lower the risk of cancer. The objectives of prevention trials are to determine if the agents are appropriate and if the interventions prevent cancer (*Types of Clinical Trials*, NIH, 2020).

2. **Screening trials** are designed to answer the question to find new ways to detect cancer in the early stages when treatment may be more successful. Examples of screening trials are chest x-rays for former or current smokers to detect lung cancer, prostate exams with PSA evaluation to detect prostate cancer or routine mammograms. Screening trials are attempting to answer questions about whether finding the disease early saves lives, if there is a screening test that is superior to detecting disease in early stages, and if the people receiving the screening tests are subjected to costly and unnecessary tests or procedures.

3. **Quality-of-life (QOL) trials** can either be conducted independently or contained within a phase I-IV investigational drug trial. Quality-of-life trials are designed to find out

how cancer treatment affects patients and how can patients' quality of life or comfort be improved. Due to innovations in oncology treatment, patients are living longer lives; QOL trials seek to find out if length of time is complemented by the quality of time, symptom relief, comfort, pain, and stress relief. Patients participate in QOL trials by anonymously answering questionnaires developed specifically to ask questions about symptom management and the data is compiled for review. An example of a questionnaire a patient completes is the FACT-Lym; the questionnaire gives specific instructions to the patients to mark how they are feeling within the last seven days. The patients are asked questions about their physical, social, emotional, and functional well-being. The FACT-Lym and other questionnaires like it can be completed on paper or by electronic device.

⬤ THE CLINICAL TRIAL PROCESS

Oncology patients presently have vast treatment options due to the availability of clinical trials. Clinical trials are available in different phases and stages of development that can provide patients with an opportunity to receive cutting-edge treatment that is not currently FDA approved. The difference between standard treatment options and clinical trials is there is no guarantee that the investigational agent or device will be beneficial. Historically, clinical trials have not been the first treatment choice for patients. Unfortunately, clinical trials have been noted to have a negative context, and patients often viewed themselves as "guinea pigs." Due to unethical treatment of patients during trials in the past, regulations for clinical trial execution are strict and have oversight from multiple governing bodies.

For patients to fully appreciate their commitment to the clinical trial as well as risks, the patients must undergo a thorough informed consent process, which includes meeting with the principal investigator and several members of the clinical and research team.

To date, clinical trials are subject to Institutional review board (IRB) review, FDA oversight, and approval from the data safety monitoring board review (DSMB) to ensure trial participants are receiving ethical treatment. It is imperative that patients are fully aware of all their treatment options, research, and standard of care, before deciding to pursue a clinical trial.

Clinical trials are an opportunity for patients to gain access to promising medical advances that may have a meaningful impact on their life. Patients are becoming very savvy and have access to medical information through the internet, print media, publications, and television. Patients start disease-specific support groups that discuss pertinent relevant research and provide resources to each other for treatment options.

▸ INSTITUTIONAL REVIEW BOARDS

Clinical research trials are subject to strict review and approval processes to protect the health, safety, and welfare of participants. Institutional review boards (IRB) are a group of individuals who oversee the research process to ensure the protection of human subjects. The FDA mandates according to the code of federal regulations (CFR) in 21 CFR subpart 56 gives the standards for the composition, operation, and responsibilities of an IRB (FDA, 21 CFR 56, 2020). "An IRB is defined as a board or group to review, to approve the initiation of, and to document periodic review of, biomedical research involving human subjects. The primary purpose of such review is to assure the protection of the rights and welfare of human subjects" (FDA, 21CFR56, 2020). IRBs are required to have at least five members with diverse backgrounds; each member must have adequate knowledge to review research proposals and make recommendations regarding study conduct. The members must also be diverse with respect to race, gender, and cultural backgrounds; the IRB members may not all come from the same profession. A community member, or nonscientific member, must also be present to bring a nonmedical perspective to the board. The IRB must also have a board member that is not affiliated with the institution in any capacity. IRB members, like principal investigators, must disclose any potential conflict and cannot vote on any agenda items for which they have conflict. The IRB must do a review of the research trial at least once yearly.

To approve clinical trials, the IRB must review the criteria as dictated in 21 CFR 56. The IRB must ensure the risks to subjects are minimized, risks to subjects are reasonable, the selection of subjects is equitable, informed consent is provided and the process appropriately documents, subject privacy is protected, protections for vulnerable subjects is provided, and data monitoring is conducted to ensure subject safety (FDA, 21 CFR 56, 2020).

The IRB is responsible to review the informed consent, protocol, and data used for trial development to determine whether the clinical trial is appropriate to move forward to human subjects testing. During the review of the research trial submission, the IRB can determine that the trial is approved, disproved, or needs modifications. If the documents require modifications before resubmission, the IRB will provide feedback to the investigator. The investigator can be called upon to discuss trial relevance, including preclinical and clinical data, known or suspected risks to subjects, or data safety monitoring plans.

The IRB can be classified as local or central. Local IRBs review studies on site where the research will be conducted. Central IRBs are used to review large multicenter trials; 21 CFR 56 allows for multi-institutional studies to avoid duplication on local IRBs, which would slow down the research process. There are benefits and issues to central and local IRBs (Wandile, 2018).

LOCAL INSTITUTIONAL REVIEW BOARD

A local IRB will review studies on site where the research is going to be conducted. The advantage of utilizing a local IRB is that most of the members are likely employed by the institution and understand the culture and standards that are important to the institution and community. The review process is controlled locally, and the IRB members are familiar with the process and familiar with each other. Conversely, some drawbacks to using a local IRB are high startup costs and maintenance salaries as well as high demand for work, especially at academic institutions. Small hospitals conducting research risk maintaining the required five members for a quorum. Local IRBs can also function as external IRBs for investigators at outside institutions to offset the institutional financial burden and therefore their caseload may be time consuming (Wandile, 2018).

CENTRAL INSTITUTIONAL REVIEW BOARD

A central IRB is beneficial for large multicenter trials and prevents duplication of work and IRB function. IRBs are expensive to maintain and centralized IRBs help offset the institutional costs while also providing a more streamlined approach to opening potentially lifesaving clinical trials. Central IRBs adhere to the same FDA guidelines as a local IRB. An academic institution with its own IRB may opt to have both local and central IRB oversight, which is also allowed by FDA guidelines. A drawback to central IRB utilization is that if there is an error in oversight it could affect all the sides for the large multicenter trial and risk subject safety or affect data integrity. Central IRBs also do not have the benefit of being on site at the institution and having a personal relationship with the investigators or members of the research team (Wandile, 2018). Central IRBs have access to large panels of experts and can guarantee a quorum of at least five members, as per 21 CFR 56 guidelines (2020); it is the responsibility of the principal investigator to ensure that the board has an expert that is pertinent to the proposed research material to satisfy the IRB directives.

▶ DATA SAFETY MONITORING COMMITTEE

DSMC, also known as DSMB (Data Safety Monitoring Boards), is a group of individuals separate from an IRB that review ongoing data from the trial to make determinations that subjects are protected, and that the data gathered has scientific merit (Guidance of Clinical Trial Sponsors, 2006). Not all clinical trials require a DSMC, and early phase trials also do not require a DSMC. Trials conducted at the NIH and the VA are required to have DSMCs in certain trials, but the FDA does not require the use of DSMCs except for emergency use trials.

DSMCs are usually implemented for large multicenter trials that implement investigational agents that impact morbidity and mortality. Oncology trials frequently utilize DSMCs for intervention trials as the objectives in later phase trials are frequently remission and survival focused. Utilizing a DSMC does lengthen the trial timeline because the DSMC must pause trial enrollment to review data and make recommendations regarding their findings. Trials that will enroll and close quickly are unlikely to benefit from a DSMC due to the short time frame.

A DSMC is beneficial because it increases collaboration between industry and government, provides heightened awareness within the scientific community about the risk of inaccurate or biased research results, protects human subjects by reviewing data and terminating problematic trials, and addresses the IRB concerns of oversight and monitoring outside of the investigator and sponsor levels to promote patient safety. The guidelines for DSMC meetings are usually outlined in the protocol (Guidance of Clinical Trial Sponsors, 2006). Planned and unplanned pauses in clinical trial enrollment and dose escalation are possibilities. Patients should be educated that safety review is a standard part of clinical trials and a pause is not indicative of unexpected serious events. If unexpected events are related to the investigational product, and the side-effect profile is updated or changed patients will be made aware. Notifying the patients of changes in the protocol or the clinical trial are documented in the patient's medical record.

Drugs and products that are being developed and tested have a path that is followed to determine safety and efficacy. The process to find a successful drug from bench to market can take years or decades. Factors like barriers to enrollment, patient population, access to clinical trials, product safety and efficacy, and data integrity will affect how quickly investigational products progress through the phases. There are five phases that a drug needs to pass through to be FDA approved and available for marketing.

▶ **EXAM TIP**

Review and understand the clinical trials approval process.

⬤ PHASES OF CLINICAL TRIALS

▶ PHASE 0: FIND THE MOLECULE

Phase 0 clinical trials are conducted prior to any large-scale testing using small doses of the proposed agents. Phase 0 trials are intended to ascertain which new products may be successful in a clinical trial with human subjects. Phase 0 trials have the smallest number of human subjects participants at approximately 10 to 15 (Gupta et al., 2010) and the shortest time of administration of about 7 days. Phase 0 trials can be conducted quickly, and multiple compounds can be tested under a single IND. Once a molecule of the drug has shown promise, the trial will move forward into phase 1 testing.

▶ PHASE I

Phase 1 studies are early phase clinical trials that serve to find a recommended dose for potential escalation to a phase 2 trial. Phase 1 clinical trials are dose escalating and aim to find the maximum tolerated dose (MTD) by algorithms and cohorts. For example, a 3 + 3 is a common design for phase 1 cohorts; a small number of patients (3) are enrolled at each dose level and monitored. After a period of monitoring and then review without safety concerns, the trial may proceed to the next dose level. If adverse outcomes are noted at a specific dose level, additional patients are added to the dose level for continued monitoring. Doses can be decreased if there are safety concerns of the patient, concerns from industry scientists or administrators and/or clinical investigators. Once the MTD is found, the cohort often expands to compile additional safety data before moving into phase 2 trials. Historically, due to the design of phase 1 drugs, these research studies are slow to enroll patients. Often, patients who participate in a phase 1 trial have likely had systemic treatment before and do not have any standard treatment options available.

Phase 1 trials are also not designed to provide long-term overall response data; phase 1 trials are primarily to establish safety and dosing parameters for an investigational agent. Phase 1 and 2 trials can be combined to shorten the duration of the clinical trial process. Yan et al. (2018) note that the phase 1-2 combination is more efficient and can identify a phase 2 dose more optimally while meeting both the safety and efficacy criteria. The phase 1-2 trial allows for a larger patient sample size and incorporates efficacy which is not a primary or secondary outcome for phase 1 trials. Increasing the data set provides more information about the investigational product and potentially shortens the time the drug spends in trials and then to market. If a phase 1-2 trial was completed and advances in the clinical trial process, a phase 2 trial will not be required.

An issue with the phase 1-2 trial design is that the inclusion and exclusion criteria for the trial remain the same throughout both phases. Phase 1 trials usually have an open eligibility criterion as the trial is designed to enroll extensively previously treated populations. Applying the same eligibility criteria to both phase 1 and phase 2 patients enables the data to be analyzed across phases and progress more efficiently, but the targeted patient population may not be desirable for both phases.

The FDA guidelines for phase 1 trial design and participation indicate that preclinical testing in laboratory animals must take place and then extrapolate plans for human subject participation. Based on the animal model data results, the FDA will determine if the trial should begin first-in-human testing. Once phase 1 testing is approved, the trial can project treating approximately twenty to eighty patients in the trial. This number will be larger if the trial is a phase 1-2 combination, but for phase 1 only designs the enrollment will be smaller than any other clinical trial phase. Phase 1 trials are designed to determine if a product is safe to use; phase 1 trials are not designed to determine if a drug is going to be efficacious for the condition under study.

▶ PHASE 2

Phase 2 studies can be considered once an MTD or acceptable dose based on pharmacodynamics and pharmacokinetic studies if an MTD is not achieved and if the phase 1 trial does not demonstrate unacceptable toxicities. Phase 2 trials enroll more patients than a phase 1 trial to have a larger data sample to analyze if the product will be effective. The goal for phase 2 trial enrollment is up to several hundred patients. Safety and adverse events are continuously evaluated in the larger sample size, so long-term and short-term data can be collected and augment the information gleaned from the phase 1 trial. Jung (2015) states phase 2 trials are used to weed out experimental therapies that will not be efficacious in the targeted population; phase 2 trials most commonly use a single-arm treatment group, and the results are compared to information about currently available and approved treatment regimens. A common endpoint of phase 2 trials is tumor response which can be measured by RECIST, Lugano, or Cheson criteria depending on the diagnosis. Small samples sizes and short study periods are common for phase 2 trials as the primary goal is efficacy as safety has previously been established in the phase 1 trial.

▶ PHASE 3

Phase 3 trials can proceed if phase 2 or phase 1-2 trials have shown drug efficacy. The phase 3 trial will gather more data regarding efficacy, safety (long and short term) and study the product in combination with other drugs. The gold standard for phase 3 trials is randomized controlled trials. For example, Bhatt and Mehta (2016) discuss how RCT is the standard for clinical research trials and have been the established method for moving drugs through to market. RCT enrolls large numbers of patients and offers a comparison with the drug under study against the approved standard of care treatment. For example, Connors et al. (2018) discuss the trial design for Echelon 1, a randomized trial for patients diagnosed with stage III or IV Hodgkin's lymphoma. The standard therapy for patients with Hodgkin's for stage III–IV was ABVD for six cycles given every 15 days as per NCCN guidelines. ABVD has been the most used frontline regimen since 1975. Bleomycin has the potential to cause pulmonary fibrosis, and patients who develop intolerable side effects to bleomycin cannot continue to receive it through the duration of their treatment. A phase 2 trial predated the large-scale phase 3 RCT; A+AVD was administered to 25 patients with newly diagnosed advanced Hodgkin's lymphoma and showed a 96% complete response rate and a 5-year overall survival rate of 100%. Based on the findings in the phase 2 trial, the combination was approved to move into a phase 3 RCT.

The patients in the Echelon 1 trial were randomized into two groups: ABVD (doxorubicin, bleomycin, vinblastine, and dacarbazine) or A+AVD (doxorubicin, vinblastine, dacarbazine, and brentuximab vedotin). The trial design was an open-label format, meaning the patients, providers, and sponsors would be aware of the combination assignment. The patients were randomly assigned 1:1 by a computer program to ensure the arm assignments were randomized. A total of 1334 patients were treated in the study with 664 patients in the investigational arm and 670 patients in the standard therapy arm. The phase 3 trial enrolls more patients than phase 1 and 2 trials. The data collected for each arm were more robust than previous trials with smaller numbers. The trial had a successful outcome in that "A+AVD had superior efficacy to ABVD in the treatment of patients with advanced-stage Hodgkin's lymphoma, with a 4.9 percentage-point lower combined risk of progression, death, or incomplete response and use of subsequent anticancer therapy at two years (Connors, 2018).

▶ PHASE 4 (POST-MARKET)

Post-market, or expansion trials, are performed when a drug receives an abbreviated approval through either priority review, breakthrough therapy, accelerated approval, or fast track. The rapid approval trials are usually conducted on a smaller number of patients either due to available sample size, superior response to the therapeutic agent, or treatment needed for the disease under study. Phase 4 trials are jointly conducted with commercial approval of the drug and are designed to gather more data about the drug. Rapid approval trials do not usually have long-term data analysis based on their time frame, and phase 4 trials can provide the drug to patients who meet an inclusion/exclusion criterion based on the product labeling with the intent of long-term and larger-scale data collection. The inclusion/exclusion criteria are shorter than a phase 2-3 trial and reflect the FDA-approved labeling, so the data gathered will be consistent with the population for whom the drug is approved. If the phase 4 trial completes and patients are still enrolled and are receiving benefits from the drug, they can be transitioned to commercial supply to prevent disruptions in therapy.

INVESTIGATOR BROCHURE

The Investigator Brochure (IB) is a collection of all the data on the investigational product that provides sponsors, IRBs, the FDA, and investigators with clinical data. The IB is required to have a table of contents, summary of the investigational product, drug formulation properties, animal model study data, clinical data on humans including pharmacokinetics and pharmacodynamics, dose response, adverse effects (serious and non-serious), marketing experience, and summary of data and guidance from the investigator (Guideline for Good Clinical Practice ICH E6(R2) Consensus Guideline, 2020). When determining if adverse events are related to the drug under study, the research team will reference the IB to verify if the adverse event has been previously reported. When the drug is in the early development stages, the adverse effect profile is rapidly evolving. The investigator is required to determine if, regardless of presence in the IB, the relationship between the adverse effect and the drug. Drugs in post-marketing have a more advanced IB and FDA labeling, and the adverse effect may already be reported. IBs are updated as new clinical information becomes available and side effect profiles change. Ensuring the most up-to-date IB is being utilized for adverse event relationship review is important to accurate clinical trial documentation and patient management. An institution performing multiple clinical trials with a pharmacologic agent will share an IB as it contains the most updated information about that product. For example, a trial utilizing Nivolumab for patients diagnosed with melanoma and a separate trial for patients diagnosed with lymphoma will use the same IRB.

▶ **EXAM TIP**

Review and understand the different phases of drug development.

INFORMED CONSENT

Informed consent is the cornerstone of patient autonomy. Patients consent prior to any voluntary procedure, which can be as innocuous blood draws or as complex as brain surgery. Clinical trials are not exempt, and the informed consent process is highly regulated for patients consenting to research. Oncology clinical trials are presented to patients, and the stakes are high because patients are concerned about their mortality. The informed consent process serves as a guide to protect the patient by guaranteeing that every effort is made to inform the patient, provide information, avoid coercion, and support the patient and family through a potentially difficult decision-making process.

▶ HISTORY OF INFORMED CONSENT

Informed consents are heavily regulated by government agencies, and the requirements of the content have evolved throughout the years. Many experiments have been conducted in the United States that did not meet the basic principles of human subject research protection. Of note, experiments performed on prisoners of war during World War II in Nazi-occupied territories are some of the most horrific examples of "research"; these assaults on human beings lead to significant changes in research regulations and guidelines. "The Medical Case" also known as "The Doctors' Trial" took place from December 9, 1946, through August 20, 1947, and tried Nazi war criminals, many who were prominent physicians, for war crimes due to executing nonvoluntary research (Capron, 2018, p. 19). The prisoners in concentration camps were utilized as unwilling human subject participants in unethical trials. The experiments exposed the prisoners to illness, disease, poisons, saltwater ingestion, immersion in freezing water, subjected them to high altitude conditions, and performed unnecessary experimental surgeries in inhumane conditions.

Former prisoners testified against the Nazis, and some were executed for their participation in sadistic and immoral experiments. The Nuremberg Code was developed because of "The Doctors' Trial" in August 1947. There are ten statements in the code that apply to human subject's research, the most important being, "the voluntary consent of the human subject is absolutely essential" (Nuremberg, 2018, p. 10). In summary, the other statements require that the patient be of sound mind to provide informed consent that is not influenced by bias or coercion, the experiment is intended to provide results that will benefit society, the experiment is based on animal models, the trial is designed to avoid any unnecessary physical or mental harm, no experiment will be conducted if death or disabling injury is suspected, the risk must outweigh the benefits, subjects must be protected and accommodations to care for them if they are injured must be arranged, the experiment will be carried out by qualified individuals, the subject can end participation in the experiment at any time, and the scientist in charge of the trial can terminate the experiment to avoid any injury or death to the subjects.

The horrors of the experiences of innocent men, women, and children in Nazi Germany seem far removed from the American medical system. Unfortunately, during the same period, Macon Country, Alabama, conducted its own unorthodox research on patients in Tuskegee, Alabama. A clinical trial for African American males diagnosed with syphilis ran for an unprecedented forty years. The Tuskegee trial is credited with causing radical changes to enhance human subject's protection (Brown, 2017).

In 1932 an observational research study began with participants who were coerced into believing they were receiving free medical visits. The study enrolled a total of 600 African American men; of the 600 men, 399 were diagnosed with syphilis and 299 compromised the control group. Participants recount that they were told they had "bad blood" but were never informed they had contracted syphilis. Thirteen years after study enrollment began, penicillin was approved to cure primary, secondary, and early latent syphilis. Health centers opened in high-risk areas to provide access to penicillin for positive patients. The men unwillingly participating in the Tuskegee study were not given penicillin to treat their syphilis and continued to be observed without intervention until 1972. The CDC in the Sexually Transmitted Diseases Fact sheet (2017) states syphilis is curable, but in later stages treatment cannot reverse the damage that has been done secondary to untreated infection. Tertiary syphilis, although rare, can occur from untreated syphilis and develop 10–30 years after initial infection. End-organ damage, brain damage, and neurologic symptoms like blindness and paralysis can result from tertiary stage syphilis.

A study designed to withhold treatment for American citizens diagnosed with a curative condition for observation purposes continued from 1932 to 1972. Ultimately, a public health investigator leaked details of the study to a reporter who wrote an article that was published on the front page of *The New York Times*. The study was discontinued, and the government provided a $10 million settlement, lifetime medical benefits, and funeral services to the patients and families involved in the study (Brown, 2017). In response to the human violations discovered in the Tuskegee experiment President Richard Nixon and the U.S. Congress passed the National Research Act of 1974. The National Research Act is intended to prevent the exploitation of human research subjects (Brown, 2017). The legislature also identified that basic ethical principles should be the backbone of any research involving human subjects (National Research Act, 1974).

The Declaration of Helsinki (1974), which has had multiple amendments through October 2013, is a document that was created to reinforce ethical principles for research involving human subjects. The Declaration of Helsinki reinforces that consent provided by subjects participating in medical trials must be voluntary; subjects must be made aware that they can refuse to participate in a research trial and that they can withdraw from the trial at any time without repercussion. Patients must be given the opportunity to be informed of trial outcomes when data is available. Patients who participate in trials, regardless of their clinical outcomes, are frequently curious about the trial outcomes. Many patients feel that, even if they did not get the benefit they were seeking, that they helped someone else by generating data.

Helsinki also dictates that if subjects cannot competently provide consent to participate in trial themselves that a physician can obtain consent from a legally authorized representative (LAR). In an emergency, research can proceed without obtaining consent, and the study was approved by a research ethics committee. Consent from a conscious patient or from the LAR is an emergent situation that must be obtained as soon as possible (Declaration of Helsinki, 1974).

The Belmont Report was published on April 18, 1979, by the Department of Health, Education, and Welfare. The Belmont Report defines the ethical principles most important to basic rights for human research subjects: respect for persons, beneficence, and justice (Belmont Report, 1979).

▶ INFORMED CONSENT PROCESS

Informed consent is a process that requires detailed information regarding the study to the patient and family members. Informed consent is more than a document described hastily to a patient who is faced with making a decision that may alter the length and quality of their life. Patients forget 50% to 70% of the information healthcare providers provide and when that information is coupled with an unexpected diagnosis or bad news the information is likely to take a backseat to their personal concerns, worries for their own mortality, and distress about their friends and family. The informed consent must contain the specific information to meet criteria to comply with regulatory requirements (Box 8.1).

Box 8.1 Informed Consent Requirements to Meet Regulatory Requirements

1. Statement that the study involves research
2. Description of potential risks and discomforts
3. Description of potential benefits
4. Statement of alternative procedures or treatments
5. Confidentiality commitment plan
6. Explanation regarding compensation for medical injuries if incurred on trial
7. Contact information for study team

▶ **KEY POINT**

Regardless of the background or level of education of the patients, information should be provided at the sixth- to eighth-grade comprehension level.

▶ ETHICAL CONCEPTS RELATED TO INFORMED CONSENT

There are several key ethical elements that are imperative to clinical trials and informed consent:

- **Respect for persons:** Requires that individuals should be treated as autonomous agents; persons with diminished autonomy are entitled to protection. Individuals who meet the criteria for reduced or diminished autonomy may have diminished capacity, are incarcerated, and are younger than the age of legal consent.
- **Beneficence:** Ensures that people are treated in an ethical manner in that their decisions are supported, and they are protected from harm. Scientists or medical professionals executing clinical trials must ensure human subjects are not harmed and that the possible benefits of participation or trial design are maximized while simultaneously minimizing any possible harms.
- **Justice:** Refers to fairness or distribution of benefits in that everyone is entitled to an equal share. Human subjects should receive fair and equal access to clinical trials that may provide a medical benefit. Subjects should not unjustly be discriminated against and not be provided access to care that is accessible to others.

The Code of Federal Regulations title 21 (21 CFR) subpart 50 from the FDA includes further guidelines for requirements of informed consent of human subjects (2019). The 21 CFR includes the important guidelines noted in the research act, Belmont report, Nuremberg code, and declaration of Helsinki by requiring voluntary consent for all research subjects. Allowances to waive consent in life-threatening situations are accounted for; if a patient requires the use of an investigational drug or product that is confirmed to be appropriate by two physicians the patient may be enrolled on trial. Once the patient is stable and coherent, the patient may sign the consent for continued trial participation if desired.

The 21 CFR details the required elements of informed consent; there are two categories that are broken down into basic elements and additional elements of informed consent. The required elements of a basic consent are statement that the study involves research, description of risks or discomforts, description of benefits, statement of alternative procedures or treatments, description of how confidentiality will be maintained, explanation regarding compensation (if applicable) or medical treatments for injuries, contact information for study team, and a statement regarding voluntary research participation. Additional elements of informed consent are risks to embryo or fetus, circumstances which would lead to the subject being terminated from the study without their consent, costs to the participant, consequences of withdrawing, statement about communicating new findings to participants, and approximate number of subjects in the study (FDA, 21 CFR, 2019).

The informed consent requires a vast amount of information that can be overwhelming to patients, especially if they do not have the educational or emotional fortitude to make an informed and rational treatment decision. Informed consent is a process. The document should be discussed with the patient or LAR, and their understanding of the process must be documented. The informed consent is written at a grade school level. A translator must be provided if the patient does not speak or read in the language the consent is written in. The FDA requires that the consent must then be translated into their preferred language, and the patient should resign as soon as the translation is complete. The study must be presented to the patient by a qualified and informed individual without any implication of coercion (Manti & Licari, 2018). The patient must have adequate time to process the option of enrolling on a clinical trial and understand that participation is voluntary. Patients refusing to participate in a clinical trial must be assured that the type of care they receive will not be influenced by their decision. Patients are concerned their physician may be upset with them for refusing or not be interested in their treatment because they opt to receive standard therapy. Enforcing the voluntary aspect of clinical trials is key to maintaining trust with patients. The patient is provided with a copy of the informed consent after agreeing to participate in the trial. The patient must be made aware who to contact for questions or concerns as the informed consent process is ongoing, and the patient should contact the study team with any questions or concerns.

> ▶ **EXAM TIP**
>
> Understand the ethical concepts related to informed consent.

▶ CLINICAL TRIAL PROTOCOL

The clinical trial protocol is the document that outlines the plan for conducting the clinical trial. The initial protocol submitted to the FDA by the sponsor is part of the IND (Investigational New Drug) Application (FDA, Title 21 subpart B, 2019). Any changes to the IND application require a protocol amendment, which follows separate guidelines. Protocols for phase I clinical trials are less detailed and are mainly an outline for safety review and plan for dosing, number of patients participating, methods of reviewing safety, including assessments like vital signs and lab work. Phase II and III studies will have a more developed protocol which must include: statement of the study objectives, sponsor's contact information, inclusion and exclusion criteria, study design, method used to determine dosing and MTD, description of required assessments for monitoring, description of all required clinical procedures, description of drug manufacturing, IND adverse event reporting requirements, description of the drug, labeling requirements, pharmacology and toxicology information, informed consent information, and identifying information to the number of amended protocols. Compared to the informed consent, the protocol is a much larger and more comprehensive document. The patients are not provided with a copy of the protocol for review, and the protocol is considered proprietary from the sponsor to the investigator.

The protocol also contains the schedule of events or assessments (SOE/SOA) calendar, which dictates the investigator and patient responsibility on any given day during the conduct of the clinical trial. A less complex SOA is often included in the informed consent, so the patient is aware of the schedule for the clinical trial and assessments are not missed, which can lead to critical lapses in drug development information. The SOA instructs the patient and research team which lab work is required for each visit, including drug administration information, physical assessments, quality of life questionnaires (if applicable), and future visits. The SOA refers to the body of the protocol or subscripts in the SOA for more extensive explanations of clinical requirements. Table 8.1 provides a sample schedule of events for a clinical trial. Each schedule of events is unique to the specific study and drug.

Table 8.1 Sample Schedule of Events for a Study Protocol

	Screening (-28 days to Cycle 1, Day 1)	Cycle 1	Cycle 1, Day 15	Cycle 2	Cycle 2, Day 15	End of Treatment
Informed Consent						
Signing of informed consent	X					
Oncology Assessments						
Confirmation of disease	X					
Oncology history	X					
AE/concomitant meds	X	X	X	X	X	X
QOL: FACT	X	X		X		
Medical History and Physical Examination						
Medical history	X					
Surgical history	X					
Physical examination	X	X		X		X
ECOG	X	X				
Diagnostics						
BMBX and aspirate	X*					X
CBC with differential	X	X	X	X	X	
Chemistry	X**	X	X	X	X	
Core biopsy	X***					
CT	X					X
ECG	X					
ECHO/MUGA	X					
Investigational Treatment						
Administer YaNN20		X	X	X	X	
Premedicate		X****	X****	X****	X****	
Observe 1 hour		X	X	X	X	

*Must be performed if not completed within the last 90 days.

**Includes potassium, magnesium, calcium, creatinine clearance, alkaline phosphatase, total bilirubin, and lactate dehydrogenase.

***Performed for disease confirmation if tumor is in a safety accessible location per predictive index assessment.

****Patient will be premedicated with Zofran, dexamethasone, and Pepcid.

AE, adverse events; BMBX, bone marrow biopsy; CBC, complete blood count; CT, computed tomography; ECG, electrocardiogram; ECHO/MUGA, echocardiogram/multigated acquisition; ECOG, Eastern Cooperative Oncology Group Scale of Performance Status; FACT, functional assessment of cancer therapy; QOL, quality of life.

The protocol includes guidance for the following:

1. treatment interruptions,
2. instructions for restarting treatment,
3. restrictions for concomitant medications or therapies
4. duration of the study, and
5. descriptive information for required protocol procedures.

For example, a patient experiences a second occurrence of grade 4 neutropenia which the investigator deems related to the study drug. Per protocol guidelines, study drug is held for seven days and gCSF is administered. The patient returns to the clinic in seven days with a repeat CBC and differential which shows resolution of neutropenia. The protocol states the patient may restart the drug at a 25% reduced dose due to the second occurrence of grade 4 neutropenia. The research team documents the lab values, concomitant medications (e.g., gCSF), treatment interruption, and dose reduction in the clinical trial documentation system. The research team also updates the sponsor and retains the communication documentation in the clinical trial record. If the patient is required to keep a diary of adverse events and concomitant medications, the clinical trial staff are responsible for checking that the documents match the data.

▶ GOOD CLINICAL PRACTICE

Good clinical practice (GCP) is a standard that incorporates the European Union, Japan, and the United States into an ethical and scientific standard for conducting human subjects research trials on an international level. GCP incorporates the Declaration of Helsinki and ensures that subjects are protected, their rights are upheld, and the data collected from the trial is credible and has scientific merit (*Guideline for Good Clinical Practice ICH E6(R2) Consensus Guideline, 2020*). GCP was developed with input from guidelines approved by the World Health Organization. GCP principles echo the requirements of the Belmont Report, National Research Act, Declaration of Helsinki, and the Nuremberg Code in that patient protection must be provided, risks must be weighed against potential benefit, the proposed trial must be clinically sound, the investigators conducting the trial must be qualified, consent is given freely without coercion, all of the information from the trial must be recorded and stored so that is can be verified and reported accurately, confidentiality is protected, and investigational products must be handled in accordance with a good manufacturing practice. GCP also makes recommendations regarding IRB review and ethical principles, investigator and sponsor responsibilities, requirements for protocol and protocol amendments, investigator brochure contents, and how essential documents are stored and handled for the conduct of the clinical trial. GCP standardizes the conduct of clinical trials, therefore, improves the quality and consistency of trial operations (Mentz, 2016). Adhering to GCP guidelines is an FDA directive (FDA.gov, 2019), and the agency provides GCP training and works with other government agencies to provide GCP training as well. Documentation of GCP training for clinical trial investigators, sponsors, and staff is required to conduct clinical trials.

▶ BARRIERS TO CLINICAL TRIAL ENROLLMENT

ENROLLMENT

Enrollment in clinical trials drives the pace that potentially lifesaving therapies are approved; historically seventy of adult patients in the United States express an interest in clinical trials, but less than 5% of adult cancer patients enroll (Unger, 2016). Conversely, pediatric patients younger than fifteen years old have a clinical trial participation rate of at least 50%, which correlates with a decreasing mortality rate since the 1970s. Adult mortality rate has only shown a positive decline since the 1990s. The higher levels of pediatric patient involvement in clinical trials directly correlate with their decreased mortality rate. Despite interventions to increase adult clinical trial enrollment, and concordantly decreased mortality rate, the participation rate has not changed for the last several years (Unger, 2016). When a trial fails to enroll an adequate number of subjects, the drug can fail to progress through the clinical trials process. The product may be promising and could offer an important treatment option for patients, but without the required data to analyze the product and bring it further to market the venture will be terminated. When a trial quickly accrues the research, process is shortened and time from bench to market is faster.

INCLUSION AND EXCLUSION CRITERIA

Strict inclusion and exclusion criteria affect the ability for a trial to enroll quickly. If about seventy percent of adults are interested in enrolling in a clinical trial approximately fifty percent of those interested are disqualified due to exclusion criteria. Early phase trials have more generalized inclusion and exclusion criteria, and the drug is being tested for safety, not efficacy. As the trial advances in stage, the criteria become more specific as it is being tested for a defined population with preclinical and clinical data supporting the success of the disease in question.

TRUST IN THE HEALTHCARE SYSTEM

Lack of trust in medicine and healthcare at large affects trial enrollment rates as well. The unethical treatment of the Tuskegee patients has influenced how minorities feel about the research process. Patients have voiced concerns over feeling like a guinea pig and require extensive education about the risk and potential benefits of participating in a clinical trial (Nipp, 2019). Due to the breadth of understanding that is required to retain information about the drug under study and the commitment to clinical trials, patients with lower education levels and socioeconomic status are less willing to participate.

FINANCIAL IMPLICATIONS

Financial costs related to trial participation can have an impact on patient participation. Clinical trials frequently have a budget for reimbursement depending on the requirements of the protocol. Trials associated with a pharmaceutical company often have the capacity to have the largest budget, but they are bound by Medicare rules for compensation and reimbursement. Additional clinic visits are required from the patients to monitor for adverse effects, and these are often at the time and expense of the patient.

Grants and financial programs should be explored to assist with the financial responsibility of oncology care; this must be offered to clinical trial patients as well. The budget for the clinical trial may allow for travel reimbursement under certain circumstances to help offset cost as well. The reimbursements must be handled with care to ensure the patients do not feel coerced or bribed to enroll in the trial at any point. Institutions that implemented a financial program to assist with research-related costs saw increased enrollment and retention rates in clinical trials (Nipp, 2019, p. 109).

RETENTION STRATEGIES

Research-specific staff like patient navigators, research nurses, and clinical trial associates have demonstrated positive patient retention strategies as these positions are dedicated to following the patients on trial. Research-specific staff decrease the likelihood of patient protocol-specific visits, falling outside of required time windows to complete diagnostic testing, and improve compliance with participation. The staff is an experienced conduit that patients can contact for questions or concerns and decrease delays in therapy and increase the percentage of patients who complete treatment (Nipp, 2019, p. 109).

CLINICAL TRIAL ACCESS

Another barrier to clinical trials enrollment is access for patients. In large metropolitan areas, patients have more options for treatment due to the availability of large academic medical institutions. In rural areas, the availability of clinical trials may be limited to facilities that are not accessible to patients. Patients with financial means to travel outside of their immediate area are disproportionately advantaged.

Utilization of nonprofit groups, like the American Cancer Society, can provide housing or travel assistance for patients and families to have the opportunity to explore clinical trials as a treatment option. The oncology nurse serves as a resource for patients who express interest in clinical trials. The oncology nurse provides patients with information for resources like Hope House from ACS.org, information on how to search for treatment opportunities at clinicaltrials.gov, and assist with referrals in conjunction with the provider if appropriate.

▶ ADVERSE EVENTS

Adverse events are medical occurrences that are recorded and potentially reported while patients are on trial. These events do not have to be related to meeting the criteria for documentation. The FDA defines an adverse event as "any untoward medical occurrence associated with the use of a drug in humans, whether or not considered drug related." This means that any event that occurs while the patient is on trial must be documented and reported to the sponsor. The sponsor in large multicenter trials has global oversight and can recognize trends in the data that individual investigators do not see. Adverse events are further classified as serious or non-serious and suspected or unexpected. The relationships of adverse events are determined by the site investigator and the sponsor. The site investigator is responsible for the primary relationship between the patient and the event; the sponsor may be able to provide additional information either at the time of the event or when more data is available, and the relationship between the event and the drug can change with the receipt of additional information.

Patients who have enrolled on a clinical trial must be made aware they are responsible for reporting any side effects they are experiencing, and the research team and investigator will decide as to whether the information is related to the drug under study. Patients can report this information in person or via telephone. For example, a patient may contact the research nurse and complain of increasing diarrhea. Diarrhea is listed as a potential side effect in the consent and the investigator determines that this is related to the drug and the information is documented in the data capture system for the sponsor. The patient can be medically managed as per the investigator's discretion and in conjunction with protocol guidelines. For example, the patient may also contact the research nurse and notify the team that they fell at home and broke the left wrist and requires surgery with pin placement. This event meets reporting criteria as an adverse event that is unrelated to the drug under study. The adverse event will be documented and reported to the sponsor in the data capture system just as the related adverse event is.

SERIOUS ADVERSE EVENTS

An adverse event meets the criteria for "serious" when it causes any of the following: death, a life-threatening adverse event, inpatient hospitalization, or prolongation of existing hospitalization, a persistent or significant incapacity or substantial disruption or the ability to conduct normal life functions, or a congenital anomaly/birth defect (FDA, CFR 21, 2019). Events that do not meet these criteria, but the investigator or sponsor believes they should be reported fall under the important medical event criteria. Examples of important medical events may be related to an emergency room visit that did not require hospital admission, events related to multiple outpatient procedures or visits, or any event that jeopardizes the patients' safety that is not listed in the serious definition.

SUSPECTED ADVERSE REACTION

A suspected adverse reaction is a side effect or event that is likely caused by the drug under study. If the drug has an investigator's brochure or a side-effect profile developed the adverse event is likely listed in the developing drug profile. An investigator that has experience with the drug under study can also decide whether the event is suspected or unexpected based on their knowledge. If an investigator brochure is not available, the events should be consistent with the available information listed as potential risks in the consent form.

UNEXPECTED ADVERSE EVENT

Unexpected adverse events are not listed in the investigator's brochure as possible side effects from a drug; they are also events that are not consistent with the product and are unanticipated. If an investigator brochure is not available, the events are not consistent with the available information listed as potential risks in the consent form.

REPORTING

An individual site investigator is required to notify the sponsor of any serious adverse events within twenty-four hours of notification from awareness of the event. The investigator decides as to whether the event is suspected or unexpected; choices, for example, may be possibly related, probably related, and unlikely to be related, possibly related, related, or unrelated. The sponsor then reviews this information in conjunction with all the available information from preclinical studies, animal models, and submitted information from other institutions, both foreign and domestic (if applicable).

If the event meets reporting criteria, the sponsor then notifies the FDA and all participating investigators within fifteen calendar days in a document called an IND safety report. The form utilized for the IND safety report is the FDA Form 3500A, which is also known as a MedWatch form. The sponsor and investigator are responsible for updating the report within twenty-four hours of awareness when new information is made available. An updated report should also be submitted if the level of seriousness increases or the hospitalization is prolonged. This information is processed by the sponsor and submitted to the FDA as a follow-up report, which is also sent to investigators as an IND safety report.

Post-Marketing Adverse Event Reporting

Post-marketing reporting occurs after a clinical trial has likely concluded and the drug is available commercially. The reporting criteria definitions are the same for commercially available agents. The reporting time frame for post-marketing reports is also the same as for drugs under study; the FDA should receive reports within 15 days of notification of the event. Unlike drugs under study adverse events that are not related to the product do not require reporting. Post-marketing adverse event notification is specifically concerned with serious adverse events and unexpected adverse events. During post-marketing for an approved drug, an FDA label will exist for the product. Any potential side effect that is not listed in the current labeling and meets the criteria for serious or unexpected should be reported to the FDA on an ICSR (individual case safety report). The ICSR is HIPAA compliant, and any identifiable patient information is not included. The FDA will further redact the report and remove names of the institution and health care providers who completed the form when distributing information if necessary.

▶ CONCOMITANT MEDICATIONS

Any medication the patient is taking during the conduct of the clinical trial must be recorded and reported to the sponsor. If the patient is taking any medications prior to enrolling in the trial, the date, or best-known date, of the initiation of the medication must also be documented. These criteria apply to both prescription and over-the-counter medications. Concomitant medications in relationship to any adverse event must also be reported. The concomitant medications must always have a documented purpose, for example: acetaminophen 325 mg po q6 hours for headache. The concomitant event must reflect on either an adverse event or a diagnosis in the patient's medical history. Concomitant medications must be reviewed during patient interactions and amended anytime there is a change in the patient's medication regimen. If the patient who reported the left wrist break initiates ketorolac 10 mg po q4 hours post-surgery this will be documented in the concomitant medication record and associated with the unrelated adverse event of left wrist break. Although the wrist break and the ketorolac are not related to the drug or clinical trial, they meet FDA guidelines for reporting. The information, although unrelated, needs to be documented in case any additional adverse events occur from the wrist break or initiation of Toradol so the side effect profile from the drug under study can be accurately developed. If the patient experiences increased diarrhea and the investigator determines the diarrhea is from the ketorolac and not the drug under study, this is an important distinction and can affect potential labeling of the drug if it is approved for market.

▶ CLINICAL PEARL

Ask the patient to bring in all of their prescribed and over-the-counter medications so that they may be documented accurately.

▶ MEDICATION ADMINISTRATION AND COMPLIANCE

Adherence to medication compliance and proper administration of investigational products are key to drug development, adverse effect attribution, and efficacy benefit to patients. Patients who do not take their medication as prescribed risk losing a positive benefit from therapy. Medication noncompliance is estimated to cause 30% to 50% of chronic disease treatment failures (FDA, 2016). Adverse effects can be present with suboptimal dosing without derived positive response. Patients need to be educated about strict medication compliance and understand why directions on medication administration are important to them and to the clinical trial. Investigational products are often provided gratis to the patients as part of the trial as insurance companies do not approve investigational agents for treatment. The additional elements in an informed consent dictate the necessity of patients adhering to protocol requirements to ensure their safety and data integrity. Patients who do not follow directions and practice unsafe behaviors may not be permitted to continue as a clinical trial participant.

Medication administration diaries are a tool to assist with medication compliance. The diaries are completed on paper or via electronic device. Ancillary tools like cell phone alarms, pill cap or box alarms, and apps are assistive devices that can be implemented to increase medication compliance.

Oncology nurses must be vigilant when speaking with patients to ascertain medication compliance. Patients who report an adverse effect that is intolerable and prevents them from taking their medication as prescribed must be supported. For example, a patient complains of grade 2 diarrhea that is disruptive to their normal schedule. The oncology nurse must review diet, medication administration schedule, medication dosing, rule out viral or bacterial illness, and supportive medications with the provider to determine a potential relationship from the investigative agent. If the investigational agent is determined to be the causative factor, the patient can be treated with antidiarrheal medications or, if ineffective or not an option, dose reduction of the medication. The protocol must be reviewed for guidance to determine the dose reduction. Dose reductions can improve adverse effects while providing therapeutic benefit. The patients must be provided extensive and continuous education to understand the importance of taking their investigational agents, and all medications, as prescribed and verbalize the necessity of speaking to their treatment team before making any changes to their regimen.

● CONCLUSION

Research is a delicate and necessary process for oncology nurses and practice; see summary in Box 8.2. Using clear and concise communication skills, providing adequate time and ethical principles the patient and families can make an informed decision regarding the clinical trial regardless of what phase is being recommended. Ensuring that the patient fully understands the consent form is crucial to all parties involved. The oncology nurse is instrumental in providing the education regarding the protocol schedule as well as clarifying any misconceptions and questions.

Box 8.2 Research Process: Step-by-Step

1. Informed consent process including signing an informed consent
2. Begin screening procedures
3. Review inclusion/exclusion criteria
4. Determine eligibility
5. Begin treatment
6. Adhere to protocol specified visits and assessments
7. Document and report applicable adverse events, serious adverse events, important medical events, and concomitant medications
8. Review and audit trial as specified in the protocol
9. Retain records per FDA guidelines
10. Update patients with additional information as received

The bibliography and references for this chapter are available on ExamPrepConnect; see inside front cover for access instructions.

1. Informed consent is BEST described as:

   A. A document the patient signs with the clinical team
   B. A process that includes a document, discussion of potential treatment options, and discussion of voluntary participation
   C. A document that can be discussed only with the physician or the principal investigator of the trial
   D. Guidelines that were developed by the National Institutes of Health

2. A patient enrolled in a clinical trial contacts the research nurse to say that they broke their hand in a skiing accident. The patient was admitted to a local hospital, underwent surgery, and is now discharged home on antibiotics. The nurse understands that:

   A. The event must be recorded as a serious adverse event (SAE) and submitted to the sponsor with attribution to the investigational agent identified
   B. The medications do not need to be recorded in the patient's medical record
   C. The event is not related to the investigational product or the clinical trial and does not need to be submitted
   D. The concomitant medications must be recorded, but the serious adverse event does not

3. A patient is considering enrollment in a clinical trial. The patient was deemed potentially eligible by the principal investigator who is also the patient's primary oncologist. All of the following statements made by the patient to the nurse indicates that they understand their options, EXCEPT:

   A. "My doctor believes this is a good option for me. I will read the information, talk it over with my family, and come back to ask questions before I make a decision."
   B. "I am worried my doctor will be upset if I do not participate in the trial."
   C. "I know that I can change my mind at any time during the clinical trial and choose to receive standard treatment."
   D. "I know that even if I agree to participate in the study that there is a chance that I will not be eligible based on information found during the screening process."

1. B) A process that includes a document, discussion of potential treatment options, and discussion of voluntary participation

Informed consent is a process. The procedure for embarking on a clinical trials journey with a patient is more than just signing the informed consent document. Obtaining informed consent is a task that can be delegated from the principal investigator to other members of the clinical research team if adequate training has been provided and documented. Informed consent guidelines are provided by the Nuremberg Code, Declaration of Helsinki, National Research Act, Belmont Report, GCP, and FDA.

2. A) The event must be recorded as a serious adverse event (SAE) and submitted to the sponsor with attribution to the investigational agent identified

The patient's broken hand must be recorded as an adverse event. An adverse event is any event associated with a drug in humans that may or may not be related. Any medications the patient has taken during the clinical trial and in relationship to any adverse event should be documented. Unrelated events do need to be reported, and medications connected to an unrelated event should be documented.

3. B) "I am worried my doctor will be upset if I do not participate in the trial."

Options A, C, and D demonstrate that the patient understands that adequate time is provided to understand the clinical trial before agreeing to participate, the voluntary aspect of participation, and that there is potential that they may be deemed ineligible during the screening process. The patient's physician will not tell the patient they must participate or face retribution, as that is coercive.

4. A patient has returned to speak with the primary oncologist about enrolling in a clinical trial. The patient has decided to sign consent and begin the screening process to determine further eligibility. All of the following statements made by the patient to the nurse indicates that they understand the research process, EXCEPT:

   A. "I know the risks are listed in the consent form, and I understand that more information may be available in the future, and I will be made aware of it."
   B. "I see the schedule for the tests, procedures, and visits I have to make listed in the consent form. I will miss a lot of these because I have a busy work schedule."
   C. "I will let my research nurse know about any side effects, hospital admissions, and other doctor appointments that happen at any time."
   D. "I know I had some of the required screening tests done in the past, but I understand I have to have them performed again to make sure that I am eligible for the study."

5. Which of the following is the most accurate statement regarding post-marketing research trials (phase 4)?

   A. In post-marketing research trials, a drug receives abbreviated approval, and more data is required to continue to support the expedited approval
   B. Post-marketing research trials are the final step in the drug approval process to bring a new product to market
   C. Every new drug product must complete a post-marketing research trial
   D. Post-marketing research trials are utilized only for drugs that were never tested in animals

(See answers next page.)

4. B) "I see the schedule for the tests, procedures, and visits I have to make listed in the consent form. I will miss a lot of these because I have a busy work schedule."

In option A, the patient is verbalizing understanding that the known risks are listed in the consent form and if more information is available in the future the patient will be made aware. Although the risks in the consent form are cumulative and may not all occur the patient must understand that the possibility of the risks occurring are real. The more experience an investigator has with an investigational agent and the further along the clinical trial phases process an agent is, the more information there is about the side effect profile. The participants must inform the clinical trial staff about any doctor appointments, hospital visits, or new medications during the trial. The protocol for required procedures must be completed. A window for screening procedures (e.g., within 28 days of starting investigational therapy) is provided for guidance when obtaining diagnostic, laboratory, or clinical testing. If a test was performed prior to the patient signing the informed consent but falls within the specific screening window, the test will not have to be repeated (e.g., bone marrow biopsy).

5. A) In post-marketing research trials, a drug receives abbreviated approval, and more data is required to continue to support the expedited approval

Post-market studies are not utilized in every journey a new product makes from bench to approval. Abbreviated approval brings an investigational agent to market early and long-term data as well as larger data subsets are required to continue to support approval and substantiate efficacy. Animal model testing is required prior to investigational agents being trialed in humans.

Part III
Disease-Specific Cancers

Section I: Solid Tumors
Skin Cancers

INTRODUCTION

Skin cancer is the most common type of cancer. The main types of skin cancer are basal cell carcinoma, squamous cell carcinoma, and melanoma. Skin cancer statistics are not readily available because basal cell carcinoma and squamous cell carcinoma are not regularly tracked by national cancer registries. Basal cell carcinoma is the most common type of skin cancer, followed by squamous cell carcinoma. Melanoma is less common (approximately 15% of skin malignancies diagnosed in 2019), but it is more likely to metastasize (ACS, 2020).

STRUCTURES AND FUNCTION OF THE SKIN

▶ EPIDERMIS

Skin cancer is the abnormal growth of the outer layer of skin, the epidermis. The abnormal growth is directly related to the DNA changes of the skin that cause the skins cells to grow out of proportion. The skin is composed of three layers: the epidermis, the dermis, and subcutaneous tissue (Figure 9.1). Each layer consists of sublayers. The five sublayers of the epidermis include the following:

- **Basal cell layer:** It is responsible for constantly producing new cells and housing the melanocytes and Merkel cells, which can develop into a malignancy of the skin.
  - Melanocytes: Cells that make melanin, which is the pigment that gives skin its color. Melanoma can develop when the melanocytes undergo malignant transformation.
  - Merkel cells: These are responsible for light touch sensation on the skin and are also referred to as *tactile epithelial cells*. Merkel cells can develop into an aggressive malignancy.
- **Squamous cell layer:** It is responsible for producing keratin, which is a protein that is necessary for skin, hair, and nails to grow. The squamous layer develops as the basal cells mature.
- **Stratum granulosum and stratum lucidum layers:** It is responsible for the migration of squamous cells to the top of the skin, creating the toughness of the exterior of the skin.
- **Stratum corneum layer:** It is responsible for shedding of the skin and allows for new cells to grow and develop. The shedding process slows down with age.

The bibliography and references for this chapter are available on ExamPrepConnect; see inside front cover for access instructions.

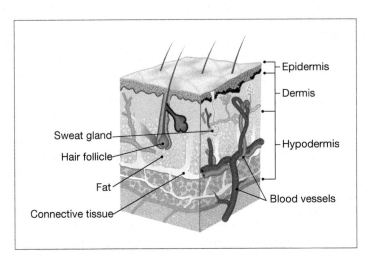

Figure 9.1 Anatomy of the skin

Source: From Gawlik, K.S., Melnyk, B.M., & Teall, A.M. (2021). *Evidence-based physical examination: Best practices for health and well-being assessment.* Springer.

▶ DERMIS

The dermis, the second layer of the skin, is responsible for temperature regulation and supplying nutrients to the skin. The dermis houses important structures such as:

- Blood vessels
- Lymphatic vessels
- Hair follicles
- Sweat glands
- Sebaceous glands
- Nerve complex
- Collagen and elastin

The dermis has two sublayers: the papillary layer, which consists of collagen and is responsible for temperature control and consists of collagen, and the reticular layer, which is responsible for the strengthening of the skin.

▶ SUBCUTANEOUS TISSUE

The subcutaneous tissue layer, or hypodermis, is composed of fat and collagen. This layer is responsible for insulation, fat storage, and the production of energy.

RISK FACTORS FOR SKINS CANCERS

Risk factors for skin cancers include the following:

- Age: The risk increases with age
- Gender: More common in males than females

- Fair skin
- Family history of skin cancer, specifically melanoma
- History of multiple and excessive sunburns
- Exposure to UV rays (natural and man-made)
- Living closer to the Equator
- Multiple moles on the body
- Decreased immune systems
- Genetic predisposition: Xeroderma pigmentosum, which is a rare genetic skin condition that can cause melanoma

▶ **EXAM TIP**

Identify and recognize the differences between benign and precancerous skin lesions (Box 9.1).

Box 9.1 Benign and Precancerous Skin Lesions

Benign Skin Lesions

- Hemangiomas
- Lipomas
- Moles
- Seborrheic keratoses
- Warts

Precancerous Skin Lesions

- Actinic keratosis
- Bowen's disease (squamous cell carcinoma in situ)
- Keratoacanthoma

TYPES OF SKIN CANCERS

There are several different types of skin cancers, ranging from non-life-threatening to life-threatening:

- **Basal cell carcinoma:** It originates from the basal cells, which are located at the base of the epidermis and are continually replicating to replace new cells. The new cells are replacing the dying and shedding cells, particularly the squamous cells, which are at the top layer of the epidermis.
- **Squamous cell carcinoma:** It originates from the squamous cells, which are flat top cells of the epidermis. They are also rapidly dividing and continually shedding.
- **Melanoma cancer:** It originates from melanocytes, the cells that make melanin, which is the pigment that gives skin its color. Melanin is the natural form of skin protection from the sun. Melanocytes can be damaged and develop a malignancy. Melanoma is considered an aggressive and deadly cancer.

■ **Merkel cell cancer:** It is an extremely rare skin cancer that is a form of neuroendocrine cell cancer because it involves nerve endings, which are located at the top layer of the skin and responsible for the light-touch sensation.

▶ BASAL CELL CARCINOMA

Basal cell carcinoma is the most common skin cancer. It is treatable and unlikely to cause death to a patient. Many patients may have more than one basal cell carcinoma. There has been an increase in basal cell and squamous cell skins cancers due to enhanced and diligent skin detection practices, increased exposure to sunlight, and the aging population.

▶ SQUAMOUS CELL SKIN CANCER

Squamous cell carcinoma is the second most common type of skin cancer. It occurs from damage related to ultraviolet light from the sun and tanning salons. Like basal cell carcinoma, it is treatable and unlikely to cause death to a patient. Squamous cell cancer tends to be a slower growing malignancy when discovered at the earliest stage; however, it has the propensity to invade lymph nodes and surrounding tissues, including bone, making it much more difficult to treat.

▶ MELANOMA

Melanoma is an extremely aggressive and the most serious and deadly form of skin cancer. The exact causes of melanoma are not accurately understood; however, the sun and UV rays are major contributing factors. Melanoma can be classified as non-invasive or invasive. As with any solid tumor, the more invasive and advanced the cancer, the harder to treat and obtain a cure. Melanoma follows the same path—the more advanced the disease, the worse the prognosis. Melanomas do not only originate from moles; they can develop from different layers of the skin. There are four subsets of melanoma:

1. **Superficial melanoma:** Located on the top layer of the skin with minimal or no invasion into the skin. Usually identified with an abnormal mole. Equally identified in both sexes. Most commonly found on the trunk in males and on the legs of females.
2. **Lentigo malignant melanoma:** Develops in the elderly population on the face, arms, and trunk and can have a bluish to black hue. This type of melanoma has the propensity to become more invasive.
3. **Acral lentiginous melanoma:** Tends to involve patients with darker skin tones. Appears as black/brown lesions in unexposed areas, such as the nails and soles of the palms and feet.
4. **Nodular melanoma:** Considered the most life-threatening and aggressive because it grows deep into the skin. This type of melanoma is responsible for approximately 10% to 15% of cases. Nodular melanoma is typically discovered on the trunk, arms, legs, and scalp and appears bluish-black in color or can present with pink to red bumps.

IMPORTANCE OF MOLE IDENTIFICATION

Examining moles is a vital part of determining a malignancy, especially when diagnosing melanoma. Moles are normal for many individuals and are developed in childhood. Most individuals can have between 10 and 40 moles. The literature supports that the presence of moles throughout the body can be an increased risk factor for developing a malignancy. Many moles are benign and will never cause any problems, while others have the potential to become malignant. The following moles can develop into malignancies:

- **Dysplastic Nevi:** Similar features as melanoma.
- **Dysplastic Nevus Syndrome:** Inherited disease in which family members have numerous dysplastic nevi and an increased chance of developing melanoma.
- **Congenital Melanocytic Nevi:** Moles identified at birth that have 0–5% chance of developing melanoma; however, that is dependent upon the size of the congenital melanocytic nevi. For example, if a small congenital nevus is found on the sole of the foot, the risk of melanoma is much lower than if a large congenital nevus is found on the back or buttocks.

Moles can be evaluated using the ABCDE rule. Table 9.1 reviews the rule for identifying changes within moles.

Table 9.1 ABCDE Rule for Melanoma Identification

A = Asymmetry	Moles normally are symmetrical. Asymmetry occurs when the mole has an irregular shape, and the mole can look different, especially from one side of the mole to the other
B = Border	Moles normally have regular borders. Irregular borders have notches and/or scalloped borders. This is a typical characteristic of melanoma
C = Color	Moles normally have even color of shades of tan, brown, and black. Uneven color and distribution are concerning for a malignancy
D = Diameter	Normal moles are usually approximately 6 mm in diameter (no larger than the width of a pencil eraser). Moles larger than 6 mm can be concerning for a melanoma; however, melanoma can present in a normal-sized mole based upon the other ABCDE factors
E = Evolving	Evolving, or changing, is a major factor in melanoma development. A normal mole will not change its size, color, or contour; if it does, it requires evaluation and biopsy

⬤ SIGNS AND SYMPTOMS

Signs and symptoms of skin cancer involve areas of the body that have been exposed to direct sunlight, as well as areas that do not receive direct sunlight and UV rays. Each form of skin cancer has targeted areas of involvement. Table 9.2 describes the specific body sites related to the different types of skin cancer.

Table 9.2 Skins Cancers: Types, Body Sites, Lesions, and Metastatic Sites

Type of Skin Cancer	Affected Body Sites	Description of Lesions	Sites of Metastasis
Basal cell carcinoma	Face, neck, back; can develop on any part of the body	Wound that does not heal and continues to bleed for an extended period; crusting and oozing wound Itchy red raised patches; red patches which with blue, tan, and black areas; red patch that has extensions like wheel spokes (typically blood vessels) Scar-like lesion with white, yellow, or waxy color and flat, shiny, and taut with irregular borders (sign of advanced cancer)	Usually does not spread to other sites; local lymph nodes and skin if left untreated
Squamous cell carcinoma	Ears, lips, face, genital area (less common)	Red, rough, scaly patches that can bleed and become crusty Lesions that resemble warts Wounds that do not heal and bleed (like basal cell cancers)	Lungs, liver, bone
Melanoma	Scalp, face, neck, arms, legs, back, nails, in between fingers and toes; may also affect organs in eyes, nose, throat, gastrointestinal tract, vagina, anus (rare)	Darkened or lightened brownish spots Change in mole size, shape, and contour Moles that bleed Small lesion red, pink, white, blue, or blue/black in color Painful or itchy lesion	Lymph nodes, skin, brain, lung, liver, bone, intestines
Merkel cell carcinoma (rare and aggressive)	Face, head, neck; can develop on any part of the body	Lesions can be normal skin color or have shades of red, blue, or purple	Lymph nodes, brain, lung, bone

▶ HISTOLOGY GRADING

Histology grading is the ability to determine how much the cancer cell looks like the original skin cell. Skin cancers are graded on a scale of 1 to 3:

- Grade 1: Low grade; resembles a normal skin cell
- Grade 2: Medium grade; looks somewhat like a normal skin cell
- Grade 3: High grade; does not resemble a skin cell, and it concerned abnormal

● DIAGNOSIS

▶ SCREENING

Screening for skin cancer includes an annual physical examination, self-skin examination, especially of multiple moles on the body.

▶ BIOPSY OPTIONS

There are multiple options available to obtain a tissue sample of the skin. The location, size, and depth of the area in question will determine the best biopsy method. Different biopsy methods include:

- **Skin biopsy:** Removal of mole(s)
- **Shave biopsy:** Removal of the top layer of the skin
- **Punch biopsy:** A crucial diagnostic test to examine skin disorders such as cancers. It can penetrate the layers of the skin to produce a full-thickness skin specimen. A special tool is used, which has a circular blade that rotates into the layers of the skin and obtains a round thick tissue sample. Requires sutures due to the depth of the biopsy.
- **Excisional biopsy:** Removal of the tumor and a small amount of surrounding tissue to obtain clear margins.

▶ DIAGNOSTIC TESTS

Skin cancer, primarily melanoma, has the ability to spread to other organs. Chest x-ray, CT scans (head, chest, abdomen, and pelvis), and MRI may be used to determine if the disease has spread to other parts of the body. Imaging location is determined by the original location of the skin cancer. For example, a patient diagnosed with vaginal melanoma would have a CT of the abdomen and pelvis.

LABORATORY TESTING

There are no specific blood tests that are ordered which are directly related to skin cancers. However, there are several genetic tests that can be performed on the blood and/or on tissue samples of the skin to assess the genetic makeup of the skin cancers and assist with the appropriate treatment options.

Genetic Testing

The majority of cancers have a link to the identification of a genetic mutation. Although not all the factors related to genetics are completely understood, the literature suggests that there is a relationship between tumor suppressors genes and basal and squamous cell cancers. Mutations are as follows:

- P53 mutation: Seen with squamous cell carcinoma. A tumor suppressor gene; with this mutation, the cell loses the ability to die, meaning it inhibits apoptosis.
- PTCH1 and PTCH2 mutations: Seen with basal cell carcinoma; also, tumor suppressor genes.
  - Gorlin Syndrome: An autosomal dominant inherited basal cell nevus syndrome that can affect numerous areas of the body. Carries an increased risk of both cancerous and non-cancerous lesions. Lesions can develop in early adulthood and often are discovered on the face, chest, and back.
- CDKN2 mutation: Tumor suppressor gene mutation that has been attributed to approximately 35–40 of familial melanomas.
- MITF mutation: Seen with melanoma. Responsible for creating melanocyte-inducing transcription factor and is directly involved with DNA replication. The exact mechanism is not completely understood.

- BAP1 mutation: Germline mutation that has been associated with melanoma of the skin and eye and basal cell carcinoma.
- BRAC2 mutation: BRAC1 and 2 mutations are directly related to breast cancer. BRAC2 is also associated with melanoma.

STAGING

As with other solid tumors, skin cancers use the AJCC TNM (tumor, node, metastasis) Staging System. Once the TNM factors are identified, the stage can be addressed and treated. For staging information for skin cancers, visit https://www.cancer.org/. Metastatic sites depend on the type of skin cancer (see Table 9.2).

▶ EXAM TIP

Review the AJCC TNM Staging System for skin cancers: https://www.cancer.org/.

TREATMENT

As with many cancers, there are usually several treatment options to eradicate cancer. More times than not, multiple treatment options will be provided to reach a cure of the disease. The choices depend on the type of skin cancer, location, age and genetic makeup of the patient, and comorbidities.

▶ SURGICAL PROCEDURES

Surgery is the first form of defense against skin cancers and primary treatment for skin cancers. The initial goal is to remove the diseased skin and surrounding tissues and to determine if lymph nodes are involved. Surgical treatment options include:

- **Cryosurgery:** A procedure performed to freeze the cancer cells using liquid nitrogen. Used to remove precancerous lesions and/or exceedingly small lesions.
- **Curettage and Electrodesiccation:** A special instrument that resembles a spoon is used to remove the lesion(s). Performed on small superficial squamous cancers. It is **not** recommended for large tumors.
- **Excision:** Removal of the lesion and surrounding tissue. Used for many types of skin cancer.
- **Lymph Node Dissection:** Lymph nodes may be removed with squamous and melanoma skin cancers if suspicious of involvement (e.g., enlarged or hard to palpation). To determine if cancer has spread or extended to the lymph nodes, they are removed and examined by a pathologist.
- **Mohs Surgery:** Invasive surgery performed with larger and/or recurrent skin cancers. The procedure allows the provider to remove each layer of skin at a time and stop when no more cancer cells are identified. Typically performed on the area of the nose to preserve as much healthy tissue as possible.

- **Skin Grafting and Reconstruction:** In some cases, the cancer is extensive and deep and requires a skin graft and or reconstruction of the skin. This is especially common after Mohs surgery and procedures on the nose and legs.
- **Amputation:** In severe or rare cases, amputation of a digit has been used for the extensive invasion of melanoma.

▶ RADIATION THERAPY

Depending on the location and stage of cancer, the following radiation treatments may be used:

- **External Beam Therapy/Superficial Radiation Therapy:** Used for basal cell carcinoma to stop the multiplication of the cancer cells. It does not penetrate beyond the skin, limiting the damage from radiation therapy.
- **Stereotactic Radiosurgery (SRS; also known as Gamma Knife):** Delivers high doses of radiation to specific parts of the brain; used to treat brain metastases.
- **Stereotactic Body Radiation (SBRT):** Used to treat metastatic sites of skin cancer.

> ### ▶ KEY FACT
>
> Stereotactic radiosurgery does not involve any surgical procedure. The name is misleading. The procedure is performed in the radiation department.

▶ CHEMOTHERAPY

Chemotherapy is not as successful with basal and squamous cell skin cancers as it is with other malignancies. However, chemotherapy is used to treat various stages of melanoma and Merkel cell cancer. Table 9.3 describes the chemotherapy agents used to treat skin cancers.

Table 9.3 Common Chemotherapy Agents Used to Treat Skin Cancers

Chemotherapy Agents	Type of Skin Cancer	Monitoring and Other Considerations
Dacarbazine (DTIC)	Melanoma	Myelosuppression, nausea/vomiting Irritant properties; can cause burning during administration, especially with peripheral access
Etoposide (VP-16)	Merkel cell	Hypotension, myelosuppression
5FU (5-Fluorouracil; Efudex, Carac, Fluoroplex)	Basal cell, squamous cell, actinic keratoses	Redness, pain, and swelling of the skin; may weaken the immune system and cause other infection processes such as upper respiratory conditions Applied as a topical agent; double gloves should be worn when applying the medication

(continued)

Table 9.3 Common Chemotherapy Agents Used to Treat Skin Cancers (*continued*)

Chemotherapy Agents	Type of Skin Cancer	Monitoring and Other Considerations
Albumin-bound paclitaxel (Abraxane)	Melanoma	Myelosuppression (can be dose-limiting), peripheral neuropathy
Paclitaxel (Taxol)	Melanoma	Anaphylaxis/infusion reaction, peripheral neuropathy (can be dose limiting) Use of pre-medications; use of non-PVC tubing and 0.22-micron filter for administration
Paraplatin (Carboplatin)	Melanoma, Merkel cell	Input and output, kidney function Dosing based upon area under the curve (AUC)
Platinol (Cisplatin)	Melanoma and Merkel cell	Kidney function, strict input and outputs, hydration and fluid replacement, nausea/vomiting, myelosuppression
Temozolomide (Temodar, Temodal, Temca; oral)	Melanoma	Myelosuppression, kidney and liver function Double glove during the administration
Topotecan (Hycamtin)	Melanoma	Myelosuppression, nausea/vomiting

▶ BIOTHERAPY/IMMUNOTHERAPY

Immunotherapy utilizes the patient's immune system to help destroy the cancer cells. Immunotherapy such as immune checkpoint inhibitors is a newer treatment for Merkel cell carcinoma that has shown promising results.

- **Immune Checkpoint Inhibitors:** Immune checkpoint cells are responsible for turning cells on and off to initiate the immune response. The primary role of immune checkpoints is to activate the cells to replicate appropriately. When the checkpoint flow is interrupted, it provides an opportunity for the growth of abnormal cells to develop. Immune checkpoint inhibitors block PD-1 and PD-L1 and are used to treat melanoma. Side effects include flu-like symptoms, fatigue, cough, decreased appetite, rashes, and diarrhea/constipation.
  - Avelumab (Bavencio): Focuses on the PD-L1 mechanism
  - Pembrolizumab (Keytruda) and Nivolumab (OPDIVO) IV infusions: Focuses on the PD-1 mechanism
- **CTLA-4 Inhibitors:** Used to initiate the immune system. CTLA-4 targets a protein that is located on the T-cells
- **Ipilimumab (Yervoy):** Used to treat melanoma; can be used in combination with other targeted medications. IV Infusion; requires 0.22-micron filter for administration
- **Interleukin-2 (IL-2):** Interleukins are chemicals that are produced in the body to maintain and spark the immune system.

▶ TARGETED THERAPY

Targeted therapy is an advancement in oncology therapies that has aided in directly attacking cancer cells at the cellular level. The following are skin cancer targeted therapies.

HEDGEHOG PATHWAYS INHIBITORS

Hedgehog pathways are a signaling mechanism that develops in utero and is responsible for adult tissue development and maintenance. The pathway allows for communication between one cell to another. When there is a disruption in the signaling system, the cells do not respond appropriately, which leads to the malfunction and opportunity of abnormal cell growth. The literature supports that hedgehog pathway activation has been associated with basal cell carcinoma and medulloblastoma. Hedgehog inhibitors block the pathways that create abnormal cell development. These medications are used for advanced basal cancer. It is important to remember that advanced basal cancer is much less common than the other skin cancers discussed in this chapter. Hedgehog pathway oral medications include vismodegib (Erivedge) and sonidegib (Odomzo), which should be taken on an empty stomach and has a risk of embryo/fetal toxicity. Side effects include muscle spasms, decreased appetite, fatigue, nausea, and diarrhea.

EGFR INHIBITORS

Epidermal growth factor (EFGR) protein helps cells to grow. Agents such as EGFR inhibitors interfere with the cellular proteins to stop cell growth. In relationship to squamous cell cancer, these medications can prevent the proteins from replicating and thus decrease the cancer cell multiplication. The exact mechanism is not fully understood, and the true benefit is still under investigation. Cetuximab (Erbitux) is an oral agent that has been shown to decrease tumor size with squamous cell cancer. Side effects include rashes (most common), diarrhea, fatigue, sunlight sensitivity, and the development of secondary skin cancer.

BRAF INHIBITORS

BRAF inhibitors are oral medications that directly combat the BRAF protein and are used to treat melanoma. Agents include vemurafenib (Zelboraf), dabrafenib (Tafinlar), and encorafenib (Braftovi). Side effects include rashes, fatigue, nausea, and joint pain.

MEK INHIBITORS

These medications block the MEK proteins on cells and are used to treat melanoma. Agents include Trametinib (Mekinist), cobimetinib (Cotellic), and binimetinib (Mektovi). Side effects include rashes, nausea, diarrhea, sunlight sensitivity, and the development of secondary skin cancer.

▶ OTHER TREATMENT OPTIONS

- **Photodynamic Therapy:** Photodynamic therapy (PDT) is the use of direct light therapy. It is used to treat local/superficial skin cancers such as basal cell and squamous cell carcinomas. Medications used in this type of therapy include perfumer sodium (Photoprint), which is a known photosensitizer and activated with a red light laser, and aminolevulinic acid (ALA or Levulan), which is used to treat actinic keratosis. It is applied directly to the skin and is activated by a specific blue light. Side effects of PDT include skin damage (may cause new skin cancer, comprised immune system, and sunlight sensitivity.
- **Laser Surgery:** It can be used to treat affected areas in superficial skin cancers under certain circumstances. It is not used for aggressive skin cancers.

■ **Chemical Peels:** The use of chemicals to remove the damaged skin cancer with a chemical called trichloroacetic acid (TCA). Although chemical peels are less common, they may be used to treat actinic keratosis.

🌑 SURVIVAL INFORMATION

The literature suggests that patients do not die directly from squamous and basal cell carcinoma; however, melanoma is a significant cause of death, according to the ACS (2020) 5-year survival rates specific for melanoma. The information was based upon the Surveillance, Epidemiology, and End Results (SEER) Program, which is governed by the National Cancer Institute that collects and monitors cancer statistics. SEER examined patients diagnosed with melanoma from 2009 to 2015; the 5-year survival rates are:

■ Local disease: 99%
■ Regional disease: 65%
■ Distant disease: 25%
■ All stages: 92%

The bibliography and references for this chapter are available on ExamPrepConnect; see inside front cover for access instructions.

1. A patient presents with a 2-cm scaly red bleeding lesion on the right side of the face, close to the ear, which will not heal. The nurse suspects:

    A. Merkel cell cancer
    B. Melanoma
    C. Basal cell carcinoma
    D. Squamous cell carcinoma

2. Which type of surgical procedure would the nurse expect for a patient with a diagnosis of invasive melanoma of the left thigh?

    A. Cryosurgery
    B. Excisional with lymph node removal
    C. Excisional without lymph node removal
    D. Mohs surgery

3. Which of the following targeted therapies has been successful in treating squamous cell carcinoma?

    A. Vemurafenib (Zelboraf)
    B. Cetuximab (Erbitux)
    C. Dabrafenib (Tafinlar)
    D. Encorafenib (Braftovi)

4. A melanoma patient with an advanced disease called the oncology clinic nurse complaining about a red rash all over their face and chest. The nurse's BEST response is:

    A. "Don't worry; it's related to your skin cancer."
    B. "It is most likely a side effect of the targeted therapy treatment; you should be seen by the provider."
    C. "It is most likely a side effect from the radiation therapy; you should be seen by the provider."
    D. "Don't worry, it's a normal reaction; there is nothing to do."

5. Which of the following chemotherapy agents would be used to treat a patient diagnosed with actinic keratosis?

    A. Cisplatin
    B. DTIC
    C. 5-Fluorouracil
    D. Carboplatin

(See answers next page.)

1. D) Squamous cell carcinoma
Red rough scaly patches that bleed, become crusty, and do not heal are indicative of squamous cell carcinoma. Melanoma is not isolated to the face and follows the ABCDE rule. Basal cell carcinoma is usually located closer to the forehead. Merkel cell cancer can be normal skin color or have hues of red, blue, and purple.

2. B) Excisional with lymph node removal
Invasive melanoma requires removal with the examination of lymph nodes to stage and determine the appropriate treatment options. If the melanoma were not invasive, then the lymph nodes would not be removed and examined. Cryosurgery is not used to treat melanoma, and Mohs surgery is used for delicate areas of the body such as the face and nose.

3. B) Cetuximab (Erbitux)
Cetuximab (Erbitux), an EFGR inhibitor, has been successful in treating squamous cell carcinoma. Dabrafenib (Tafinlar), Encorafenib (Braftovi), and Vemurafenib (Zelboraf) are BRAF inhibitors, which are used to treat melanoma.

4. B) "It is most likely a side effect of the targeted therapy treatment; you should be seen by the provider."
The nurse should recognize that an advanced melanoma patient would be prescribed a targeted therapy, in which rash is a common side effect. The patient needs to be evaluated by the healthcare provider to determine if additional treatment is required, such as an antibiotic. Radiation may be a potential treatment option but would not cause a rash on the face and chest. A rash would be a local reaction to the area radiated. Telling the patient not to worry and minimizing their concerns are not appropriate as they are not therapeutic responses.

5. C) 5-Fluorouracil
5-Fluorouracil topical cream that is recommended for the treatment of actinic keratosis. Cisplatin, DTIC, and carboplatin are chemotherapy agents used for advanced skin cancers such as melanoma.

Brain Cancer

INTRODUCTION

As with any solid malignancy, a brain lesion is the abnormal growth of non-healthy cells. Tumors can occur in the brain and spinal cord, and there are several types of brain lesions. Not all brain lesions are malignant; many are benign. Although a brain lesion may be benign, it can cause lifelong disabilities. The ACS (2020) does not account specifically for benign lesions in the statistics. Approximately 24,000 malignant brain and spinal cord tumors were diagnosed in 2020—approximately 14,000 males and 11,000 females. Unfortunately, the death rates for brain and spinal cord lesions are quite high, and long-term survival success is low. To fully understand brain and spinal cord lesions, one must understand the structure and function of the brain and nervous system.

BRAIN AND NERVOUS SYSTEM

The brain is a complex organ and lies within an intricate nervous system. The brain serves as the foundation of the nervous system and provides numerous conscious and unconscious functioning. The nervous system is divided into the central nervous system (CNS) and peripheral nervous system (PNS).

- **Central Nervous System:** Includes the brain, which sends messages via neurons to the rest body, and the spinal cord, which sends sensory information to the brain and neuronal information to organs of the body as well.
- **Peripheral Nervous System:** Comprises cranial and spinal nerves. Cranial nerves are 12 nerves responsible for vital functions visual acuity, sense of smell, swallowing and taste, hearing, and facial expressions. Spinal nerves are responsible for identifying pain and temperature. The PNS is further subdivided into:
  - Somatic nervous system: Responsible for voluntary muscle control.
  - Autonomic nervous system: Responsible for automatic functioning of the heart and lungs.
  - Sympathetic nervous system: Responsible for the fight-or-flight mechanisms.
  - Parasympathetic nervous system: Responsible for rest and digestion mechanism.

▶ BRAIN FUNCTION

The brain is composed of anatomical structures such as the cerebellum and lobes, which each play a specific role in the functioning of the body (Figure 10.1):

- **Cerebellum (or Brainstem):** Controls coordination, motor learning, and the autonomic nervous system.

The bibliography and references for this chapter are available on ExamPrepConnect; see inside front cover for access instructions.

- **Frontal Lobe:** Controls personality, emotional traits, behavior, and intelligence. *Broca's area* resides in the left frontal lobe and is responsible for motor speech production.
- **Occipital Lobe:** Controls visual functioning.
- **Parietal Lobe:** Controls sensations and spatial and body awareness.
- **Temporal Lobe:** Controls memory and auditory mechanisms. *Wernicke's area* resides in the left temporal lobe and is responsible for language comprehension and deciphering of sounds.

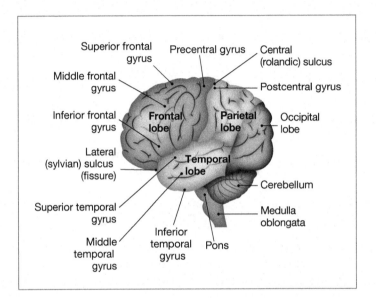

Figure 10.1 The cerebellum and brain lobes.
Source: From Gawlik, K.S., Melnyk, B.M., & Teall, A.M. (2021). *Evidence-based physical examination: Best practices for health and well-being assessment.* Springer.

BRAIN TUMORS

Lesions in the brain are categorized as either primary tumor or metastatic tumor. **Primary tumors** are tumors that originate in the brain and/or spinal column. Types of primary tumors include gliomas, which develop from the glial cells within the brain. Glial cells are non-neuronal brain cells that account for close to 80% of primary brain cancers. Gliomas are further subdivided into:

- **Astrocytomas:** Derived from astrocytes, which are star-shaped glial cells. Primarily affects the cerebrum of the brain and are responsible for half of brain tumors. They are more prevalent in middle-aged men. They tend to be diagnosed as high-grade lesions in adults.
- **Ependymoma:** Ependymal cells are another form of glial cells, which line the cerebral spinal fluid-filled ventricles. Responsible for 2% to 3% of primary brain tumors. Majority tend to be more well-defined tumors.
- **Glioblastoma Multiforme (GBM):** The most invasive, aggressive type of glial cell brain malignancy.

- Prevalent in individuals aged 50 to 70 years
- Affects more men than women
- Yields a poor prognosis
- Can involve multiple glial cell malignancies such as astrocytes and oligodendrocytes
- **Oligodendrogliomas:** Derived from the glial cells that make myelin, which insulates the wiring system of the brain.
- **Medulloblastomas:** High-grade tumors that develop in the cerebellum. Most common in children.
- **Hemangioblastomas:** Tumors that develop in the cerebellum and are created from the blood vessels of the brain. They can be accompanied by a cyst. They are most prevalent in men aged 40 to 60 years of age.
- **Rhabdoid brain tumors:** Tend to affect young children, although they can involve adults and metastasize via the central nervous system.

Metastatic tumors are tumors that have originated from cancers within another part of the body and spread to the brain. For example, breast cancer that spreads to the brain results in brain lesions, but they are breast cancer cells. Close to half of lung cancer patients have metastatic disease to the brain. Brain metastases is usually associated with poorer prognosis and decreased long-term survival rates.

▶ BENIGN AND MALIGNANT BRAIN TUMORS

Benign and malignant brain lesions include:

- **Chordomas:** Benign, rare, and slow-growing; occurs in individuals aged 50–60.
- **Craniopharyngiomas, or Rathke's pouch tumor, craniopharyngeal duct tumor, or adamantinoma tumor:** This is benign and develops adjacent to the pituitary gland, which makes removal difficult. Mostly occurs in children; however, they can be seen in the adult population.
- **Glomus jugular:** Rare and usually located at the base of the brain and above the jugular vein.
- **Meningiomas:** Evolve from the meninges. Primarily benign, but a small number can be malignant.
- **Pineocytomas:** Mostly benign, slow growing, and primarily affects adults.
- **Pituitary adenomas:** Mostly benign but can be malignant as well. Affects adults aged 30 to 40 years years. Both benign and malignant lesions are slow growing and tend to be treated successfully.
- **Schwannomas:** Benign; the most common lesions in adults. Schwannomas are lesions of the nerve cells and can develop on the face, arms, legs, and torso. As the lesions grow, they impede the nerves, which results in acute symptoms. The grade of symptoms is dependent upon the location and amount of pressure placed on the nerves. Symptoms include pain, numbness, and tingling sensation, as well as a visible lesion. Acoustic neuromas are the most common form of schwannomas and involves the eighth cranial nerve (vestibular). Although it is benign, this type of lesion can be fatal due to the amount of pressure that is placed on the nerves.

RISK FACTORS

The exact cause of brain malignancies is not identified; however, as with any solid cancer development process, the common concepts include chromosomal changes, deletions, replications, and malformations. Not understanding the rationale for brain cancers lends to the poor prognosis. Risk factors include:

- Radiation exposure: Cell phone usage and exposure
- Family history of brain cancer
- Genetic disorders:
  - Neurofibromatosis type 1 (NF1), or von Recklinghausen disease: Correlated with brain and spinal cord cancers, as well as benign brain lesions.
  - Neurofibromatosis type 2 (NF2): Less common than NF1; linked to bilateral vestibular schwannomas.
  - Tuberous sclerosis: Disorder of the *TSC1* or *TSC2* gene. Related to giant cell astrocytoma as well as at other benign tumors within the body such as skin, heart, and kidneys.
  - Von Hippel-Lindau disease: Inherited disorder of the VHL gene. Corelated with several benign and malignant tumors of the brain and spinal cord, as well as other parts of the body.
  - Li-Fraumeni syndrome: Disorder caused by the *TP53* gene. Associated with gliomas and numerous other malignancies, including breast cancer, sarcomas, leukemias, and adrenal tumors.
- Comprised immune system
- Angiogenesis properties that cause brain cancer to create new blood vessels.

SIGNS AND SYMPTOMS

Signs and symptoms of brain tumors include:

- Headache (results from increased intracranial pressure [ICP])
- Nausea and vomiting
- Blurred vision
- Unsteady gait (balance issues)
- Loss of function either motor or sensation of upper or lower extremities
- Personality and behavioral changes
- Seizures
- Altered speech patterns
- Altered mental status (can result in coma)

DIAGNOSIS

Currently, there are no screening recommendations or tests for brain malignancies. Unfortunately, brain cancers are diagnosed after a patient presents signs and symptoms. Diagnostic tests used to diagnose and determine if the disease has spread from/to other parts of the body include:

- CT scans: Depending on the original location of the cancer, CT scans of head, chest, abdomen, and pelvis may be ordered. Several areas may be imaged as well.
- MRI: May be ordered to determine if advanced disease is present. Imaging location will be determined by the original location of the cancer.
- EEG: Used to determined brain function and presence and/or absence of seizure activity.
- CXR: Chest x-ray is used to identify if there is a lung lesion that has spread to the brain versus primary brain cancer.
- PET scan: Used to determine the stage of the brain lesion, as well as the progression of the disease.

STAGING

Brain cancers are no longer included in the American Joint Committee on Cancer (AJCC) staging manual. Brain lesions are categorized as localized or the ability to cross the midline and/or metastasize. The histological grade of brain lesions is the most important factor in determining the aggressiveness of the cancer. It also aids in treatment planning.

▶ HISTOLOGICAL GRADING

A grading system describes how much the malignant cell resembles the cell of origin. The World Health Organization (WHO) has developed the grading system for central nervous system tumors (Louis, 2016). See Table 10.1 for the histological grading of brain tumors.

Table 10.1 Histological Grading of Brain Tumors

Grade	Characteristics
I	■ Slow growing ■ May be a benign lesion ■ Prognostic indicator ■ Closely resembles the original brain cell
II	■ Relatively slow growing ■ Has the potential to recur ■ Tendency to spread to local areas within the brain ■ Abnormalities in the original brain cell
III	■ Malignant ■ Higher grade ■ Increased propensity to recur ■ Spreads to adjacent brain tissue ■ Little resemblance to a brain cell
IV	■ Most aggressive ■ Spreads to adjacent brain tissue ■ Does not resemble a brain cell ■ Brain tumor can create blood vessels and contain areas of necrosis

Source: From Louis, D.N., Ohgaki, H., Wiestler, O.D., & Cavenee, W.K. (2016). *WHO Classification of Tumours of the Central Nervous System WHO Classification of Tumours, Revised 4th Edition*. World Health Organization.

TREATMENT

There are multiple treatments options for brain cancers. The appropriate treatment is determined based upon the age of the patient, the location of the lesion, and the histology of the cancer.

▶ SURGICAL PROCEDURES

Surgery is often the first approach with solid malignancies. The primary goal is to determine if the tumor can be removed to ensure the best possible result for cure. Surgical options for brain lesions include:

- **Stereotactic biopsy:** Hole drilled into the skull to access the brain to obtain a tissue sample to diagnose the brain lesion.
- **Craniotomy:** Skull is opened to remove the brain lesion in its entirety or as much as can be removed safely. In some cases, an external ventricular drain (EVD) is placed to measure and monitor the flow of cerebrospinal fluid (CSF).
- **Ventriculoperitoneal shunting:** Used to prevent the CSF from clogging the ventricles of the brain and causing hydrocephalus. If the CSF is blocked, a permanent internal shunt placed in the brain drains the fluid into the abdomen so that it will be reabsorbed by the body.
- **Surgical navigation system:** Equipment such as computers and cameras used to guide the removal of lesions in difficult and hard-to-reach portions of the brain.

▶ RADIATION THERAPY

Radiation has been shown to be an effective treatment option for many malignant brain cancers. Options include:

- **External beam therapy/superficial radiation therapy:** External radiation rays are directed to a specific area and location of the brain without causing damage to the surrounding tissue. Types include 3-dimensional conformal radiotherapy and intensity-modulated radiotherapy (IMRT).
- **Proton beam radiation:** Uses protons to target the brain cancer; prevents damage to the adjacent tissues in the brain.
- **Stereotactic radiosurgery (SRS):** Used to treat brain metastases. Delivers high doses of radiation to specific parts of the brain with the goal of preventing as much damage as possible to the surrounding brain tissue. SRS products include Gamma knife, Novalis, and Cyberknife.

▶ CHEMOTHERAPY

Chemotherapy is typically not an effective treatment option due to its inability to cross the blood–brain barrier. It can be used after brain surgery, in combination with radiation, or administered alone for advanced brain cancer disease. Table 10.2 describes common chemotherapy agents used in the treatment of brain cancers.

Table 10.2 Common Chemotherapy Agents Used in Brain Cancers

Chemotherapy Agent	Monitoring Considerations
Carmustine (BCNU)*	Nausea/vomiting, facial flushing, risk for seizures Delayed nadir (5–6 weeks)
Cyclophosphamide (Cytoxan; oral/IV)	Myelosuppression, nausea/vomiting, hemorrhagic cystitis
Etoposide (VP-16)	Hypotension, myelosuppression
Irinotecan (Camptosar and Onivyde)	Acute-/late-onset diarrhea (teach patient the use of loperamide), risk for bleeding (monitor CBC)
Lomustine (CCNU)*	Nausea/vomiting, risk for pulmonary toxicities Delayed nadir (6–8 weeks)
Carboplatin (Paraplatin)	Input and output, kidney function
Methotrexate (oral/IV/IM)	Kidney function, myelosuppression, nausea/vomiting
Procarbazine (Matulane)	Myelosuppression, food interactions (fermented cheeses, alcoholic and non-alcoholic beverages, herbs, processed meats, and fish)
Platinol (Cisplatin)	Kidney function, input and output, hydration and fluid replacement, ausea/vomiting, myelosuppression
Temozolomide (Temodar and Temodal and Temca; oral)	Myelosuppression, kidney and liver function Double glove during administration
Vincristine (Marqibo and Vincasar PFS)	Vesicant, severe constipation Does not affect blood counts

*Crosses the blood–brain barrier.

> ▶ **KEY FACT**
>
> Most chemotherapy agents do not cross the blood–brain barrier; therefore, chemotherapy is not the best treatment option for brain lesions.

Another treatment that has been used for brain cancers is Gliadel, which are chemo-infused wafers with carmustine that dissolve over time. They are placed in the brain after the removal of the tumor. The most common side effects include N/V, constipation, abdominal pain, headaches, and insertion site reactions.

▶ BIOTHERAPY/IMMUNOTHERAPY

Anti-angiogenesis drugs block the ability of cancer cells to create a blood supply to obtain nutrients from the body. These agents have been shown to be effective in the treatment of aggressive gliomas. The two angiogenesis inhibitors are bevacizumab (Avastin) and ramucirumab (Cyramza). They are used in combination with chemotherapy and should be administered 4 weeks post-surgical procedure. The patient should be monitored for bleeding and proteinuria. Bevacizumab should be stopped 28 days prior to any surgical procedure.

▶ TARGETED THERAPY

The oral drug Everolimus (Afinitor) blocks the mTOR protein on brain cancer cell, preventing it from creating new blood supply. It has been shown to be effective in treating astrocytomas that cannot be surgically removed. Side effects include myelosuppression, mucositis, diarrhea, fatigue, and N/V.

▶ SUPPORTIVE MEDICATIONS

There are several medications that are used as supportive medications during cancer treatments to combat the side effects of the disease:

- Corticosteroids: Used to reduce the inflammation and swelling within the brain which can cause severe headaches. Most common is dexamethasone (Decadron).
- Anticonvulsants: Brain malignancies can inherently cause seizure activity; therefore, patients are placed on anticonvulsants medications to prevent seizures.
- Hormonal therapy: If the tumor affects the pituitary gland, replacement hormones may be administered.

⬤ SURVIVAL INFORMATION

Survival rates for brain and spinal cord malignancies are much lower than other solid-tumor cancers. The 5-year survival rates for brain tumors after diagnosis are quite poor and are highly dependent on the time of lesion, age of the patient, and treatment.

The bibliography and references for this chapter are available on ExamPrepConnect; see inside front cover for access instructions.

1. What type of brain tumor has the highest incidence of affecting the cerebrum?

   A. Glioblastoma
   B. Astrocytoma
   C. Medulloblastoma
   D. Hemangioblastoma

2. Which of the following benign brain lesions has the potential to be fatal?

   A. Pituitary adenoma
   B. Pineocytoma
   C. Meningiomas
   D. Schwannomas

3. A patient with advanced glioma called the oncology clinic nurse complaining that their face is red and swollen, and they have been unable to sleep for the past three nights. The nurse recognizes that the patient is experiencing side effects from:

   A. Procarbazine
   B. Keppra
   C. BCNU
   D. Decadron

4. What targeted therapy has been successful in treating astrocytoma cell carcinoma?

   A. Vemurafenib (Zelboraf)
   B. Everolimus (Afinitor)
   C. Cetuximab (Erbitux)
   D. Encorafenib (Braftovi)

5. Which of the following statements BEST describes why chemotherapy is not the most effective treatment for brain cancers?

   A. Chemotherapy does not interfere with angiogenesis
   B. Chemotherapy does not cross the blood–brain barrier
   C. Chemotherapy causes significant decreases in blood counts
   D. Chemotherapy destroys cells during different parts of the cell cycle

1. B) Astrocytoma
Astrocytomas primarily affect the cerebrum of the brain and are responsible for half of the brain tumors. Glioblastomas involve multiple glial cells. Medulloblastomas and hemangioblastomas develop in the cerebellum.

2. D) Schwannomas
Acoustic neuromas are the most common form of schwannomas and involve the eighth cranial nerve (vestibular). Even though it is a benign tumor, this type of lesion can be fatal due to the amount of pressure that is placed on specific nerves. Pituitary adenomas, pineocytomas, and meningiomas are slow growing and usually responsive to treatment.

3. D) Decadron
Corticosteroids such as Decadron are used as a supportive medication to treat headaches in patients being treated for brain cancer. Side effects include difficulty sleeping and facial flushing and swelling. Patients taking procarbazine for chemotherapy should be monitored for food–drug interactions. Keppra is used to treat seizures and infections; side effects include behavioral changes. BNCU has a delayed nadir.

4. B) Everolimus (Afinitor)
Everolimus blocks the mTOR protein on brain cancer cell, preventing the creation of new blood supply. Cetuximab, an epidermal growth factor agent, has been successful in treating squamous cell carcinoma. Dabrafenib (Tafinlar), Encorafenib (Braftovi), and Vemurafenib are BRAF Inhibitors used to treat melanoma.

5. B) Chemotherapy does not cross the blood–brain barrier
Chemotherapy does not cross the blood–brain barrier, which makes it the least successful treatment option. Chemotherapy does not act on angiogenesis; biotherapy is responsible for angiogenesis. Chemotherapy does affect blood counts. While it does destroy cells during different parts of the cell cycle, this is no reason for them being less effective for brain cancers.

Lung Cancer

INTRODUCTION

Lung cancer is the second-leading cause of cancer in men and women. There were approximately 229,000 new cases and approximately 136,000 deaths from lung cancer in 2020 (American Cancer Society [ACS]). Although lung cancer is a leading cause of death, there has been a decline in incidence decline in both men and women and a decrease in death rates since the 1990s due to changes in smoking patterns and smoking cessation programs (ACS, 2020).

▶ KEY FACTS

Lungs are divided into lobes. The right lung has three lobes, and the left lung has two lobes. Lungs are highly vascular.

RISK FACTORS

Black men have a higher risk of lung cancer than white men (ACS, 2020). The average age at diagnosis for lung cancer is above 65 years. Lung cancer develops from abnormally growing lung cells from gene malformations and/or exposures to carcinogens such as:

- Smoking
- Secondhand smoke
- Radon
- Asbestos
- Arsenic
- Air pollution
- Radiation to the chest

SIGNS AND SYMPTOMS

Signs and symptoms of lung cancer include:

- Persistent cough
- Bloody sputum
- Voice changes/hoarseness
- Chest pain
- Shortness of breath (SOB)/dyspnea
- History of pneumonia and bronchitis

The bibliography and references for this chapter are available on ExamPrepConnect; see inside front cover for access instructions.

■ Unexplained weight loss (advanced lung cancer)
■ Bone pain (advanced lung cancer; related to bone metastases)
■ Headache (advanced lung cancer; related to brain metastases)

TYPES OF LUNG CANCER

There are two types of lung cancer: non-small cell lung cancer (NSCLC) and small cell lung cancer (SCLC). There are significant differences between the two types of lung cancer, and each requires different treatment options and/or combination of treatments.

▶ NON-SMALL CELL LUNG CANCER

According to the ACS (2020), NSCLC accounts for 80% to 85% of lung cancers and can affect both smokers and nonsmokers. NSCLC is an umbrella term; there are several subtypes based upon the cell type involved:

■ **Adenocarcinoma:** Often found in the outer portion of the lung and has a better prognostic indicator.
■ **Squamous cell carcinoma:** Often found inside the bronchus and lung and is correlated with smoking.
■ **Large cell carcinoma:** Can be found in any portion of the lung and is known to be aggressive.

▶ SMALL CELL LUNG CANCER

SCLC, which is also referred to as *oat cell carcinoma*, accounts for only 10% to 15% of lung cancers (ACS, 2020). It has the potential to be more aggressive than NSCLC and has a poorer prognosis.

MESOTHELIOMA

Mesothelioma is a type of cancer that involves the lining of the chest wall, the mesothelium. It most commonly affects the pleural mesothelium and has been directly related to asbestos exposure. Signs and symptoms are similar to lung cancer:

1. Chest pain
2. SOB/dyspnea
3. Painful coughing
4. Unexplained weight loss
5. Uncommon lumps under the skin of the chest

DIAGNOSIS

▶ SCREENING

The United States Preventive Services Task Force (USPSTF, 2021) recommends annual screening with low-dose spiral computed tomography (LDCT) for adults aged 50 to 80 years who have a 20 pack-year smoking history and currently smoke or have quit within the past 15 years. LDCT has shown to be more effective in the screening process than annual chest x-rays.

▶ BIOPSY

To confirm a diagnosis of lung cancer, a tissue sample is required. The location of the nodule or lesion will dictate the best diagnostic approach. Biopsy options include:

- CT-guided needle biopsy of the lung
- Bronchoscopy transtracheal/transbronchial fine-needle biopsy
- Mediastinoscopy
- Thoracoscopy and video assisted thoracoscopy (VAT)

▶ LABORATORY TESTING

Sputum cytology is used to identify cancer cells within the sputum. Genetic testing is also used to identify gene mutations, which can aid in the determination of appropriate targeted therapies to treat lung cancer. Genetic mutations include:

- *EGFR* **gene:** Present in both healthy tissues and some lung cancer cells, specifically non-small lung cancer. Most common in women, non-smokers, and Asian individuals.
- *KRAS* **gene:** Known as the G protein and is responsible for the intracellular guanine nucleotide binding proteins, which belong to the group of small GTPases. G protein translates signals from information from the outside of the cell to the inside. *KRAS 12C* is one of the most common mutations in lung cancer and accounts for approximately 12% to 13% of adenocarcinomas.
- *ALK* **gene:** A rearrangement mutation that is found in adenocarcinomas; also found in non-smokers and light smokers.
- *ROS1* **gene:** A rearrangement mutation that is found in a small number of adenocarcinomas; also found in non-smokers and light smokers.
- *RET* **gene:** A rare genetic mutation that has been found in NSCLC cancer patients.
- *BRAF* **gene:** A mutation found in a small number of NSCLCs. Has led to the use of immunotherapy to treat lung cancer.

> ▶ **EXAM TIP**
>
> Review genetic testing for lung cancer as it will assist in the understanding of targeted therapies.

▶ DIAGNOSTIC TESTS

Once a tissue sample is confirmed for lung cancer and histology identified, additional diagnostic tests are ordered to determine accurate staging and extent of disease.

- Pulmonary function tests (PFTs): Used to measure lung function, especially prior to lung surgery
- MRI
- CT of the chest, abdomen, and brain (if metastasis is suspected)
- PET
- Bone scan (if bone metastasis is suspected)

STAGING

The TNM (tumor, node, metastasis) staging is based upon the American Joint Committee on Cancer (AJCC), which analyzes the tumor size, lymph node involvement, and metastatic site/sites. Lung cancer has the potential to spread to other areas of the body. The most common sites are local lymph nodes, liver, brain, bone, and adrenal glands.

For complete staging information, visit https://www.cancer.org/cancer/lung-cancer/detection-diagnosis-staging.

> ### ▶ EXAM TIP
>
> Review the AJCC TNM Staging System for lung cancers: https://www.cancer.org/cancer/lung-cancer/detection-diagnosis-staging.

TREATMENT

Like most solid tumors, surgery is the first treatment option for lung cancer, followed by radiation, chemotherapy, biotherapy/immunotherapy, and targeted therapy or any combination of these options.

SURGICAL PROCEDURES

Surgery can provide the best opportunity for cure in patients with lung cancer. There are multiple surgical options, which are determined based upon the size and location of the tumor/lesion.

- **Wedge Resection:** Removal of the tumor/lesion and a small amount of lung tissue to obtain clear margins. Can be performed robotically
- **Lobectomy:** Removal of one of the lobes of the lung on either the right or left lung.
- **Segmentectomy:** Removal of a portion of the lung.
- **Bilobectomy:** Removal of two contiguous lobes that are both positive for cancer; only performed with right-sided lung tumors.
- **Sleeve Resection:** Removal of the tumor, lobe, and corresponding main bronchus, which is then attached to the un-diseased bronchus.
- **Pneumonectomy:** Removal of the whole diseased lung on either the right or left side.

▶ RADIATION THERAPY

Depending on the location and stage of the cancer, the following radiation treatments are potential options.

- External Beam Radiation (EBRT)
- Stereotactic Body Radiation (SBRT)
- Stereotactic Ablative Radiotherapy (SABR)
- Three-Dimensional Conformal Radiation Therapy (3D-CRT)
- Intensity Modulated Radiation Therapy (IMRT)
- Volumetric Modulated Arc Therapy (VMAT)

- Stereotactic Radiosurgery (SRS; used for brain metastases)
- Brachytherapy

▶ CHEMOTHERAPY

There are several chemotherapy agents used for lung cancer (Table 11.1). These agents can be used in combination and/or as single agents.

Table 11.1 Common Chemotherapy Agents Used to Treat Lung Cancer

Chemotherapy Agent	Monitoring and Other Considerations
Albumin-bound paclitaxel (nab-paclitaxel, Abraxane)	Blood counts Administered in a small volume
Carboplatin (Paraplatin)	Input and output, kidney function Dosing is based upon area under the curve (AUC)
Cisplatin (Platinol)	Strict input and output, kidney function, blood urea nitrogen/creatine Replace electrolytes
Docetaxel (Taxotere)	Infusion reaction (less intense than paclitaxel), neuropathies
Etoposide (VP-16; oral/IV)	Hypotension, myelosuppression
Gemcitabine (Gemzar)	Thrombocytopenia; monitor platelets counts Can cause vein irritation if administered peripherally
Paclitaxel (Taxol)	Infusion reaction/anaphylaxis, neuropathies Administer via non-PVC tubing
Pemetrexed (Alimta)*	Administer vitamin B12 and folic acid concurrently to decrease side effects
Vinorelbine (Navelbine)	Vesicant, constipation, neuropathies Vinca alkaloid

*Used to treat mesothelioma.

▶ BIOTHERAPY/IMMUNOTHERAPY

Biotherapy is a broad term that encompasses immunotherapy. Treatment options for NSCL include several immune therapies such as immune check point inhibitors, which block either PD-1 and PD-L1 proteins, to decrease tumors and growth and boost the immune system to attack cancer cells.

- Nivolumab (OPDIVO, Pembrolizumab, Keytruda): Targets PD-1 protein
- Atezolizumab (Tecentriq): Targets PD-L1 protein
- Durvalumab (Imfinzi): Targets PD-L1 protein; used to treat stage III NSCLC in patients who are not surgical candidates

▶ TARGETED THERAPY

Targeted therapy is an advancement in oncology therapies, which directly attacks cancer cells at the cellular level. Targeted therapies for lung cancer include:

- **Antiangiogenetic Drugs:** Block the ability of cancer cells to create a blood supply to obtain nutrients from the body. The monoclonal antibody targets the VEGF receptor protein on the cancer cell. The two angiogenesis inhibitors are bevacizumab (Avastin) and ramucirumab (Cyramza), which are used in combination with chemotherapy. They should be administered 4 weeks post-surgical procedure. Bevacizumab should be stopped 28 days prior to any surgical procedure Patients should be monitored for bleeding and proteinuria.

- *EGFR* **Inhibitors (Oral):** The following agents are provided in oral form and are usually administered as single agents as first-line treatment for advanced NSCLC with the *EGFR* gene mutation. Necitumumab (Portrazza), which is administered via an IV infusion, is used to treat advanced squamous cell lung cancer.
  - Erlotinib (Tarceva): Can be administered in patients without the EGFR gene mutation
  - Afatinib (Gilotrif)
  - Gefitinib (Iressa)
  - Osimertinib (Tagrisso)
  - Dacomitinib (Vizimpro)
- *ALK* **Gene Drugs (Oral):**
  - Crizotinib (Xalkori)
  - Ceritinib (Zykadia)
  - Alectinib (Alecensa)
  - Brigatinib (Alunbrig)
  - Lorlatinib (Lorbrena)
- *ROS1* **Gene Drugs (Oral):**
  - Crizotinib (Xalkori): Possible first-line treatment
  - Ceritinib (Zykadia): Possible first-line treatment
  - Lorlatinib (Lorbrenca): Second-line treatment when crizotinib and ceritinib are no longer being effective
  - Entrectinib (Rozlytrek): Patients with ROS1 gene change
- *BRAF* **Gene Drugs (Oral):**
  - Dabrafenib (Tafinlar): BRAF inhibitor; directly attacks the BRAF protein
  - Trametinib (Mekinist): MEK inhibitor; directly attacks the MEK proteins
- *NTRK* **Gene Drugs (Oral):**
  - Larotrectinib (Vitrakvi)
  - Entrectinib (Rozlytrek)

ONCOLOGIC EMERGENCIES

Lung cancer can cause multisystem issues. Patients with lung cancer are at high risk for oncologic emergencies. These conditions are discussed in more detail in Chapter 27.

- Syndrome of inappropriate antidiuretic hormone secretion (SIADH)
- Hypercalcemia
- Cardiac tamponade
- Spinal cord compression
- Superior vena cava syndrome

SURVIVAL INFORMATION

Survival rates depend on factors such as time of diagnosis, patient age, comorbidities, stage, and treatment. Five-year survival rates for lung cancer in general are 16% for men and 22% for women. Five-year survival rates NSCLC and SCLC are 23% and 6%, respectively (ACS, 2020).

The bibliography and references for this chapter are available on ExamPrepConnect; see inside front cover for access instructions.

1. The nurse is caring for a patient in the immediate postoperative period after a wedge resection. Which of the following is the priority nursing measure for the nurse to carry out at regular intervals?

   A. Monitor pupillary responses
   B. Monitor the chest tube drainage
   C. Monitor Input and Output
   D. Monitor blood glucose levels

2. Which targeted therapy drug attacks the BRAF gene mutation?

   A. Gefitinib (Iressa)
   B. Crizotinib (Xalkori)
   C. Dabrafenib (Tafinlar)
   D. Larotrectinib (Vitrakvi)

3. A patient calls the oncology clinic nurse complaining about painful swelling of right side of their face, neck, and arm. The nurse should be concerned about which of the following oncologic emergencies?

   A. Hypersensitivity reaction
   B. Pneumonitis
   C. Superior vena cava syndrome
   D. Extravasation

4. Which of the following chemotherapy agents is used to treat lung cancer?

   A. Vincristine (Marqibo)
   B. Gemcitabine (Gemzar)
   C. Doxorubicin (Adriamycin)
   D. Eculizumab (Soliris)

5. A patient presents with a 3-cm lesion in the left lung, with invasion to the surrounding pleura and one hilar lymph node. What is the correct TNM staging for this lung cancer?

   A. T1b N1 M0
   B. T2a N1 M0
   C. T1c N1 M0
   D. T4 N1 M0

1. B) Monitor the chest tube drainage
After a wedge resection, a chest tube can be placed for 24 to 48 hours and monitoring the amount of drainage is imperative. Pupillary response is not essential to a wedge resection. Monitoring I&O is important, but secondary to monitoring chest tube drainage. Blood glucose would not be an issue unless the patient is a diabetic.

2. C) Dabrafenib (Tafinlar)
Dabrafenib (Tafinlar) is a *BRAF* gene mutation inhibitor gene drug. Gefitnib (Iressa) is an *EFGR* inhibitor gene drug, crizotinib (Xalkori) is a *ROS1* gene drug, and laratrectinib (Vitrakvi) is a *NTRK* gene drug.

3. C) Superior vena cava syndrome
Superior vena cava syndrome is a common oncologic emergency for lung cancer patients. In this condition, the tumor occludes the vena cava and causes swelling of the face, neck, and arm. If left untreated, it can cause acute respiratory distress. Hypersensitivity is related to acute reaction from the administration of chemotherapy and biotherapy agents. Pneumonitis can be caused by a reaction to chemotherapy agents; however, it would not present with facial, neck, and arm swelling. Extravasation is caused by vesicant chemotherapy agents seeping into healthy tissue and out of the vein in which the agent is being administered. While it can cause swelling at the insertion site, it would not cause swelling to the face and neck.

4. B) Gemcitabine (Gemzar)
Gemcitabine (Gemzar) is a chemotherapy agent used to treat non-small cell lung cancer. Vincristine (Marqibo) is used to treat lymphoma and prostate cancer. Doxorubicin (Adriamycin) Adriamycin is used to treat breast cancer and lymphoma. Eculizumab (Soliris) is used to treat leukemia.

5. B) T2a N1 M0
TNM staging as follows: Tumor is 3 cm, which is T2a; one lymph node involved, which is N1; and no distant sites, which is M0. Complete staging info for lung cancer can be found on the ACS website: https://www.cancer.org/cancer/lung-cancer/detection-diagnosis-staging.html.

Breast Cancer

INTRODUCTION

The breast is composed of milk ducts, lobules (lobes), lymphatic system, and breast tissue, subcutaneous tissue, and skin (Figure 12.1). Breast cancer is a tumor that has developed from cells in the ducts, milk glands, lobes, and nipples. There are several types of breast cancer, which behave differently and require different treatments. According to the American Cancer Society (ACS, 2020), there are approximately 268,600 new breast cancer cases diagnosed, including approximately 2,670 male breast cancers, which account for roughly 1% of the total number of breast cancer patients. Breast cancer is the second-leading cause of death in women (ACS, 2020). The incidence of breast cancer has declined since 2007 due to early-detection practices, as well as continuing research for advanced treatment options.

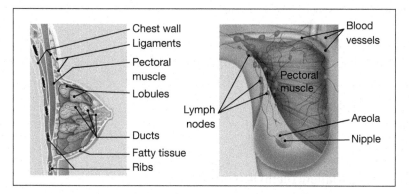

Figure 12.1 Breast anatomy, lateral (left) views and front (right) views.
Source: From Gawlik, K. S., Melnyk, B. M., & Teal, A. M. (2021). *Evidence-based physical examination: Best practices for health and well-being assessment.* Springer.

RISK FACTORS

Breast cancer is more likely to occur in White women than African American women; however, the margin is decreasing. Breast cancer is more prevalent in African American women younger than 45 years of age. Generally, breast cancer is diagnosed between the ages of 55 and 64 years, with a median age of 62 years (Howlander et al., 2019). Risk factors for breast cancer include:

The bibliography and references for this chapter are available on ExamPrepConnect; see inside front cover for access instructions.

- Age: Females over the age of 50
- Height: Taller women
- Early menstruation/late menopause: Related to estrogen factor; 80% to 90% of breast cancers are estrogen receptor positive and can promote the growth of breast cancer cells.
- Previous breast cancer: For example, if a patient had right-sided breast cancer and kept the left breast, the left breast is at risk for cancer, as well as the scar of the original breast cancer site.
- Breastfeeding factors:
  - Women who have not breastfed
  - Woman who have had mastitis (an inflammatory process of the breast tissue)
- Benign breast disease and breast density:
  - Phyllodes tumor (benign)
  - Papilloma
  - Fat necrosis
  - Duct ectasia
  - Periductal fibrosis
  - Squamous and apocrine metaplasia
  - Epithelial calcifications
  - Benign tumors: lipoma, hemangioma, neurofibroma, adenomyoepithelioma, fibrosis, atypical ductal or lobular hyperplasia, ductal hyperplasia, adenosis (non-sclerosing), fibroadenoma, radial scar
- Family history of breast cancer: First-degree relative (3× risk if >1 first-degree relative); paternal
- Genetic factors: *BRAC1* and *BRAC2*
- Use of hormones: Contraception and fertility medications
- Physical Inactivity
- Environmental factors
- Diet/obesity
- Alcohol usage
- Tobacco usage
- Exposures: Radon, radiation, diethylstilbestrol (DES)
- Working night shifts

TYPES OF BREAST CANCERS

There are numerous types of breast cancer, including:

- Lobular carcinoma in situ (LCIS) and invasive lobular carcinoma (ILC)
- Ductal carcinoma in situ (DCIS) and invasive ductal carcinoma (IDC)
- Inflammatory breast cancer
- Triple-negative breast cancer
- Paget's disease of the breast
- Male breast cancer

▶ LOBULAR CARCINOMA IN SITU AND INVASIVE LOBULAR CARCINOMA

LCIS are cancer cells of the lobes of the breast, which produce milk. *In situ* means the cancer is encapsulated and stays within a specific area of the body. In this case, the majority of LCIS cancers tend to stay within the lobes; however, the cancer cells do have the potential to become invasive and spread through the wall of the lobes. ILC refers to cancer penetrating the walls of the lobes, and it is important to understand that ILC can be seen and discovered bilaterally.

When comparing mixed ILC to IDC, some have a better prognosis than others. Table 12.1 describes the different types of ILC compared to IDC.

Table 12.1 Types of Invasive Lobular Carcinoma and Prognosis Compared to Invasive Ductal Carcinoma

Type of Invasive Lobular Carcinoma	Prognosis Compared to Invasive Ductal Carcinoma
Adenoid cystic carcinoma	Improved outcome
Low-grade adenosquamous carcinoma	Improved outcome
Medullary carcinoma	Improved outcome
Papillary carcinoma	Improved outcome
Tubular carcinoma	Improved outcome
Mucinous (or colloid) carcinoma	Improved outcome
Metaplastic carcinoma (adenosquamous carcinoma)	Potentially poorer outcome
Mixed carcinoma	Potentially poorer outcome
Micropapillary carcinoma	Potentially poorer outcome

▶ DUCTAL CARCINOMA IN SITU AND INVASIVE DUCTAL CARCINOMA

The most common form of breast cancer is ductal carcinoma, which is cancer that originates in the breast ducts (Figure 12.2). DCIS is referred to as stage 0 because the abnormal cells are contained in the ducts and have not spread out of the duct cell walls into the breast tissue. The literature suggests that most women diagnosed with DCIS can be cured of the disease with proper treatment. DCIS has less potential to spread to other parts of the body; however, it does have the potential to invade the breast tissue and move out of the duct walls, which is then referred to as IDC. This typically occurs when DCIS is undiagnosed and untreated. According to the ACS (2020), 8 out of 10 breast cancers are IDC.
Ductal carcinoma can be further divided into four uncommon forms of breast cancer:

1. **Medullary Ductal Carcinoma:** Occurs in approximately 3% to 5% of ductal breast cancers. Usually found on a mammogram; has the texture of a sponge within the breast, instead of presenting as a lump.

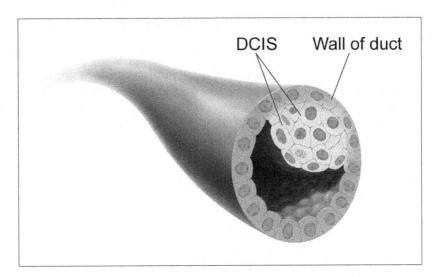

Figure 12.2 Ductal carcinoma in situ.
Source: Courtesy of National Cancer Institute, Don Bliss (Illustrator).

2. **Mucinous Ductal Carcinoma:** The ductal cancer cells produce mucus; better prognosis than other ductal breast cancers.
3. **Papillary Carcinoma:** Often seen in women over the age of 60 years; has a good prognostic indicator.
4. **Tubular Ductal Carcinoma:** Comprises a small percentage (~2%) of breast cancers; has an excellent prognosis. The cancer cells resemble tubes when viewed under the microscope.

▶ INFLAMMATORY BREAST CANCER

Inflammatory breast cancer is less common (~1% to 5% of breast cancers) but extremely aggressive form of breast cancer (ACS, 2020). It is an invasive ductal carcinoma that blocks the lymph vessels within the skin of the breast. The blockage to the lymph flow causes an inflammatory response of the skin, which results in red, swollen, and inflamed breasts. It is typically identified/diagnosed at stage 3 to 4 disease. It tends to affect younger women, African American women, and obese women. In addition, inflammatory breast cancer usually is hormone receptor negative, which innately has a poor prognostic indicator because hormone therapy is not a viable treatment option. See Box 12.1 for hallmark signs of inflammatory breast cancer.

Box 12.1 Hallmark Signs of Inflammatory Breast Cancer

- Edema
- Swelling
- Peau d'orange (thickened, pitted skin that resembles an orange peel)
- Significantly and rapidly enlarged affected breast
- Nipple inversion
- Palpable axillary and clavicular lymph nodes

▶ TRIPLE-NEGATIVE BREAST CANCER

Triple-negative breast cancer is estrogen and progesterone receptor negative, meaning that the cancer cells do not respond to estrogen and progesterone, which precludes hormonal therapy from being a treatment option, yielding poorer outcomes. In addition, the cancer cells are *HER* negative, which means that biotherapy is not an option either. As a result, triple-negative is a difficult cancer to treat and has the potential to be highly aggressive and metastasize to other sites. Approximately 10% to 15% of the breast cancers are triple negative (ACS, 2020). It presents rapidly, with symptoms occurring within 6 months, and typically affects women 40 years of age and younger, African American women, and individuals with the *BRAC1* mutation.

▶ PAGET'S DISEASE

Paget's disease is a rare form of breast cancer involving the nipple. It originates in the duct of the nipple and can spread to the rest of the nipple, causing an inflammatory response. Commonly, another form and site of breast cancer can be found with Paget's disease of the nipple. It accounts for less than 5% of breast cancers (NCI, 2019), is usually diagnosed after the age of 50 years, and affects men as well as women.

▶ MALE BREAST CANCER

Men can also be diagnosed with breast cancer; however, it is not common and typically affects older men. Most male cancers are ductal carcinomas. The exact causes are unknown; however, it is linked to inherited breast cancer genes, such as the presence of the *BRAC1* mutation, which increases the risk for male breast cancer and prostate cancer. Risks also include family history and Klinefelter's syndrome, which is a genetic malformation of the X chromosome. There is an extra copy of the X chromosome, resulting in decreased levels of male hormones and increased levels of female hormones, especially estrogen, which promotes breast cancer growth. Other risk factors include liver disease, obesity, and testicular disease.

● SIGNS AND SYMPTOMS

Breast cancer can present with both subtle and gross changes such as:

- Palpable lump
- Change in size or shape of the breast
- Inverted nipple
- Thickening and dimpling of breast tissue
- Crusting, peeling, scaling, and flaking of the skin around the nipple and breast
- Redness, peeling, or pitting breast resembling an orange rind (Peau d'orange; inflammatory breast cancer)
- Unexplained weight loss (advanced breast cancer)
- Headache (advanced breast cancer; related to brain metastases)
- Abdominal pain (advanced breast cancer; related to liver metastases)
- Bone pain (advanced breast cancer; related to bone metastases)

HISTOLOGICAL GRADING

Grading describes how much the cancer cell resembles the original breast cell. The more the cancer cell resembles the breast cell, the lower grade; the less it resembles the breast cell, the greater the grade. Grading is divided into three categories:

- **Grade I—Well-Differentiated (Score 3–5):** Resembles breast cell; less aggressive
- **Grade II—Moderately Differentiated (Score 6–7):** Somewhat resembles breast cell; moderately aggressive
- **Grade III—Poorly Differentiated (Score 8–9):** Does not resemble breast cell; more aggressive and travels more quickly

Another important factor when reviewing the grading system is the presence of tumor necrosis. *Tumor necrosis* is the collection of dead cancer cells. Tumor necrosis may be identified to describe breast cancer tumors, specifically DCIS. The following terms may be seen on pathology reports:

- Comedocarcinoma: Dead cancer cells within the tumor; indicates more aggressive cancer
- Comedonecrosis: The breast duct with dead breast cancer cells.

DIAGNOSIS

▶ SCREENING

Annual mammograms are recommended, starting between age 40 and 50, depending on risk factors (ACS, 2020). Women should also engage in clinical breast self-examination.

▶ DIAGNOSTIC TESTS

Diagnostic tests to determine if breast cancer is present include:

- Mammograms: Digital x-rays to examine the breast tissue for abnormalities, including the identification of micro-calcifications.
- Breast ultrasounds: The use of sound waves to determine if a lesion is solid or fluid filled.
- MRI of the breast: The use of magnetic fields to determine if any changes and or lesions are present; used in high-risk populations.
- PET scans: The use of radiotracers to visualize and measure changes in metabolic processes to determine if other organs are potentially involved.
- Bone scans: The use of nuclear imaging to determine if there is bone involvement.

▶ BIOPSY OPTIONS

To diagnosis if breast cancer cells are present, a biopsy is required. If the biopsy is positive, additional surgical procedures may be required (e.g., lumpectomy or mastectomy). There are several biopsy options, which depend on the size and location of the tumor:

- Fine-needle biopsy: A small needle is used to obtain a sample of breast cells on a palpable and non-palpable lesions. If non-palpable, ultrasound may be utilized to determine the appropriate site to biopsy. Performed in an outpatient setting and/or interventional radiology center. Risk for infection and not obtaining enough cells to make the cancer determination.
- Core-needle biopsy: A large-bore needle is used to obtain an adequate tissue sample on palpable tumors using. Performed in outpatient settings. Risk for infection and bruising are the most concerning factor.
- Stereotactic biopsy: Biopsies small changes such as micro calcifications seen on mammograms to determine if cancer cells are present. Performed in an outpatient setting. Risk for infection, hematoma at needle insertion site, and breast pain.
- Open biopsy: Performed in an operating room setting. This surgical procedure removes the lesion and surrounding tissue to obtain clean margins in the event the lesion is positive. Risks are infection and breast pain.

▶ LABORATORY TESTING

A breast cancer diagnosis will require different types of testing on either blood or breast cancer tissue samples. In some instances, it may be important to examine the breast cancer tissue to determine the genetic composition. Understanding the genetic makeup of the breast cancer will aid the provider in determining the appropriate treatment options.

GENETIC TESTING

ATM Gene
ATM is an inherited mutated gene. The function of *ATM* is to repair damaged DNA and/or kill the cell if repair cannot be corrected. With a mutated gene, it causes ataxia-telangiectasis, which is related to high risk of breast cancer in some families.

BRAC1 and BRAC2 Genes
BRAC1 and *BRAC2* are related to inherited breast cancer. They are known breast cancer mutated genes that can lead to a high risk of developing breast cancer by the age of 80. The risk number increases if multiple family members are positive. The mutated gene was originally discovered in the Ashkenazi Jewish population; however, many other ethnic groups have also tested positive for these mutations.

CDH1 Gene
Women who possess the inherited *CDH1* mutation have an increased risk of invasive lobular breast cancer. It is also associated with a rare diffuse gastric cancer.

CHEK2 Gene
CHEK2 genes are DNA repair genes. When a *CHEK2* mutation occurs, the DNA damage is not corrected, which causes an increased risk of breast cancer.

Mamma Print
Mamma print is a newer test that can help determine if breast cancer will recur in different body areas after the designated treatment. This test does not have specific parameters like the Oncogene DX. The mamma print examines 70 different genes. Scoring is based upon low and high risk.

Oncotype DX

The Oncotype DX test examines the breast tumor for the 21 genes in cancer cells to determine the recurrent score. The scoring is graded between 0 to 100. The score will determine the risk of recurrent disease over the next 10 years. A score of 26 to 100 is considered high and is associated with an elevated risk of recurrence. A score of 0 to 25 is considered a lower score and associated with a lower risk. Parameters for testing include stage I, II, IIIA although it may also be performed with DCIS or stage 0; hormone receptor positive; involvement of fewer than three lymph nodes; and *HER2* negative.

PALB2 Gene

PALB2 gene mutation is associated with *BRAC2* gene and creates an elevated risk of breast cancer.

Prosigna

Prosigna examines 50 genes and can assist in predicting the risk of recurrence within 10 years in women who have completed menopause, had an invasive cancer, and are hormone receptor positive. The stage of the tumors to be tested are stage I and II cancers with no more than three positive lymph nodes. Results are based upon low-, intermediate-, or high-risk scoring.

PTEN Gene

PTEN is associated with Cowden syndrome, which is a rare inherited mutation that places individuals at greater risk for breast cancer, as well as benign breast and other cancers. Cowden syndrome can also affect areas of the digestive tract, thyroid, uterine, and ovaries.

STK11 Gene

STK11 is a gene mutation that causes Peutz-Jeghers syndrome, which is an autosomal disorder that presents with benign hamartomata's polyps within the digestive tract and hyperpigmentation macules on the lips and buccal mucus. This defect has been associated with several different types of cancer including, breast cancer.

TP53 Gene

TP53 genes are engineered to stop the growth of damaged DNA cells. This gene mutation is related to Li-Fraumeni syndrome (LFS), which is an inherited gene mutation found in families and generations. *TP53* gene mutation is rare in breast cancer, but it is found in a wide range of other common malignancies.

● STAGING

Breast cancer is described in five stages, stage I to V. To determine the correct stage, the following factors should be assessed:

■ **TNM (Tumor, Node, Metastasis) Staging:** TNM staging is based on the American Joint Committee on Cancer (AJCC) TNM system, which analyzes tumor size, lymph node involvement, and metastatic site(s). The higher the number, the greater the disease present and potential poorer prognosis (ACS, 2021). For complete breast cancer staging information, https://www.cancer.org/cancer/breast-cancer/understanding-a-breast-cancer-diagnosis/stages-of-breast-cancer.html

- **Tumor status:** The size of the tumor
  - TX: No primary tumor that can be assessed
  - T0: No primary tumor identified
  - Tis: DCIS/Paget disease (nipple involvement only)
  - T1: ≤2 cm
  - T1: 2 to 5 cm
  - T3: >5 cm
  - T4: Tumor spreading into skin and/or chest wall; size does not matter (inflammatory breast cancer)
- **Node status:** Lymph node involvement
  - NX: Node status cannot be determined (e.g., prior removal)
  - N0: No involvement of local lymph nodes
  - N1: Cancer cells in 1 to 3 axillary lymph nodes
  - N2: Cancer cells in 4 to 9 axillary lymph nodes
  - N3: Cancer cells in 10 or more axillary lymph nodes, with at least one spread >2mm or spread to infraclavicular nodes, with at least one spread >2mm
- **Metastasis status:** Spread to other organs
  - M0: No evidence of distant metastasis either by diagnostic tests and/or physical exam.
  - M1: Spread to distant organs (e.g., bones, lung, brain, and/or liver)
- **Estrogen (ER) and progesterone (PR) status:** Whether the breast cancer is ER and PR positive or negative.
- *HER2* **Status:** Whether the breast cancer is *HER2* positive or negative.
- **Grade of cancer:** The histological grade of breast cancer, which specifies aggressive characteristics.

▶ EXAM TIP

Review the AJCC TNM Staging System for breast cancer: https://www.cancer.org/cancer/breast-cancer/understanding-a-breast-cancer-diagnosis/stages-of-breast-cancer.html.

Once these factors are assessed, the stage of breast cancer can be confirmed (ACS, 2021). Stage 0 is DCIS with no other evidence of disease present in lymph nodes or surrounding tissue.

i. **Stage I:** Invasive lobular or ductal breast cancer
   a. Stage IA: Tumor 2 cm with no lymph node involvement
   b. Stage IB: Tumor 0.2 mm to 2 cm with lymph node involvement
ii. **Stage II**
   a. Stage IIA:
      i. No tumor; however, cancer cells present in 1 to 3 lymph nodes *or*
      ii. Tumor <2 cm with cancer cells present in 1 to 3 lymph nodes *or*
      iii. Tumor 2 to 5 cm with no lymph node involvement
   b. Stage IIB: Tumor 2 to 5 cm with cancer cells present in one to three lymph nodes *or* tumor >5 cm but with no lymph node involvement

iii. **Stage III**

    a. Stage IIIA: Any tumor size with four to nine positive lymph nodes *or* tumor sized 2 mm to 5 cm with one to three positive lymph nodes

    b. Stage IIIB: Any tumor size with up to nine positive lymph nodes, especially near the breastbone, and signs of inflammation (e.g., inflammatory breast cancer)

    c. Stage IIIC:

        i. Any tumor size or not present; involvement with the chest wall, skin, and collarbone; and 10 or more positive lymph nodes under arm *or*

        ii. Any tumor size or not present and positive lymph nodes in collarbone area *or*

        iii. Any tumor size or not present and positive lymph under arm or near the breastbone

iv. **Stage IV:** Involvement of other organs within the body such as bone, lung, liver, and brain

▶ METASTATIC DISEASE

Breast cancer has the potential to spread to other areas of the body. The most common breast cancer metastasis sites are the bones, lungs, brain, and liver.

● TREATMENT

Like most solid tumors, surgery is the first treatment option for breast cancer, followed by radiation, chemotherapy, immunotherapy/or biotherapy, hormonal therapy, and /or any combination of any of these treatments. Another factor that dictates treatment choices are the female patient's hormonal status—pre- or postmenopausal.

▶ EXAM TIP

It is most common to use multiple treatment modalities to treat breast cancer. For example, a premenopausal patient with IDC with lumpectomy and ER position will likely be treated with surgery, radiation, chemotherapy, and hormonal treatments.

▶ SURGICAL PROCEDURES

Surgery can provide the best opportunity for cure for breast cancer. There are several surgical options, which are based upon the size and location of the tumor. The options include:

- **Lumpectomy:** Removal of the tumor and surrounding tissue to obtain clear margins where the cancer was present.
- **Mastectomy:** Removal of cancer and entire breast.
- **Bilateral Mastectomy:** Removal of cancer and both breasts.

■ **Prophylactic Mastectomy:** Removal of breasts before the identification of breast cancer cells. Performed with high-risk patients, such as those who are BRAC 1 and 2 positive.

■ **Sentinel Lymph Node Biopsy (SLNB):** Removal of only the lymph nodes that are known to have positive cancer cells.

■ **Axillary Lymph Node Dissection (ALND):** Removal of axillary lymph nodes, regardless of whether they are positive for cancer cells; usually no more than 20. Can result in lymphedema, which can lead to lifelong complications.

■ **Breast Reconstruction:** There are numerous options, and results vary based on the surgeon. The following are the most commonly performed and recommended:
  ● Breast implants: saline or silicone
  ● Autologous breast reconstruction: Using tissue from other areas of the body to create new breasts:
    ● Tram Flap: Uses skin and muscle from the abdomen. Extensive surgery with risk for surgical complications such as fever, bleeding, and blood clots.
    ● Latissimus Dorsi: Uses skin and muscle from the back and shoulder. Patient must have enough tissue in this area to be used. Extensive surgery with risk for surgical complications such as fever, bleeding, and blood clots.

▶ RADIATION

As with all treatments, there are multiple options, which depend on the location and stage of cancer:

■ **External Beam:** Performed after lumpectomy and, in some cases, after mastectomy—specifically the mastectomy scar and potential axilla—if lymph nodes involved. Performed in areas of bone metastases.

■ **Brain Irradiation:** Performed if brain metastases are present.

> ### ▶ CLINICAL PEARL
>
> A patient cannot have radiation in the same area; therefore, it is imperative to determine the prior field of radiation before treatment begins. For example, if the patient had lumbar spine irradiated and develops a new bone metastasis in the hip, the nurse must ensure that the hip area was not exposed in the previous radiation field. If it was exposed, it could cause permanent damage to the bone.

▶ CHEMOTHERAPY

There are several chemotherapy agents used for breast cancer. Chemotherapy can be administered neo-adjuvant, adjuvant, as well as for advanced/metastatic disease. Table 12.2 describes the most common chemotherapy agents used for adjuvant and advanced breast cancer.

Table 12.2 Common Chemotherapy Agents Used to Treat Adjuvant and Advanced Breast Cancer*

Chemotherapy Agent	Adjuvant or Advanced Disease	Monitoring and Other Considerations
Doxorubicin (Adriamycin) *Used in combination with Cytoxan and plus or minus Taxol*	Neoadjuvant, adjuvant	Myelosuppression, mouth sores, nausea/vomiting Use of vesicant precautions during the administration Potential to be cardiotoxic; requires a MUGA scan prior to administration of first dose Lifetime max of drug: 550 mg/m²; 450 mg/m² with commitment radiation Red urine 24 to 48 hr post infusion
Cyclophosphamide (Cytoxan; oral/IV) *Used in combination with Adriamycin and plus or minus Taxol*	Neo adjuvant, adjuvant	Myelosuppression, nausea/vomiting, hemorrhagic cystitis
Paclitaxel (Taxol)	Neo adjuvant, adjuvant, advanced	Anaphylaxis/infusion reaction, peripheral neuropathy (can be dose limiting) Use of pre-medications; use of non-PVC tubing and 0.22-micron filter for administration
Docetaxel (Taxotere)	Neo adjuvant, adjuvant, advanced	Infusion reaction
5-Fluorouracil (5FU)	Neo adjuvant, adjuvant	Diarrhea, skin and nail changes, myelosuppression
Albumin-bound paclitaxel (Abraxane)	Advanced Disease	Myelosuppression (can be dose limiting), peripheral neuropathy
Doxorubicin pegylated liposomal (Doxil)	Advanced	Hand and foot syndrome, myelosuppression, nausea/vomiting Vesicant precautions
Platinol (Cisplatin)	Advanced	Kidney function, strict input and outputs, hydration and fluid replacement, nausea/vomiting, myelosuppression
Vinorelbine (Navelbine)	Advanced	Constipation Vesicant precautions Administer over 6 min using the upper port
Carboplatin (Paraplatin)	Advanced	Kidney function, thrombocytopenia, nausea/vomiting Drug dosing based upon area under the curve (AUC)
Capecitabine (Xeloda; oral)	Advanced	Hand and foot syndrome, myelosuppression
Gemcitabine (Gemzar)	Advanced	Myelosuppression (specifically platelets), nausea/vomiting
Ixabepilone (Ixempra)	Advanced	Allergic reaction, myelosuppression, peripheral neuropathy
Eribulin (Halaven)	Advanced	Myelosuppression, prolonged QT intervals, liver and kidney function Do not mix with dextrose

*Many of these chemotherapy agents are used in combination; they are rarely administered as a single agent, except in advanced disease.

> ▶ **KEY FACT**
>
> Chemotherapy agents can be used in combination and/or as single agents.

▶ HORMONAL THERAPY

Hormonal therapy is a common treatment option for breast cancer patients who are ER positive. The majority of breast cancers are ER positive, which means that hormonal therapy can be an effective treatment. Breast cancers that are ER and PR positive have the propensity to thrive and grow with estrogen; therefore, the hormonal therapy is designed to block the production and absorption of estrogen to the breast cancer cells. There are several hormonal therapies available:

- **Tamoxifen:** The gold standard hormone treatment, which blocks the estrogen receptors of the breast cancer cell. Recommended duration of therapy is 5 years post-surgery, radiation, and chemotherapy (if received). Side Effects include weight gain, hot flashes, and risk for endometrial cancer and blood clots.
- **Selective Estrogen Receptor Modulators (SERMS):** Work similarly to Tamoxifen and have the same side effect profile. Mostly used in metastatic settings. SERMS include Raloxifene (Evista) and Toremifene (Fareston).
- **Selective Estrogen Receptor Degrader (SERD):** Used for advanced disease with postmenopausal patients. Administered after failed previous hormone therapy. Fulvestrant (Faslodex) is injected into the buttocks. Side Effects include hot flashes, bone pain, mild nausea, and injection site reaction and pain.
- **Aromatase Inhibitors (AIs):** Stop the production of estrogen, rather than blocking it, in postmenopausal women. Used in the adjuvant setting and taken for 5 to 10 years after and the 5-year treatment duration of Tamoxifen. AIs include letrozole (Femara) and anastrozole (Arimidex), exemestane (Aromasin). Side effects include muscle and joint pain and osteoporosis, for which a bone strengtheners such as denosumab (Xgeva or Prolia) is ordered.
- **Ovarian Suppression:** Completely shuts down the production of estrogen from the ovaries. Achieved with oophorectomy, which is the removal of the ovaries, or IM administration of luteinizing hormone releasing hormone (LHRH) analogs, goserelin (Zoladex) and leuprolide (Lupron)

CHEMOPREVENTION HORMONAL THERAPY

Chemoprevention drugs are used to treat patients who have the potential to develop a cancer. Tamoxifen and Raloxifene are used as chemotherapy prevention medications for breast cancer. In addition, SERMs are administered in high-risk populations, such as *BRAC* positive and patients with multiple family members with breast cancer.

▶ TARGETED THERAPY

Biotherapy and immunotherapy are forms of targeted treatments designed to work via the immune system. Table 12.3 describes the most common forms of targeted and biotherapy.

Table 12.3 Common Forms of Biotherapy/Target Therapy for Breast Cancer

Agent(s)	Indications	Side Effects
Monoclonal Antibodies*		
Herceptin (Trastuzumab)	*HER2* positive	Congestive heart failure, diarrhea (especially with combination therapy), hand and foot syndrome
Pertuzumab (Pejeta) *Can be used in combination with herceptin*	*HER2* positive; neoadjuvant, adjuvant, advanced	
Ado-trastuxumab emtansine (Kadcyla or TDM-1)	*HER2* positive patients; neoadjuvant, advanced; failed herceptin or taxane therapy	
Kinase Inhibitors (Oral)		
Lapatinib (Tykerb)	Advanced	Congestive heart failure, diarrhea (especially with combination therapy), hand and foot syndrome
Neratinib (Nerlynx)	Early-stage post–herceptin therapy	
Everolimus (Afinitor)	Postmenopausal, *ER* positive, *HER2* negative patients	Myelosuppression, mucositis, diarrhea, fatigue, nausea/vomiting
CDK4/6 inhibitors (Oral)*		
Palbociclib (Ibrance), Riociclib (Kisqali), Anemically (Verzenio)	*ER* positive, *HER2* negative patients; advanced; failed aromatase inhibitor therapy	Myelosuppression, fatigue, nausea/vomiting, mucositis
PARP Inhibitors (Oral)**		
Olaparib (Lynparza), Talazoprib (Talzenna)	*BRAC* gene mutation, advanced; failed chemotherapy or hormonal therapy	Nausea/vomiting, diarrhea, fatigue, myelosuppression
PI3K Inhibitor (Oral)***		
Alpelisib (Piqray)	*ER* positive, *HER2* negative patients; failed AIs and chemotherapy	Increases blood glucose levels; decreases calcium levels; kidney, liver, and pancreatic function changes; skin reactions; nausea/vomiting, weight loss, fatigue

*Attach to the *HER2* protein on cancer cells, stopping the cells from growing.
**Block kinase enzymes, preventing cancer cell division.
***Block CDK4 and CDK6 proteins on cancer cells.
****Block PARP proteins, which are seen in BRAC 1 and 2 gene mutated breast cancer, leading to cell death.
*****Target the *PIK3* CA gene mutation.

SURVIVAL INFORMATION

According to the ACS (2020), breast cancer survival rates are approximately 91% after 5 years, 84% after 10 years, and 80% after 15 years.

The bibliography and references for this chapter are available on ExamPrepConnect; see inside front cover for access instructions.

1. The nurse is caring for a patient during the immediate postoperative period after a bilateral mastectomy. The nurse's priority intervention is to:

   A. Monitor Jackson-Pratt drainage every 8 hours
   B. Monitor pain every 2 hours
   C. Monitor dressing for drainage every 4 hours
   D. Monitor vital signs every 8 hours

2. Which targeted therapy drug attacks PARP proteins?

   A. Alpelisb (Piqray)
   B. Everolimus (Afinitor)
   C. Lapatinib (Tykerb)
   D. Olaparib (Lynparza)

3. A breast cancer patient calls the oncology clinic nurse, complaining of right-hand swelling post doxorubicin (Adriamycin) administration. The nurse suspects which of the following complications?

   A. Lymphedema
   B. Superior vena cava syndrome
   C. Extravasation
   D. Infection

4. Which of the following chemotherapy agents would you expect a breast cancer patient to receive in the adjuvant setting?

   A. Vinorelbine (Navelbine)
   B. Cyclophosphamide (Cytoxan)
   C. Cisplatin (Platinol)
   D. Paclitaxel protein bound (Abraxane)

5. A breast cancer patient is diagnosed with T2 N0 M0. The correct breast cancer staging is:

   A. Stage IIB
   B. Stage IIA
   C. Stage IIIA
   D. Stage IIIB

1. B) Monitor pain every 2 hours

Monitoring for pain is the most important nursing intervention in the immediate postoperative mastectomy patient. Jackson-Pratt and dressing are also important but secondary to pain. Dressings should be monitored every 8 hours, and vital signs should be monitored every 4 hours.

2. D) Olaparib (Lynparza)

Olaparib (Lynparza) is a *PARP* inhibitor, which are seen in *BRAC1* and *BRAC2* gene mutated breast cancer. Alpelisb (Piqray) is a PIK3 inhibitor, Everolimus (Afinitor) is a *CDK4/6* inhibitor, and Lapatinib (Tykerb) is a kinase inhibitor.

3. C) Extravasation

Doxorubicin (Adriamycin) is a vesicant, which, if administered peripherally, can cause an extravasation leading to a chemical burn. Extravasation is caused by vesicant chemotherapy agents seeping into healthy tissue and out of the vein in which the agent is being administered. Doxorubicin (Adriamycin) is a vesicant, which, if administered peripherally, can cause an extravasation leading to a chemical burn. Lymphedema would cause the patient's arm to swell, not just the hand. Supervisor vena cava syndrome can occur with breast cancer but is more common with lung cancer. It would present with swelling of the hand, arm, and neck.

4. B. Cyclophosphamide (Cytoxan)

Cyclophosphamide (Cytoxan) is a chemotherapy agent commonly used in the adjuvant setting. It is typically administered in combination with doxorubicin (Adriamycin). vinorelbine (Navelbine), cisplatin (Platinol), and paclitaxel protein bound (Abraxane) are used in the advanced setting of breast cancer.

5. B) Stage IIA

Stage IIA is a tumor between 2 and 5 cm in size (T2), no lymph node involvement (N0), and distant metastasis cannot be assessed (M0).

Gastrointestinal Cancers

INTRODUCTION

Gastrointestinal cancers comprise alterations in any portion of the gastrointestinal (GI) tract. A cancer can originate in the esophagus, stomach, colon, and rectum, as well as the accessory glands of the GI tract, which include the liver and pancreas. Each malignancy presents its own signs and symptoms as well as the disease-specific treatment options. Often, multiple treatment modalities are used with GI cancers. This chapter will provide a general overview of each of the most common GI malignancies.

COLORECTAL CANCER

Colorectal cancers (CRC) affect both men and women and are considered the second most common cancer with a high mortality rate in the United States (Centers for Disease Control and Prevention, 2020). Adenocarcinomas comprise more than 90% of colorectal tumors. CRC may be a result of numerous genetic alterations. According to the NIH (2020), the most common sites of colon cancer include the sigmoid colon and anus (Figure 13.1). It is reported that approximately 70% of all colon cancers arise in the large intestine.

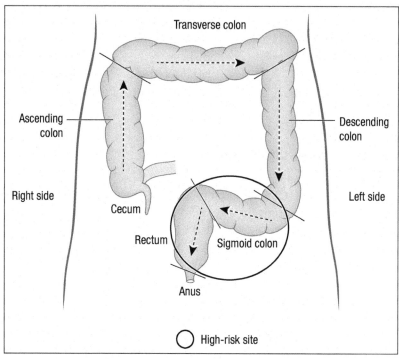

Figure 13.1 High-risk sites for colon cancer.

The bibliography and references for this chapter are available on ExamPrepConnect; see inside front cover for access instructions.

CRC is a GI malignancy originating either in the colon or rectum and is usually created from certain types of colon polyps. It is important to understand that not all polys can lead to malignancy; however, polyps that are aggressive and have atypical cells with genetic mutations can become cancerous. Polyps grow in the inner lining of the colon and, if they are left or undetected, can develop into a malignancy.

▶ RISK FACTORS

Causes and risk factors are numerous when related to colorectal cancers. The risk factors can be divided into two groups—modifiable and nonmodifiable—which are described in Table 18.1. Additionally, genetic mutations and malformations are associated with colorectal cancers. This includes loss of heterozygosity with chromosomes 8p, 17p, and 18q. The 17p deletion accounts for the loss of *p53* function, and 18q contains tumor suppressor genes deleted in the colon cancer gene, as well as the defects in the DNA mismatch repair system. Adenomatous polyposis adenomatous coli (*APC*) is a tumor suppressor gene that can occur early in tumor progression. Mutations of *K-RAS* and *N-RAS* are also seen in early tumor development (Abraham & Gulley, 2019). Studies have shown that patients with deficient DNA mismatch repairs tumors (dMMR) had more favorable outcomes than those with proficient DNA mismatch repair tumors (pMMR) (Abraham & Gulley, 2019). In addition, *B-RAF* mutation is associated with a worse prognosis.

Table 13.1 Modifiable and Nonmodifiable Risk Factors for Colorectal Cancer

Modifiable Risk Factors	Nonmodifiable Risk Factors
Obesity	Over the age of 50 years
Sedentary lifestyle	History of colorectal polyps and/or colorectal cancer
Smoking	Family history of colorectal cancer
Alcohol consumption	Personal history of inflammatory bowel
Diet with a large amount of red meat consumption	Inherited syndromes such as Lynch syndrome and familial adenomatous polyposis (FAP)
Decreased vitamin D levels	Cultural origin: African Americans, Eastern European Jews
Large amount of sugary drinks	

EARLY DETECTION AND SCREENING

One of the reasons there is a decrease in deaths of CRC is due to screening methods. According to the American Cancer Society (2020), it is recommended that colorectal screening begins at age 45 through the age of 75 with either a stool-based testing or visual exams via colonoscopy. For people aged 76 to 85, the decision to proceed with testing should depend on preferences, life expectancy, overall health performance, and screening history. Testing is not recommended for those who are over 85 years of age. Screening includes:

1. Stool-based tests
   a. Fecal immunochemical test every year
   b. Guaiac-based fecal occult blood test (gFOBT) every year
   c. Multi-targeted stool DNA test (mt-sDNA) every 3 years
2. Visual exams
   a. Colonoscopy every 10 years
   b. CT colonography (virtual colonoscopy) every 5 years
   c. Flexible sigmoidoscopy (FSIG) every 5 years

▶ SIGNS AND SYMPTOMS

Signs and symptoms of CRC can resemble other forms as cancer as well; therefore, it is important to have a complete history and physical and determine the risk of disease. In addition, the presence of anemia without an apparent source of active bleeding should be investigated with further workup, including an endoscopic study. The signs and symptoms include:

- Weight loss
- Early satiety
- Abdominal pain
- Fatigue
- Changes in bowel habits (constipation, diarrhea, or both)
- Pencil-like stool formation
- Cramping rectal pain
- Bowel obstruction
- Perforation

▶ DIAGNOSIS

Diagnostic tests include laboratory, imaging, and procedures:

- Complete blood count
- Complete metabolic panel
- Carcinoembryonic antigen (CEA) level
- Endoscopic studies (colonoscopy, sigmoidoscopy)
- CT scan of chest/abdomen/pelvis
- PET/CT (useful for staging)
- MRI (especially if suspected liver lesion)
- Endoscopic rectal ultrasound (rectal cancers)

▶ STAGING

The system most often used to stage colorectal cancer is the American Joint Committee on Cancer (AJCC) TNM (tumor, node, metastasis) system. For complete staging information, visit https://www.cancer.org/cancer/colon-rectal-cancer/detection-diagnosis-staging/staged.html.

SITES OF METASTASIS

Cancers of all types have the potential to spread to other organs. As stated previously, the more disease noted, the more advanced the stage. CRC typically spreads to the following areas: liver, lung, and peritoneum.

> ▶ **EXAM TIP**
>
> Review the AJCC TNM Staging System for colorectal cancer: https://www.cancer.org/cancer/colon-rectal-cancer/detection-diagnosis-staging/staged.html.

▶ TREATMENT

As with all other solid tumor malignancies, the multi-modality approach is utilized, which includes surgery, chemotherapy, biotherapy, and targeted therapy, and, in some cases, the use of radiation therapy. Surgery is primarily used as the first line of defense.

- **Surgical procedures:** Depending on portion of the colon involved, the resection of the affected portion of the colon is removed.
  - **Colectomy:** Resection of the colon
    - Laparoscopic resections
    - Open abdominal
  - **Colostomy:** The cancerous portion of the colon is removed, and an artificial opening for the stool to drain is created on the abdomen. Can be temporary or permanent.
  - **Colon anastomosis:** A portion of the colon is removed, and then the remainder of the colon is reconnected.
- **Radiation therapy (RT):** External beam radiation therapy is primarily used to treat rectal cancers adjuvant or to manage pain with advanced disease (Abraham & Gulley, 2019)
- **Chemotherapy:** Can be adjuvant or advanced diseases. Table 13.2 describes the most common chemotherapy agents used to treat the different stages of colorectal cancers.

Table 13.2 Common Chemotherapy Agents Used to Treat Adjuvant and Advanced Colorectal Cancers

Chemotherapy Agent	Monitoring Considerations	Adjuvant or Advanced Disease
Capecitabine (Xeloda; oral)	Hand/foot syndrome, myelosuppression	Advanced disease
5-Fluorouracil (5FU)	Diarrhea, skin and nail changes, myelosuppression	Neoadjuvant/adjuvant disease
Irinotecan (Camptosar)	Acute-onset diarrhea, myelosuppression, nausea/vomiting	Neoadjuvant/adjuvant disease and advanced disease
Oxaliplatin (Eloxatin)*	Neuropathy (peripheral); cold sensitivity usually 3–5 days, but may be longer	Neoadjuvant/adjuvant disease and advanced disease

*Can be mixed only with D5W.

TARGETED THERAPY

There are several types of targeted therapies that work well against CRC, including vascular endothelial growth factor (VEGF), epidermal growth factor receptor (EGFR), BRAF agents, and kinase inhibitors. These are proteins that aid tumors to form and create new blood vessels to obtain nutrients from the host to continue to grow, as well as connect to mutated genes. Targeted therapies are agents that stop the creation of blood vessels.

Targeted therapy has been a great advancement to the treatment regimen of colorectal cancers. The most common **VGEF agents** include:

- Bevacizumab (Avastin)
- Ramucirumab (Cyramza)
- Ziv-aflibercept (Zaltrap)

Side effects of VEGF inhibitors include:

- Hypertension
- Fatigue
- Bleeding
- Low white blood cell counts
- Headaches
- Mouth sores
- Loss of appetite
- Diarrhea

Common **EGFR agents** include:

- Cetuximab (Erbitux)
- Panitumumab (Vectibix)

Common side effects of EGFR include:

- Acne-like rash on the face and chest during treatment, which can sometimes lead to infections, treated usually with Clindagel and an oral prophylactic antibiotic such as Minocycline daily dosing
- Fever
- Fatigue
- Headache
- Diarrhea

BRAF agents are usually combined with other treatment options. Encorafenib (Braftovi) is a drug that targets the abnormal BRAF protein directly. The most common side effects include:

- Skin thickening
- Diarrhea
- Rash
- Loss of appetite
- Abdominal pain
- Joint pain and fatigue
- Nausea

Kinase inhibitors block several kinase proteins that decrease the ability for the cancer cell to grow and stop the growth of new blood vessels that help tumor cells grow or help form new blood vessels to feed the tumor. Regorafenib (Stivarga) is used with advanced disease. Common side effects of kinase inhibitors include:

- Rash
- Hand/foot syndrome (HFS)
- Diarrhea
- Fatigue
- High blood pressure
- Weight loss
- Abdominal pain

IMMUNOTHERAPY

PDL1- inhibitors and CTLA- 4 inhibitors use the patient's own body immune system to help recognize the cancer cells as abnormal and start the cascade of cancer cell death. These agents can be used in combination with each other for many types of cancers. The two most common immunotherapy agents are Pembrolizumab (Keytruda) and Nivolumab (OPDIVO). Ipilimumab (Yervoy) is a CTLA-4 inhibitor that blocks CTLA-4, a protein on T cells. Side effects of immunotherapy include:

- Fatigue
- Cough
- Nausea
- Diarrhea
- Skin rash
- Loss of appetite
- Constipation
- Joint pain
- Itching
- Autoimmune reactions: The immune system can start attacking parts of their own body:
  - Lungs: Pneumonitis
  - Intestines: Colitis
  - Liver: Immune-related hepatitis or reactivation of hepatitis
  - Thyroid: Hypo/hyperthyroid
  - Kidneys: Renal insufficiency
  - Pancreas: Diabetes
  - Skin: Rash

PANCREATIC CANCER

Most pancreatic cancers are located at the head of the pancreas, which lives within the duodenal curvature, the body located behind the stomach, and the tail that is near the spleen. The primary function of the pancreas is to aid in digestion and assist in managing blood glucose levels by the release of pancreatic enzymes.

▶ PANCREATIC CANCER CELLS

Each of the pancreatic cancer cells can be further identified as subtypes. Some are more prevalent than others.

- Exocrine pancreatic: Accounts for 95% of all cancers of the pancreas
  - Adenocarcinoma: The most common cancer, which typically occurs in the lining of the ducts.
- Acinar cancer cells: Occurs in 1% to 2% of pancreatic cancers.
- Squamous cell: Exceedingly rare in pancreatic cancers.
- Colloid carcinoma: Usually develop from benign cysts.
- Neuroendocrine: Referred to as islet cell cancers; not common.

▶ RISK FACTORS

The common risk factors for pancreatic cancer include:

- Family history: Plus or minus hereditary syndromes such as:
  - Peutz-Jeghers syndrome: An inherited autosomal disease that produces intestinal polyps. This polyp has a significant risk of developing intestinal and pancreatic cancers.
  - Hereditary breast/ovarian cancers
  - Familial adenomatous polyposis
  - Hereditary non-polyposis colon cancer
- Smoking
- Chronic pancreatitis
- Alcohol consumption
- Increased weight
- Insulin resistance
- Increased consumption of processed and red meats
- Chronic infections such as hepatitis B and C and *Helicobacter pylori*

▶ SIGNS AND SYMPTOMS

Pancreatic cancer is an insidious disease because in the early stages there are often no symptoms. Unfortunately, symptoms usually begin when the disease is advanced and has spread to other organs, causing multisystem failure. In addition, there are no screening tests for pancreatic cancers, and those that find a lesion in early stages are usually incidental findings. Those with a first-degree relative with pancreatic cancer are recommended to undergo screening with MRI or endoscopic ultrasound (EUS), although no specific guidelines have been established regarding the age at which to start and the frequency of screening.

The most common signs and symptoms include.

- Fatigue
- Weight loss
- Anorexia
- Abdominal pain, sometimes radiating to the back
- Jaundice (with advanced disease)
- Itchy skin
- Tea-colored urine
- Back pain
- Ascites in advanced disease
- Loose, foul smelling, greasy stools
- Late-onset diabetes

▶ DIAGNOSIS

Diagnostic and laboratory testing vary depending on the symptoms at diagnosis. The most common initial diagnostic evaluation includes:

- Ca 19.9
- Triple-phase CT, which is a pancreatic protocol CT scan. It includes arterial phase, portal venous phase, and a late washout phase, which are useful to distinguish between normal parenchyma and tumor as well as tumor and nearby by venous structures and any liver metastasis.
- Endoscopic ultrasound with a fine-needle biopsy has extremely high sensitivity and specificity for diagnosing pancreatic cancer (Abraham & Gulley, 2019).

▶ STAGING

Staging for pancreatic cancer is based on the TNM (tumor, node, metastasis) system of the American Joint Committee on Cancer (AJCC). For complete staging information, visit https://www.cancer.org/cancer/pancreatic-cancer/detection-diagnosis-staging/staging. html. In addition, pancreatic cancers are also divided into four different categories:

1. Resectable
2. Borderline resectable
3. Unresectable
4. Metastatic

> **▶ EXAM TIP**
>
> Review the AJCC TNM Staging System for pancreatic cancer: https://www.cancer.org/cancer/pancreatic-cancer/detection-diagnosis-staging/staging.html.

▶ TREATMENT

As with all other solid tumor malignancies, the multimodality approach is utilized, which includes surgery, chemotherapy, biotherapy, and targeted therapy, and in some cases, the use of radiation therapy.

- **Surgical procedures**
  - Whipple procedure: Removal of the head and potentially a portion of the body of the pancreas, as well as adjacent structures such as part of the bile duct, gallbladder, lymph nodes near the pancreas, and, in some cases, a portion of the stomach.
  - Distal pancreatectomy: Removal of the tail and a portion of the body of the pancreas, as well as the spleen.
  - Total pancreatectomy: Removal of the entire pancreas, as well as the gallbladder, part of the stomach, part of the small intestine, and the spleen.
- **Radiation therapy:** Use of external beam radiation.
- **Chemotherapy:** Can be adjuvant or advanced diseases. Table 13.3 describes the most common chemotherapy agents used to treat the different stages of pancreatic cancer.

Table 13.3 Common Chemotherapy Agents Used to Treat Pancreatic Cancer*

Chemotherapy Agents	Monitoring Considerations
Albumin-bound paclitaxel	Myelosuppression, peripheral neuropathy
Capecitabine (Xeloda; oral)	Hand/foot syndrome, myelosuppression
Taxotere (Docetaxel)	Infusion reaction
5-Fluorouracil (5FU)	Diarrhea, skin and nail changes, myelosuppression
Gemcitabine (Gemzar)	Myelosuppression (specifically platelets), nausea/vomiting
Irinotecan (Camptosar)	Acute-onset diarrhea myelosuppression, nausea/vomiting
Paclitaxel (Taxol)	Anaphylaxis/infusion reaction, peripheral neuropathy (can be dose limiting) Use of pre-medications; use of non-PVC tubing and 0.22-micron filter for administration
Platinol (Cisplatin)	Kidney function, strict input and outputs, hydration and fluid replacement, nausea/vomiting, myelosuppression
Oxaliplatin (Eloxatin)	Neuropathy (peripheral); cold sensitivity usually 3–5 days, but may be longer Use of pre-medications; use of non-PVC tubing and 0.22-micron filter for administration

*Many of these chemotherapy agents are used in combination; they are rarely administered as a single agent.
PVC, polyvinyl chloride.

TARGETED THERAPY

It has become common practice to have both chemotherapy and targeted therapy used in combination for pancreatic cancer. This includes (American Cancer Society, 2020):

- EGFR inhibitor: Erlotinib (Tarceva)
- PARP inhibitor (those with *BRCA* mutation): Olaparib (Lynparza)
- NTRK inhibitors: Larotrectinib (Vitrakvi) and entrectinib (Rozlytrek)

HEPATOCELLULAR CARCINOMA

Hepatocellular carcinoma (HCC), or primary liver cancer, is caused by direct damage to the hepatocytes. Chronic infections of the liver are the most common causes of HCC; that is, hepatitis B and C and cirrhosis.

▶ RISK FACTORS

The ACS (2020) has identified several risk factors related to HCC:

- Hepatitis B and C
- Cirrhosis and alcohol-induced cirrhosis
- Nonalcoholic fatty liver disease
- Primary biliary cirrhosis
- Hemochromatosis

- Alpha1-antitrypsin deficiency
- Aflatoxin exposure
- Smoking
- Type 2 DM
- Obesity

▶ SIGNS AND SYMPTOMS

HCC historically does not present with symptoms; if symptoms occur, it is unfortunately with advanced disease. Common sites of metastasis are regional lymph nodes, lungs, and bone. Advanced disease symptoms include:

- Unintentional weight loss
- Early satiety
- Nausea or vomiting
- Enlarged liver and spleen
- Abdominal pain or right shoulder pain
- Abdominal ascites
- Severe itching
- Jaundice of skin and sclera
- Coagulation alterations: Bruising and bleeding

▶ DIAGNOSIS

Several diagnostic tests can be ordered to confirm HCC:

1. Alpha feta protein (AFP)
2. Triple phase CT scan and/or an MRI
3. Liver biopsy (ultrasound- or CT-guided)

▶ STAGING

Staging for HCC uses the TNM system; however, there are multiple staging systems that can be utilized:

- The American Joint Committee on Cancer (AJCC): https://www.cancer.org/cancer/liver-cancer/detection-diagnosis-staging/staging.html; note that it does not include the function of the liver and overall functional status of the patient.
- The Okuda System
- The Cancer of the Liver Italian Program (CLIP) System
- Barcelona Clinic Liver Cancer (BCLC) System: Incorporates parts related to liver function, which is known as the Child-Pugh score, and determines the severity of cirrhosis.

▶ **EXAM TIP**

Review the AJCC TNM Staging System for HCC:): https://www.cancer.org/cancer/liver-cancer/detection-diagnosis-staging/staging.html.

▶ TREATMENT

SURGICAL PROCEDURES

Surgery should be the main curative option. However, to determine if surgery is the best method, the Child-Pugh score needs to be determined. The Child-Pugh score measures liver function, especially in people with cirrhosis. A patient with a score of B is usually not recommended for surgery. A patient with an A score typically has enough liver function to undergo surgery and recover without complications. Types of surgical procedures include:

- Partial hepatectomy
- Liver transplantation (if appropriate criteria are met)
- Ablation
- Hepatic artery embolization (also known as trans arterial chemoembolization [TACE])

RADIATION THERAPY

The liver is considered a radiosensitive organ; therefore, radiation can be successful in eliminating cancer cells. As with any type of solid malignancy, there are multiple treatment modalities with the field of radiation: Radioembolization uses Yttrium-90 microspheres, which are injected into the liver to cause tumor necrosis, and stereotactic body radiation therapy (SBRT).

CHEMOTHERAPY

Some chemotherapy agents can be effective for HCC; however, there is a balance of how much drug can be administered safely. Liver functions need to be monitored, and doses of agents may be adjusted based upon the liver functions. Table 13.4 describes the most common agents used for HCC.

Table 13.4 Common Chemotherapy Agents Used to Treat Hepatocellular Carcinoma

Chemotherapy Agents	Monitoring Considerations
Capecitabine (Xeloda; oral)	Hand/foot syndrome, myelosuppression
Doxorubicin (Adriamycin)	Myelosuppression, mouth sores, nausea/vomiting Use of vesicant precautions during administration Potential to be cardiotoxic; requires a MUGA scan prior to administration of first dose Lifetime max of drug: 550 mg/m^2; 450 mg/m^2 with commitment radiation Red urine 24–48 hr post infusion
5-Fluorouracil (5FU)	Diarrhea, skin and nail changes, myelosuppression
Gemcitabine (Gemzar)	Myelosuppression (specifically platelets), nausea/vomiting
Platinol (Cisplatin)	Kidney function, strict input and outputs, hydration and fluid replacement, nausea/vomiting, myelosuppression
Oxaliplatin (Eloxatin)	Neuropathy (peripheral); cold sensitivity usually 3–5 days but may be longer Use of pre-medications; use of non-PVC tubing and 0.22-micron filter for administration

MUGA, multigated acquisition.

BIOTHERAPY/IMMUNE THERAPY

Biotherapy has become highly effective with HCC. There are several agents that can be used:

- **Kinase inhibitors:** Common side effects include fatigue, loss of appetite, hand-foot syndrome, high blood pressure, weight loss, diarrhea, abdominal pain.
  - Sorafenib (Nexavar)
  - Lenvatinib (Lenvima)
  - Regorafenib (Stivarga)
  - Cabozantinib (Cabometyx)
- **Monoclonal antibodies:** Common side effects include high blood pressure, diarrhea, fatigue, bleeding, decreased/loss appetite, mouth sores, decreased white blood cell count, headaches.
  - Bevacizumab (Avastin)
  - Ramucirumab (Cyramza)
- **PDL-1 inhibitors:** Common side effects include fatigue, fever, cough, nausea, itching, rash, loss of appetite, muscle/joint pain, constipation/diarrhea, infusion reactions, autoimmune reactions.
  - Atezolizumab (Tecentriq) usually combined with bevacizumab (Avastin), pembrolizumab (Keytruda), nivolumab (Opdivo)

ANAL CANCER

Anal cancer starts in the anus can also be identified in the anal canal and the perianal skin. It is more commonly diagnosed in the female population. There are multiple types of cellular anal cancers: squamous cell carcinoma, adenocarcinoma, basal cell, and melanoma. Squamous is the most identified, while the other types are mentioned but are considered rare.

▶ RISK FACTORS

Risk factors for anal cancer include:

- Multiple sexual partners: More than 10 in lifetime
- History of sexually transmitted diseases
- HPV infection: Majority of squamous cell cancers are associated with HPV, especially HPV 16 and 18 strains
- HIV infection
- History of cervical
- Cigarette smoking

▶ SIGNS AND SYMPTOMS

Signs and symptoms for anal cancer include:

- Rectal bleeding (anemia)
- Anal itching

- Lump or mass at the anal opening
- Pain or feeling of fullness in the anal area.
- Narrow stools
- Change in bowel habits
- Discharge from the anus
- Swollen lymph nodes in anal and groin area
- Incontinent of stool

▶ DIAGNOSIS

Best method of diagnosis is the digital rectal examination (DRE) for both men and women. Men often have a rectal examination to assess and palpate the prostate but also can determine a rectal cancer or bleeding and investigate for colon cancer. Female patients have rectal examination by the gynecologist after a pelvic examination. In addition, an anoscope can be performed to visually the anal canal. Biopsy and CT of the abdomen and pelvis is used to determine the stage of the disease.

▶ STAGING

As with all solid tumors, the staging used is the AJCC TNM system. For complete staging information, visit https://www.cancer.org/cancer/anal-cancer/detection-diagnosis-staging/staging.html.

> ▶ **EXAM TIP**
>
> Review the AJCC TNM Staging System for anal cancer: https://www.cancer.org/cancer/anal-cancer/detection-diagnosis-staging/staging.html.

▶ TREATMENT

SURGICAL PROCEDURES

Surgery is typically not the first treatment used for anal cancer. The surgical procedure used depends on the type and location of the tumor. Procedures include local resection and abdominoperineal resection (APR).

RADIATION THERAPY

External beam radiation therapy and brachytherapy (internal radiation therapy) are used to treat anal cancer.

CHEMOTHERAPY

Chemotherapy is commonly used for anal cancer. The most commonly used drugs are 5FU (Fluorouracil) and mitomycin (Mutamycin), or 5FU and cisplatin (Platinol).

BIOTHERAPY/IMMUNE THERAPY

Immunotherapy options include the PDL-1 inhibitors pembrolizumab (Keytruda) and nivolumab (Opdivo). Common side effects include fatigue, fever, cough, nausea, itching, rash, loss of appetite, muscle/joint pain, constipation/diarrhea, infusion reactions, autoimmune reactions.

⬤ ESOPHAGEAL CANCER

Esophagus is the muscular structure that connects the throat with the stomach and a cancer can develop within any portion. However, most tumors occur in the lower to one-third and middle of the esophagus. The lowest numbers of tumors are in the upper one-third of the esophagus. Approximately 80% of esophageal cancers occur in less developed countries such as Asia and Africa (American Cancer Society, 2020). There are two main types: adenocarcinoma and squamous cell carcinoma.

▶ RISK FACTORS

Risk factors for adenocarcinoma include:

- Barret's esophagus: Tissue lining becomes damaged from chronic gastroesophageal reflux disease (GERD)
- GERD
- Overweight or obese
- Smoking

Risk factors for squamous cell carcinoma include (Abraham & Gulley, 2019):

- Smoking (tobacco)
- Alcohol consumption
- HPV
- Celiac disease
- Achalasia: When the muscle on the lower part of the esophagus does not relax properly, food and liquid collect, causing the muscle to stretch.
- Plummer-Vinson syndrome: Webs in the upper part of the esophagus cause food particles to get stuck, which can cause dysphagia and chronic irritation.
- Tylosis: Rare inherited disease in which papillomas form in the esophagus.
- Diet high in processed meats and drinking hot liquids frequently, which cause temperature discomfort

▶ SIGNS AND SYMPTOMS

Signs and symptoms include (Abraham & Gulley, 2019):

- Dysphagia
- Weight loss/anorexia
- Painful swallowing

- Regurgitating food that has not yet been digested
- Iron-deficiency anemia
- Hoarseness
- Hiccups

▶ DIAGNOSIS

The gold standard for diagnosing esophageal cancer is an upper endoscopy. This allows several tissue biopsies to be taken to provide an accurate diagnosis. A PET scan or CT scan can also be ordered to evaluate for any other sites of disease. Tissue testing for PDL-1, HER-2, and MSI/MMR can be ordered (American Cancer Society, 2020).

▶ STAGING

The AJCC TNM staging system is used in esophageal cancer. For complete staging information, visit https://www.cancer.org/cancer/esophagus-cancer/detection-diagnosis-staging/staging.html.

> **▶   EXAM TIP**
>
> Review the AJCC TNM Staging System for esophageal cancer: https://www.cancer.org/cancer/esophagus-cancer/detection-diagnosis-staging/staging.html.

▶ TREATMENT

SURGICAL PROCEDURES

Esophagectomy is a treatment option for esophageal cancer. It is the removal of a portion of the esophagus, as well as examination of the lymph nodes. In some cases, a small portion of the upper stomach is removed, depending on the extent of the cancer. Side effects include pain, reactions to anesthesia, bleeding, pneumonia, voice changes, leak at anastomosis site, strictures causing problems with swallowing, regurgitation, and frequent nausea or vomiting.

RADIATION THERAPY

External beam radiation is used. Usually, radiation is ordered before and after surgery, as well as in addition to chemotherapy.

CHEMOTHERAPY

Chemotherapy can be given before, after, or for advanced cancers for palliation. Chemotherapy drugs that may be used alone or in combination with or without radiation include:

- Carboplatin and Paclitaxel
- Oxaliplatin and 5FU/Capecitabine

- Cisplatin and 5FU/Capecitabine
- Cisplatin and Irinotecan
- Taxol and 5FU/Capecitabine

Other drugs include the following, but they are not usually given concurrently with radiation (American Cancer Society, 2020)

- Epirubicin (Ellence), cisplatin, and 5FU
- Docetaxel (Taxotere), cisplatin, and 5FU
- Trifluridine and Tipiracil (Lonsurf)

TARGETED THERAPY

- Herceptin (*HER2*-positive tumors)
- VEGFR2 antagonist: Ramicurumab
- NTRK inhibitors: Entrectinib (Rozlytrek) and Iarotrectinib (Vitrakvi)

BIOTHERAPY/IMMUNE THERAPY

Immunotherapy options include the PDL-1 inhibitors pembrolizumab (Keytruda) and nivolumab (Opdivo). Common side effects include fatigue, fever, cough, nausea, itching, rash, loss of appetite, muscle/joint pain, constipation/diarrhea, infusion reactions, autoimmune reactions.

GASTRIC CANCER

Gastric cancer is a direct effect of the cells lining the stomach and can tend to involve patients over 50 years of age. However, there is a rise in the younger population ranging at the age 40. In the younger population, gastric cancers are being seen at the cardiac/gastroesophageal junction (GEJ). Approximately 90% are adenocarcinoma and are further subdivided into intestinal and diffuse. Unfortunately, there is no approved or recommended screening tool in the United States for gastric cancer (Abraham & Gulley, 2019).

▶ RISK FACTORS

Risk factors for gastric cancer include:

- Increased age
- More common in males
- Cigarette smoking
- Alcohol intake
- Diet rich in salt, smoked foods
- Diet low in fruits and vegetables
- Vitamin deficiency (A, C, E): beta carotene, selenium, low fiber
- First degree relative with cancer

- Previous conditions: *Helicobacter pylori*, chronic gastritis, pernicious anemia, intestinal metaplasia, gastric polyps, Epstein-Barr virus
- Familial conditions such as familial adenomatous polyposis

▶ SIGNS AND SYMPTOMS

Signs and symptoms for gastric cancer include:

- Indigestion
- Stomach discomfort/pain
- Bloating
- Nausea/vomiting
- Early satiety
- Decreased or loss of appetite
- Weight loss
- Blood in stool

▶ DIAGNOSIS

Several diagnostic tests can be ordered to confirm gastric cancer (Abraham & Gulley, 2019):

1. Upper gastrointestinal endoscopy: Includes obtaining several biopsies within the stomach.
2. EUS: Used to assess the depth of tumor invasion.
3. Blood tests: CBC, Chem, CEA (elevated in 40%–50% of tumors, therefore not a useful screening test).
4. CT and PET/CT: Used to assess the local spread and distant metastasis.

▶ STAGING

The AJCC TNM staging system is used for gastric cancer. For complete staging information, visit https://www.cancer.org/cancer/stomach-cancer/detection-diagnosis-staging/staging.html.

▶ **EXAM TIP**

Review the AJCC TNM Staging System for gastric cancer: https://www.cancer.org/cancer/stomach-cancer/detection-diagnosis-staging/staging.html.

▶ TREATMENT

SURGICAL PROCEDURES

Surgery is the first line of defense to treat gastric cancers. Surgical procedures include:

- **Subtotal gastrectomy:** Removal of the part of the stomach with cancer, nearby lymph nodes, other tissues, and organs that are near the tumor such as the spleen.

- **Total gastrectomy:** Removal of the whole stomach, nearby lymph nodes, part of the esophagus, small intestine, tissues near tumor, and possibly the spleen. Esophagus is then connected to the small intestine.
- **Palliative surgery and stents:**
  - Stent placement: Placed in stomach or esophagus to keep the passage open to help relieve some obstructive symptoms.
  - Gastrojejunestomy: Removal of the cancerous part of the stomach. The stomach is then connected to the jejunum to allow the passage of food. Percutaneous jejunostomy/gastrostomy includes a feeding tube surgically placed directly into the stomach to the small intestine. Recommended for patients who are unable to take food orally. Usual for those suffering from nausea, vomiting, and gastroparesis.

RADIATION THERAPY

The use of external beam radiation can be utilized after surgery.

CHEMOTHERAPY

Chemotherapy is commonly used in gastric cancers. The most commonly used drugs are 5FU (Fluorouracil), usually given with leucovorin (folinic acid), and capecitabine (Xeloda).

The bibliography and references for this chapter are available on ExamPrepConnect; see inside front cover for access instructions.

1. A patient diagnosed with colon cancer says to the nurse, "I can't believe that I have to wear gloves when I remove food from the freezer." The nurse recognizes that the patient is being treated with which chemotherapy agent?

    A. Gemcitabine (Gemzar)
    B. Paclitaxel (Taxol)
    C. Irinotecan (Camptosar)
    D. Oxaliplatin (Eloxatin)

2. The most common risk factors for anal cancer include:

    A. Cirrhosis
    B. Hepatitis B and C
    C. HIV and HPV
    D. Epstein-Barr virus

3. The nurse is caring for a patient with advanced pancreatic cancer who has suspected myelosuppression from gemcitabine (Gemzar) treatment. The nurse expects which blood counts to be most affected?

    A. White blood cells
    B. Red blood cells
    C. Platelets
    D. Liver functions

4. Radioembolization utilizes which of the following radioisotopes to cause tumor necrosis?

    A. Mylotarg
    B. Yttrium-35
    C. I-131
    D. Yttrium-90

5. A 47-year-old patient with a severe intellectual disability has been diagnosed with colon cancer. The patient's provider recommends a reversible colostomy. The patient lacks decision-making capacity. The nurse expects which of the following individuals will provide consent for the surgery?

    A. The patient
    B. The healthcare provider
    C. The patient's guardian ad litem
    D. The administrator of the group home where the patient resides

1. D) Oxaliplatin (Eloxatin)
Oxaliplatin can cause acute neuropathy when a patient is exposed to cold. Gemcitabine (Gemzar) can cause myelosuppression, Paclitaxel (Taxol) can cause acute infusion reactions, and irinotecan (Camptosar) can cause acute-onset diarrhea.

2. C) HIV and HPV
HIV and HPV (strain 16) are common risk factors for anal cancer. Cirrhosis and hepatitis B and C are risk factors for liver cancers. The Epstein-Barr virus is a risk factor for lymphoma.

3. C) Platelets
Platelets are the most affected blood counts seen in patients with myelosuppression from gemcitabine (Gemzar). The platelet counts can be dose limiting.

4. D) Yttrium-90
Yttrium-90 is used with radioembolization of the liver to cause tumor necrosis. Mylotarg is used in lymphoma patients, I-131 is used for thyroid malignancies. Yttrium-35 is used to make microwaves; it is not used in healthcare.

5. C) The patient's guardian ad litem
A guardian ad litem is an individual who is assigned by a court to act in the best interest of a "ward." A ward is a person who lacks decision-making capacity, such as an individual with a severe intellectual disability. Given that the patient lacks decision-making capacity, it would not be appropriate for them to provide consent, nor would it be appropriate for the healthcare provider or the administrator of the group home to provide consent.

Genitourinary and Male and Female Reproductive Cancers

INTRODUCTION

The genitourinary system in men and women includes urinary and reproductive organs such as the kidneys, bladder, testes, ovaries, and uterus. This chapter reviews renal cancer, bladder cancer, male reproductive cancers such as testicular and penile cancer, and female reproductive cancers such as ovarian, vulvar, and endometrial.

RENAL CELL CARCINOMA

Renal cell carcinoma tends to be more prevalent in women than men, and, unfortunately, there are no screening tools available. Renal cancers are usually discovered at later stages of the disease, which decreases the chance for cure. There are several types of renal cell cancers; the most common types include:

- **Clear Cell**: The most common type, which accounts for the majority of renal cancers. These cancers can be aggressive to slow-growing tumors. These are usually treated with targeted agents.
- **Papillary Cell**: Accounts for approximately 10% to 15% of renal cancers. It is further divided into type I and type II categories. The first line of treatment is surgical resection for local papillary renal cancer. In the event papillary cancer is diagnosed with metastatic disease, anti-antigenic agents can be used.
- **Medullary Cell:** An extremely aggressive and rare form of renal cancer, it is more prevalent in the African American population and patients with sickle cell anemia trait. Chemotherapy and biotherapy agents are recommended treatment options.
- **Sarcomatoid**: An aggressive and unorganized form, which can include all the cell types mentioned earlier. When observed by the pathologist, this disorganization is called *sacromatoid*.

▶ RISK FACTORS

As with the majority of solid tumor malignancies, there are numerous risk factors that can cause renal cell carcinomas, including:

- Smoking
- Obesity
- Hypertension (controlled)
- Family history
- Exposure to trichloroethylene (TCE), a chemical used to make refrigerants and used as a degreasing agent in cleaning products (e.g., spot removers, cleaning wipes, and dry-cleaning products)

The bibliography and references for this chapter are available on ExamPrepConnect; see inside front cover for access instructions.

- Extended use of acetaminophen
- Genetic predispositions:
  - Von Hippel-Lindau disease
  - Hereditary papillary renal cell carcinoma
  - Hereditary leiomyomas
  - Birt-Hogg-Dubé syndrome
  - Cowden syndrome

▶ STAGING

Renal cell carcinoma is staged with the American Joint Committee on Cancer (AJCC) TNM (tumor, node, metastasis) staging system, which analyzes the tumor size, lymph node involvement, and metastatic site(s). For complete staging information, visit https://www.cancer.org/cancer/kidney-cancer/detection-diagnosis-staging/staging.html.

> ### ▶ EXAM TIP
>
> Review the AJCC TNM Staging System for renal cell carcinoma: https://www.cancer.org/cancer/kidney-cancer/detection-diagnosis-staging/staging.html.

▶ TREATMENT

The most common treatment options for renal cell carcinoma include the following:

- **Surgical Procedures:** As with all other solid tumors, surgery is the first line of defense. Nephrectomy and partial nephrectomy are the two best options. The location of the tumor and the extent of kidney involvement will determine if a radical or partial nephrectomy will be recommended. Advancements in robotic and laparoscopic surgeries have made them a promising option for patients to avoid the use of a large incision to remove kidney, resulting in fewer complications and shorter hospital stays.
- **Radiation:** Not used as first-line or adjuvant therapy as with other solid tumors; however, it can be used for palliation and in advanced disease when surgery is not an option.
- **Chemotherapy:** Chemotherapy agents have not been effective in treating renal cell carcinoma and are typically used in only advanced/late-stage disease. The chemotherapy agents prescribed with late cancer include:
  - Cisplatin (Platinol): Monitor for nephrotoxicity and ototoxicity
  - 5-Fluorouracil (5FU): Monitor for diarrhea and skin reactions
  - Gemcitabine (Gemzar): Monitor for myelosuppression and nausea/vomiting
- **Targeted Therapies:** Targeted therapy can be effective in treating renal cell carcinoma. The most common and successful agents include oral and IV agents:
  - Oral agents:
    - Sunitinib (Sutent)
    - Sorafenib (Nexavar)
    - Pazopanib (Votrient)
    - Cabozantinib (Cabometyx)
    - Lenvatinib (Lenvima)
    - Axitinib (Inlyta)
    - Everolimus (Afinitor)

- IV agents:
  - Bevacizumab (Avastin)
  - Temsirolimus (Torisel)
  - Pembrolizumab (Keytruda)
  - Nivolumab (Opdivo

▶ SURVIVAL INFORMATION

Treatment with a nephrectomy can yield a 94% 5-year survival rate. The 5-year survival rate for stage II disease is approximately 70%, and metastatic disease to distant areas is approximately 12% (ASCO, 2020).

◗ BLADDER CANCER

Bladder cancers are another solid tumor disease that can affect both men and women. The incidence is higher in White men, and it is typically diagnosed at 55 years or older. The most common form of bladder cancer is transitional cell carcinoma (TCC). Less common forms include squamous cell carcinoma, adenocarcinoma, small cell carcinoma, and sarcoma (extremely rare). Bladder cancer is divided into two categories, which indicate the depth of the cancer cells invading the lining of the bladder and determine the treatment options:

1. Invasive: Greater involvement of the bladder, with cancers cells extending deep into the lining of the bladder; promotes metastases. Significantly more difficult to treat.
2. Noninvasive: Cancer cells are found on only the inner layer of the bladder. It is easier to treat and less likely to spread.

▶ RISK FACTORS

Risk factors for bladder cancer are the typical risk factors for most solid tumors: obesity, smoking, family history, genetic predisposition, and age. However, the most important risk factor is exposure to chemicals, particularly the aromatic amines such as benzidine and beta-naphthylamine, which are used in the dye industry. Other occupations that carry a high risk for bladder cancer are printers, textile workers, painters, machinists, truck drivers, and hairdressers. Recurrent bladder infections, ingestion of arsenic via drinking water, and decreased fluid intake can also increase risk.

▶ STAGING

Bladder cancer is staged with the American Joint Committee on Cancer (AJCC) TNM (tumor, node, metastasis) staging system, which analyzes the tumor size, lymph node involvement, and metastatic site(s). For complete staging information, visit https://www.cancer.org/cancer/bladder-cancer/detection-diagnosis-staging/staging.html.

▶ EXAM TIP

Review the AJCC TNM Staging System for bladder cancer: https://www.cancer.org/cancer/bladder-cancer/detection-diagnosis-staging/staging.html.

▶ TREATMENT

SURGICAL PROCEDURES

Surgery is the first treatment option to cure the disease. Surgical procedures include the following:

- Transurethral bladder tumor resection (TURBT): Used both to diagnose bladder cancer and to remove cancerous tissue from the bladder.
- Cystectomy (partial or radical): Removal of all or part of the bladder. A radical cystectomy in men typically involves the removal of the bladder, prostate, and seminal vesicles. In women, it typically involves the removal of the bladder, ovaries, uterus, ovaries, and part of the vagina. When a patient receives a radical cystectomy, a urine diversion, such as an ileal conduit, is created to collect the urine (Figure 14.1). In some patients, a neobladder (new bladder) is created from the intestine and is sewn into the ureters (Figure 14.2).

RADIATION

Radiation is not the primary treatment for bladder cancer. In some instances, external radiation can be used in combination with systematic chemotherapy in advanced stages of the disease or if a patient is not a surgical candidate as primary treatment and or had partial cystectomy.

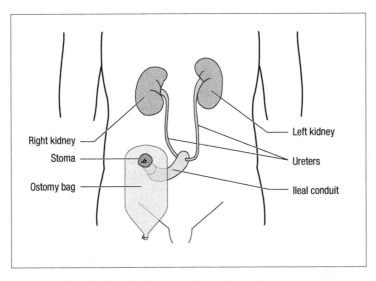

Figure 14.1 An ileal conduit created to collect the urine during a radical cystectomy.

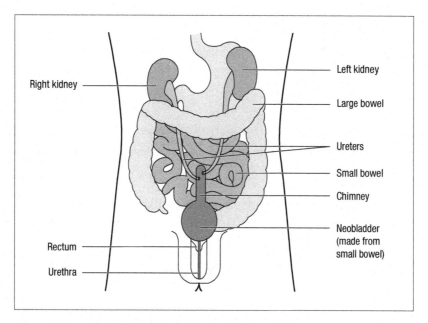

Figure 14.2 A neobladder created during a radical cystectomy.

CHEMOTHERAPY

Chemotherapy can be an extremely effective treatment with noninvasive localized bladder cancer. Chemotherapy is delivered with the use of intravesical therapy, which allows the chemotherapy and/or immunotherapy agents to be directly placed into the bladder (via a catheter) for a prescribed amount of time. The most common chemotherapy agents used for intravesical therapy include gemcitabine (Gemzar) and mitomycin (Mutamycin). Both agents can cause local irritation to the bladder. Immunotherapy agents used for intravesical therapy include:

- BCG (Bacillus Calmette–Guerin): First developed in the early 1900s as a vaccine against the tuberculosis virus. In the 1950s, it was discovered that BCG influenced cancer cells in animals, and it is now a viable treatment for noninvasive bladder cancer, prompting the immune system to kill the cancer cells within the bladder. Side effects include local reactions in the bladder, pain, urinary urgency and frequency, blood in the urine, and fatigue.
- Interferon (Roferon-A, Intron, Alferon): In some cases, it can be used in combination with BCG. It has similar side effects to BCG therapy.

Systematic chemotherapy/biotherapy agents are administered intravenously in patients with advanced bladder cancer. Agents include:

- Cisplatin (Platinol) and/or carboplatin (paraplatin) with gemcitabine (Gemzar)
- MVAC protocol for advanced disease: **M**ethotrexate, **v**inblastine, doxorubicin (**A**driamycin), **c**isplatin
- Docetaxel (Taxotere) or Paclitaxel (Abraxane)
- Pemetrexed (Alimta)
- Immune-check inhibitors: Atezolizumab (Tecentriq) or nivolumab (Opdivo)

▶ SURVIVAL INFORMATION

According to the ACS (2020), the 5-year survival rates vary based upon the stage of the disease: noninvasive disease has 96% survival rate, local disease 69%, regional disease 37%, and metastatic disease 6%.

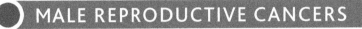

● MALE REPRODUCTIVE CANCERS

▶ TESTICULAR CANCER

Testicular cancer is the most common male reproductive cancer in men. Although it can occur at any age, it is most commonly diagnosed in the mid-30. It rarely occurs in men younger than 15 years of age and men over the age of 55 years. Germ cell malignancies, further divided into seminomas and nonseminomas, account for the vast majority of testicular cancers. Table 14.1 describes the differences between seminoma and nonseminoma testicular cancers.

Table 14.1 Differences Between Seminoma and Nonseminoma Testicular Cancers

Defining Factors	Seminomas	Nonseminomas
Average age of diagnosis	25–45 years of age	Late teens to 30 years of age
Rate of growth	Slow growing	More aggressive
Subcategories	Spermatocytic seminoma (rare)	Embryonic carcinoma Yolk sac carcinoma (responds well to chemotherapy) Choriocarcinoma (rare) Teratoma (usually benign) In some cases, there can be combination of seminoma and nonseminoma cells; however, it does not change the category or recommended treatment options
Tumor markers	Do not secrete AFP; a small percentage can secrete HCG	Increased levels of AFP and HCG (embryonic, yolk sac, and teratomas)

AFP, alfa feta protein; HCG, human chorionic gonadotropin.

TUMOR MARKERS FOR TESTICULAR CANCER

There are two specific blood tests that are used as tumor markers for testicular cancer: alfa feta protein (AFP) and human chorionic gonadotropin (HCG). They are used to measure the disease, as well as respond to chemotherapy treatments. Senominas do not secrete AFP, and only a small percentage secrete HCG. AFP and HCG levels are increased with nonsenominas (embryonic, yolk sac, and teratomas). AFP and HCG levels can be elevated with other malignancies such as lung, gastrointestinal, and hepatic cancers.

RISK FACTORS

A primary risk factor for testicular cancer is cryptorchidism, which is an undescended testicle. Other risk factors include:

- Age
- Height: Taller men are at increased risk
- Personal or family history
- HIV infection
- Race and ethnicity: White men residing in Europe and the United States are at increased risk

STAGING

Testicular cancer is staged with the American Joint Committee on Cancer (AJCC) TNM (tumor, node, metastasis) staging system, which analyzes the tumor size, lymph node involvement, and metastatic site(s). For complete staging information, visit https://www. cancer.org/cancer/testicular-cancer/detection-diagnosis-staging/staging.html.

> ▶ **EXAM TIP**
>
> Review the AJCC TNM Staging System for testicular cancer: https://www.cancer.org/cancer/testicular-cancer/detection-diagnosis-staging/staging.html.

TREATMENT

Surgery is considered the first line of defense for testicular cancer. Treatment modalities include:

- **Surgical procedures**
  - Radical inguinal orchiectomy: Removal of the involved testicle
  - Retroperitoneal lymph node dissection: Performed to determine if there is lymph node involvement and appropriate chemotherapy agents.
- **Radiation therapy**: External beam radiation is used to treat seminomas, which are highly receptive to radiation. Radiation is also frequently used post-orchiectomy.
- **Chemotherapy:** Can be a successful treatment option for early and advanced stages, as well as be used as adjuvant therapy post-surgery to reduce the risk of recurrence. Common regimens include:
  - BEP (**B**leomycin, **E**toposide, **C**isplatin)
    - Bleomycin: Monitor for pulmonary fibrosis and allergic reaction (requires a test dose).
    - Etoposide: Monitor for hypotension and myelosuppression.
    - Cisplatin: Monitor for nephrotoxicity, nausea, and myelosuppression.
  - EP (**E**toposide, **C**isplatin)
    - Etoposide: Monitor for hypotension and myelosuppression.
    - Cisplatin: Monitor for nephrotoxicity, nausea/vomiting, and myelosuppression.
  - VIP (**V**inblastine, **I**fosfamide, **C**isplatin)
    - Vinblastine: Monitor for constipation.
    - Ifosfamide: Monitor for nausea/vomiting, diarrhea, and use of Mesna (Mesnex).
    - Cisplatin: Monitor for nephrotoxicity, nausea, and myelosuppression.

SURVIVAL INFORMATION

According to the ACS (2020), the 5-year survival rates vary based upon the stage of the disease: local disease is 99%, regional disease is 96%, and advanced disease with metastases is 73%.

▶ PENILE CANCER

Penile cancer can involve the shaft and/or the glans of the penis. Penile cancers are considered a rare malignancy in the United States and Europe; however, they are more prevalent in parts of Africa, Asia, and South America (ACS, 2021).

RISK FACTORS

Uncircumcised men are at the highest risk for penile cancer. Other risk factors include HIV or HPV infection and poor genital hygiene.

TREATMENT

Surgery is the primary treatment for penile cancer, especially when it is discovered in the earliest stage, when the penis may not be disrupted. Treatment modalities include:

- **Surgical Procedures**
  - Circumcision (for uncircumcised men)
  - Simple excision: Removal of the tumor and small amount of surrounding tissue
  - Wide excision: Removal of the tumor and a significant amount of surrounding tissue to obtain clean margins. A skin graft may be used to replace the removed and damaged tissue.
  - Mohs surgery: Technique used to prevent removal of unaffected tissue and preserve the penis. It is also used with skin cancers.
  - Glansectomy: Excision of the glans penis.
  - Penectomy (partial or total): Removal of the entire penis or a portion of it. The urethra is left intact, and reconstruction is required to enable urination. While the urinary sensation is preserved, patients will have to sit while urinating and take testosterone supplements for life.
- **Radiation Therapy:** External beam and/or brachytherapy is used to treat advanced penile cancer. It can be used in combination with chemotherapy. With brachytherapy, a radioactive source is placed inside the penis with the use of a foley catheter to drain the urine. Another option is interstitial radiation, in which radioactive needles are inserted into plastic templates that are surgically placed prior to the radiation.
- **Chemotherapy:** Chemotherapy can be useful with advanced penile cancers. Agents are often used in combination; the most common agents include:
  - Capecitabine (Xeloda)
  - Cisplatin (Platinol)
  - Fluorouracil (5 FU)
  - Ifosfamide (Ifex)
  - Mitomycin C (Mutamycin)
  - Paclitaxel (Taxol)

SURVIVAL INFORMATION

According to the ACS (2020), the 5-year survival rates vary based upon the stage of the disease: localized is 80%, regional disease is 50%, and metastatic disease is 9%.

FEMALE REPRODUCTIVE CANCERS

▶ OVARIAN CANCER

Ovarian cancer typically affects women over the age of 60 years and is more common in White American women than other races. Ovarian cancer is too difficult to differentiate from other diseases because the signs and symptoms can be vague and represent non-threatening disorders. As a result, ovarian cancer is often diagnosed in later stages, leading to a poorer prognosis. The most common symptoms include decreased appetite, abdominal distention and pain, unintentional weight loss, constipation, and frequent urination.

Ovarian cancer develops from the three different cell types:

1. Epithelial cell: Accounts for the majority of ovarian cancers
2. Germ cell: Similar to the cell that produces testicular cancer in men
3. Stromal cell: Cell that produces estrogen and progesterone; causes constipation and frequent urination

RISK FACTORS

Risk factors for ovarian cancer include:

- Obesity
- Smoking
- Late or no pregnancies
- Hormone replacement therapy (especially in postmenopausal women)
- Fertility medications
- Family history of breast, ovarian, and/or colorectal cancers
- History of family cancer syndrome (breast, ovarian, and prostate)
- History of genetic disorders: BRAC1 and 2, hereditary nonpolyposis colon cancer (HNPCC), and Peutz–Jeghers syndrome
- Talcum powder usage: Some studies suggest that use of talcum powder can cause ovarian cancer, but there is not a definitive correlation.

SCREENING

There are two diagnostic tests that can be performed to help in identifying ovarian cancer:

- Transvaginal ultrasound (TVUS): An imaging test which allows visualization of the ovaries without the radiation exposure.
- CA-125 laboratory test: Measures CA-125 protein in the blood, which can be elevated with ovarian cancer. Note that CA-125 can be elevated in other disorders such at pelvic inflammatory disease and endometriosis.

STAGING

Ovarian cancer is staged with the American Joint Committee on Cancer (AJCC) TNM (tumor, node, metastasis) staging system and the FIGO (International Federation of Gynecology and Obstetrics) system, which are similar. For complete staging information, visit https://www.cancer.org/cancer/ovarian-cancer/detection-diagnosis-staging/staging.html.

> ▶ **EXAM TIP**
>
> Review AJCC and FIGO staging information for ovarian cancer: https://www.cancer.org/cancer/ovarian-cancer/detection-diagnosis-staging/staging.html.

TREATMENT

Treatment modalities for ovarian cancer include:

- **Surgical Procedures:** Surgery is the primary treatment option to treat ovarian cancer. It is used for staging and debulking.
  - Hysterectomy with bilateral salpingo-oophorectomy (BSO): Removal of both ovaries and fallopian tubes.
  - Omentectomy: Removal of the omentum, which is a common area for metastases.
- **Radiation Therapy:** External beam radiation is the best method of delivering radiation to ovarian cancer patients. It can be adjuvant and used for palliation in advanced disease.
- **Chemotherapy:** Essential for the treatment of early and advanced ovarian cancer. It is delivered intravenously (IV) and intraperitoneally (IP), which is within the peritoneal cavity. Table 14.2 describes chemotherapy agents commonly used to treat ovarian cancer.
- **Hormone Therapy:** Can be used to treat ovarian cancer, similar to breast and prostate cancers. Stromal cell ovarian cancers respond to hormonal treatment because they produce estrogen and progesterone. The goal is to block these hormones to decrease the promotion and growth of malignant stromal ovarian cancer cells. Common hormonal agents include:
  - Goserelin (Zoladex)
  - Leuprolide (Lupron)
  - Tamoxifen
  - Letrozole (Femara)
  - Anastrozole (Arimdex)
  - Exemestane (Aromasin)
- **Targeted Therapy:** Beneficial with advanced ovarian cancer. Anti-angiogenic agents such as bevacizumab (Avastin) are most commonly prescribed. Bevacizumab works by decreasing the ability of the cancer cells to develop new blood vessels and thus prevents the cancer cells from growing, as well as targeting the VEGF protein on the cancer cell.

Table 14.2 Common Chemotherapy Agents to Treat Ovarian Cancer

Agent	Monitoring and Other Considerations
Albumin-bound paclitaxel (Abraxane)	Myelosuppression (can be dose limiting), peripheral neuropathy
Altretamine (Hexalen; oral)	Myelosuppression, nausea/vomiting, peripheral neuropathy
Capecitabine (Xeloda; oral)	Hand/foot syndrome, myelosuppression
Cisplatin (Platinol)	Kidney function, strict inputs/outputs, hydration and fluid replacement, nausea/vomiting, myelosuppression
Cyclophosphamide (Cytoxan; oral/IV)	Myelosuppression, nausea/vomiting, hemorrhagic cystitis
Doxorubicin pegylated liposomal (Doxil)	Hand/foot syndrome, myelosuppression, nausea/vomiting Vesicant properties
Etoposide (VP-16; oral/IV)	Hypotension, myelosuppression
Gemcitabine (Gemzar)	Myelosuppression, nausea/vomiting
Ifosfamide (Ifex)	Myelosuppression, nausea/vomiting, neurotoxicity, kidney and liver functions, use of Mesna
Irinotecan (CPT-11, Camptosar)	Acute-onset diarrhea, myelosuppression, nausea/vomiting
Melphalan (Evomela)	Myelosuppression, nausea/vomiting, diarrhea
Pemetrexed (Alimta)	Administer vitamin B12 and folic acid concurrently to decrease side effects
Topotecan (Hycamtin)	Myelosuppression, nausea/vomiting, diarrhea
Vinorelbine (Navelbine)	ConstipationVesicant precautions; administer over 6 minutes using the upper port

SURVIVAL INFORMATION

According to the ACS (2020), the 5-year survival rates for ovarian cancer are based upon the stage of the disease. Localized disease is 93%, regional is 75%, and metastatic is 31%.

▶ ENDOMETRIAL CANCER

Endometrial cancer affects the inner portion of the uterus, which is the endometrium. It is typically diagnosed after the age of 60 years and is more prevalent in White women; however, the mortality rate is higher in Black women. There are several types of endometrial cancer cells, including:

- Adenocarcinoma
- Serous carcinoma
- Small cell carcinoma
- Transitional carcinoma

RISK FACTORS

Risk factors for endometrial cancer include:

- Age
- Obesity
- Smoking
- Family history of endometrial, ovarian, and breast cancer
- Diabetes (specifically type 2)
- Hormone medications:
  - Tamoxifen (used for treatment for breast cancer)
  - Oral contraception and use of intrauterine devices (IUDs)
- Menstrual cycle history
- Pregnancies
- Ovarian dysfunction (e.g., polycystic ovarian syndrome [PCOS])
- Previous external beam radiation to the pelvic area

STAGING

Endometrial cancer is staged with the American Joint Committee on Cancer (AJCC) TNM (tumor, node, metastasis) staging system and the FIGO (International Federation of Gynecology and Obstetrics) system, which are similar. For complete staging information, visit https://www.cancer.org/cancer/endometrial-cancer/detection-diagnosis-staging/staging.html.

> ▶ **EXAM TIP**
>
> Review AJCC and FIGO staging information for ovarian cancer: https://www.cancer.org/cancer/endometrial-cancer/detection-diagnosis-staging/staging.html.

TREATMENT

Treatment modalities for endometrial cancer include:

- **Surgical Procedures:** Like the other solid tumor malignancies for the female reproductive organs, patients are treated with surgical options first. The common surgical procedures include:
  - Hysterectomy with salpingo-oophorectomy (simple or total): Approaches include laparoscopic, robotic laparoscopic, and open abdominal. Local lymph nodes are removed.
- **Radiation Therapy:** Methods include brachytherapy via the vaginal route and external beam radiation. The stage of the disease and involvement of lymph nodes is used to determine the best delivery method for radiation.
- **Chemotherapy/Biotherapy Agents:** The most commonly used agents include:
  - Doxorubicin (Adriamycin)
  - Bevacizumab (Avastin)
  - Carboplatin (Paraplatin)
  - Cisplatin (Platinol)
  - Docetaxel (Taxotere)

- Everolimus (Afinitor)
- Liposomal doxorubicin (Doxil)
- Lenvatinib (Lenvima)
- Pembrolizumab (Keytruda)
- Temsirolimus (Torisel)

SURVIVAL INFORMATION

According to the ACS (2020), the 5-year survival rates for ovarian cancer are based upon the stage of the disease: localized disease is 95%, regional is 69%, and metastatic is 17%.

▶ VULVAR CANCER

Vulvar cancer is the cancer of the tissue surrounding the vagina. It is a less common female reproductive cancer, with only 1 in 333 women developing vulvar cancer during their lifetime (ACS, 2020). Vulvar cancer cells include:

1. Adenocarcinoma
2. Basal cell carcinoma
3. Melanoma
4. Sarcoma
5. Squamous cell carcinoma

RISK FACTORS

Risk factors for vulvar cancer include:

- Age: Women over the age of 70 years at higher risk
- HIV and HPV infection
- Smoking
- History of other reproductive cancers
- History of pre-cancerous lesions
- Lichen sclerosus (skin disorder)
- Vulvar intraepithelial neoplasia (VIN)
- Melanoma

STAGING

Vulvar cancer is staged with the American Joint Committee on Cancer (AJCC) TNM (tumor, node, metastasis) staging system and the FIGO (International Federation of Gynecology and Obstetrics) system, which are similar. For complete staging information, visit https://www.cancer.org/cancer/vulvar-cancer/detection-diagnosis-staging/staging.html.

▶ **EXAM TIP**

Review AJCC and FIGO staging information for vulvar cancer: https://www.cancer.org/cancer/vulvar-cancer/detection-diagnosis-staging/staging.html.

TREATMENT

Treatment modalities for vulvar cancer include the following:

- **Surgical Procedures:** Surgery is the first line of defense. The extent and depth of cancer will determine the surgical approach. Potential options include:
  - Laser surgery: Used to treat noninvasive cancer
  - Simple vulvectomy: An excisional surgery to remove the tumor and provide clear margins.
  - Vulvectomy: An aggressive surgical procedure to remove vulva and surrounding tissue, including the clitoris. Vulvar reconstruction can be performed. Not a commonly used procedure.
- **Radiation Therapy**: 3D-conformal radiation provides targeted radiation that decreases exposure to the surrounding tissue. Intense modulated radiation can be used as well.
- **Chemotherapy:** Used with vulvar cancer in advanced stages. The most commonly used agents:
  - Cisplatin (Platinol)
  - Carboplatin (Paraplatin)
  - Vinorelbine (Navelbine)
  - Paclitaxel (Taxol)

SURVIVAL INFORMATION

According to the ACS (2020), the 5-year survival rates for vulvar cancer are based upon the stage of the disease. Localized disease is 86%, regional is 54%, and metastatic is 19%.

The bibliography and references for this chapter are available on ExamPrepConnect; see inside front cover for access instructions.

1. Which of the following measures will the nurse include in the care plan for a patient who is 48 hours post ifosfamide (Ifex) therapy for endometrial cancer?

   A. Administer pain medication
   B. Restrict IV fluids
   C. Administer antinausea medications
   D. Monitor patient for constipation

2. Which of the following diagnostic results should a nurse recognize as a concern for a patient who was prescribed tamoxifen for breast cancer?

   A. Enlarged heart on chest x-ray
   B. Abnormal pulmonary function tests (PFTs)
   C. Fatty liver noted on CT scan
   D. Increased lining of the uterus with transvaginal ultrasound

3. A risk factor for renal cell carcinoma is:

   A. HPV virus
   B. HIV infection
   C. Exposure to trichloroethylene (TCE)
   D. Exposure to previous radiation therapy

4. External beam radiation therapy is used as adjuvant therapy to treat:

   A. Renal cell carcinoma
   B. Seminoma testicular cancer
   C. Nonseminoma testicular cancer
   D. Bladder cancer

5. The nurse is providing teaching to an ovarian cancer patient who is being treated with liposomal doxorubicin (Doxil). The nurse will advise the patient about the risk for:

   A. Lymphedema
   B. Constipation
   C. Pain
   D. Hand and foot syndrome

(See answers next page.)

1. C) Administer antinausea medications

Ifosfamide (Ifex) can cause acute and delayed nausea, so the nurse should administer antinausea medications. Ifosfamide (Ifex) causes diarrhea, not constipation. Fluids should be encouraged to protect the kidneys. Pain medication is not indicated for this chemotherapy.

2. D) Increased lining of the uterus with transvaginal ultrasound

Use of tamoxifen is a risk factor for endometrial cancer; therefore, the nurse would be concerned about increased lining of the uterus with transvaginal ultrasound. Enlarged heart, abnormal PFTs, and fatty liver are not related to tamoxifen therapy.

3. C) Exposure to trichloroethylene (TCE)

Trichloroethylene is a chemical that has been correlated with renal carcinoma. HPV virus, HIV infection, and exposure to previous radiation therapy are more specific risk factors for male and female reproductive cancers.

4. B) Seminoma testicular cancer

Seminomas are radiosensitive, and external beam radiation therapy is used following an orchiectomy to treat testicular cancer. Nonseminomas do not respond as well to radiation. Radiation is not used commonly with bladder and renal cancers in the adjuvant setting.

5. D) Hand and foot syndrome

Liposomal doxorubicin (Doxil) is a chemotherapy agent used to treat ovarian cancer. Hand and foot syndrome can be a side effect of therapy with liposomal doxorubicin (Doxil). Constipation, pain, and lymphedema are not side effects of this drug.

Prostate Cancer

INTRODUCTION

The prostate is a small gland (the size of a walnut) that is responsible for the production of seminal fluid. The gland lies in front of the rectum, and behind the prostate are the seminal vesicles (Figure 15.1). The aging process has a direct effect on the prostate; as men age, the prostate becomes enlarged and can become malignant. Androgens, which are male hormones, promote the growth of healthy prostate cells and are also responsible for the abnormal growth of prostate cancer cells. Prostate cancer is more prevalent in older men and African Americans; in rare cases, it can occur before the age of 40 years. Prostate cancer is the most common malignancy in the male population, and the second-leading cause of death for men, following lung cancer (ACS, 2020).

Although there are multiple types of prostate cancer, the most common is adenocarcinoma. The other types of prostate cancers are known as rare malignancies, including sarcoma, small cell carcinoma, neuroendocrine lesions, and transitional cell carcinomas.

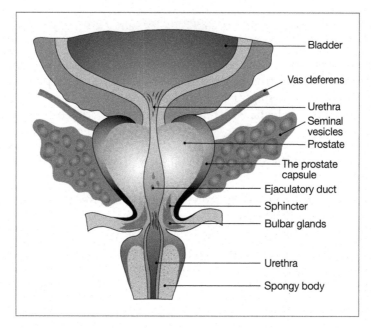

Figure 15.1 Anatomy of the prostate.
Source: From Gawlik, K.S., Melnyk, B.M., & Teal, A.M. (2021). *Evidence-based physical examination: Best practices for health and well-being assessment.* Springer Publishing Company.

The bibliography and references for this chapter are available on ExamPrepConnect; see inside front cover for access instructions.

RISK FACTORS

Risk factors for prostate cancer include:

- Age: More prevalent in individuals 65 years and older.
- Family history: First-degree relative; risk increases with younger age at diagnosis or if more than one first-degree relative develops cancer.
- Genetic factors: Positive for the inherited genes *BRAC1* and *BRAC2* gene (*BRAC2* more specifically related to prostate cancer); Lynch syndrome; or *HEK2, ATM, PALB2, RAD51D, MSH2, MSH6,* or *MLH1* gene mutations.
- Ethnicity: African American and Caribbean men with African ancestry are at higher risk.
- Geography: Although not clearly understood, it is observed that men from the Caribbean, North America, Northwestern Europe, and Australia are at higher risk than other regions.
- Diet: High-fat, including large amount of red meats; diets high in calcium
- Obesity
- Smoking
- Exposure to chemicals/toxins (e.g., Agent Orange): Farmers, firefighters, and welders at increased risk
- Inflammatory process: Prostatitis, sexually transmitted diseases (e.g., gonorrhea, chlamydia)
- Vasectomy

SCREENING

Prostate-specific antigen (PSA) levels, digital rectal examinations (DREs), and physical exams are performed to identify prostate cancer at the earliest possible stage. When a malignancy is diagnosed in stage I or II disease, the chances for cure are significantly higher. There are several new tests, which include different forms of PSA and other tumor-maker monitoring:

- Prostate Health Index (PHI): A blood test that incorporates the total PSA, free PSA, and proPSA.
- 4Kscore® test: A blood test that incorporates the total PSA, free PSA, and intact PSA, plus the human kallikrein 2 (hK2) factor.
- Progensa: A urine test that measures the PSA 3 levels (PCA3). It is administered after a DRE because the exam pushes the prostate cells into the urine.
- *TMPRSS:ERG:* A urine test that measures the *TMPRSS:ERG* gene post-DRE. The literature supports that this gene is not found in men that do have prostate cancer.
- ExoDX Prostate (IntelliScore): Also referred to as EPI, this urine test examines three biomarkers.

▶ PRECANCERS OF THE PROSTATE

There are several types of precancer cell abnormalities that have the potential to lead to prostate cancer. If a patient is found to have any of these abnormal changes of the prostate cell after a biopsy, a repeat biopsy is often recommended in a few months.

- Prostatic Intraepithelial Neoplasm (PIN): Low- or high-grade abnormalities. High-grade abnormalities tend to lead to prostate cancer.
- Proliferative inflammatory atrophy (PIA): Cellular changes that are not considered malignant; however, they should be monitored to ensure prostate cancer does not develop.
- Atypical Small Acinar Proliferation (ASAP): Glandular proliferation cells that are considered suspicious for cancer.

SIGNS AND SYMPTOMS

In its early stages, prostate cancer typically does not produce many symptoms; however, advanced prostate cancer produces multiple and often painful symptoms (Box 15.1).

Box 15.1 Signs and Symptoms of Prostate Cancer

Early Signs and Symptoms

- Asymptomatic
- Nocturnal urination
- Difficulty urinating or change in the stream of urination
- Blood in urine or semen
- Difficulty obtaining and maintaining an erection

Advanced Signs and Symptoms

- Loss of bladder or bowel function
- Pain in back, ribs, and/or hips
- Numbness and/or weakness of lower extremities

DIAGNOSIS

▶ PROSTATE-SPECIFIC ANTIGEN TEST

One of the best methods for monitoring the prostate is the use of PSA blood test. PSA is a protein that is released from prostate cells and found mostly in semen and in small amounts in the blood. PSA can be used as a diagnostic tool, as well as a tool to measure the extent of disease and response to cancer treatment. Healthcare providers use these benchmarks:

- PSA 2.5 to 3: Investigate for prostate cancer
- PSA 4 to10: Borderline positive for prostate cancer
- PSA >10: 50% chance of being positive for prostate cancer

▶ IMAGING

Imaging modalities for prostate cancer include:

- TRUS and MRI: Determines the size of the prostate and identifies lesions.
- Multiparametric MRI: Examines the anatomy of the prostate; in some cases, an endorectal coil will be placed in the rectum during the exam.
- PET, CT, bones scans: Determines if other organs are involved.

▶ BIOPSY

As with any solid tumor malignancy, a biopsy is recommended to evaluate the cells. The most common prostate biopsy is a core-needle biopsy, which can be obtained via transrectal ultrasound (TRUS) or MRI/ultrasound fusion-guided prostate biopsy. This approach requires the patient to obtain an MRI before the biopsy to guide and review the abnormal areas of the prostate.

▶ GENETIC TESTING

Several genetic tests are available to identify the risk of developing aggressive and/or metastatic disease. The tests are performed after a biopsy and/or surgery of the prostate gland and are used to determine appropriate treatment options.

- *BRAC1* and *BRAC2*: Tests for breast cancer mutated genes, which can lead to breast and prostate cancer.
- Oncotype DX Prostate: Measures the activity of specific prostate cancer genes to determine metastatic risk.
- Prolaris: Measures the activity of specific prostate cancer genes to determine metastatic risk.
- ProMark: Measures the activity of proteins in the prostate cancer cells to determine metastatic risk.
- Decipher: Performed on the surgically removed prostate to determine metastatic risk.

HISTOLOGICAL GRADING

The grading system for prostate cancer is the Gleason score, which is determined by a pathologist. The Gleason scores represent how much or how little the prostate cancer cells resemble healthy normal prostate cells. The more the cancer cells resemble the original cell, the better the prognostic indicator. Gleason scores help to determine the appropriate treatment options.

A Gleason score of <5 is typically not utilized as the cells resemble normal prostate cells and are slow-growing malignancies. Scores between 6 and 10 are moderate to aggressive prostate cancer (Table 15.1).

Table 15.1 Gleason Score for Prostate Cancer

Gleason Score	Description
5	Cannot be assessed
6	Well-differentiated; resembles a healthy prostate cell
7	Moderately differentiated; has some characteristics of a healthy prostate cell
8–10	Poorly differentiated; does not resemble a healthy prostate cell

● STAGING

Prostate cancer staging is based upon the American Joint Committee on Cancer (AJCC) TMN staging system, which analyzes the tumor size, lymph node involvement, and metastatic site/sites.

I. **Stage I:** Nonpalpable tumor; only half of one side of the prostate is involved; slow growing

II. **Stage II:** Tumor isolated to the prostate
   a. Stage IIA: Nonpalpable tumor; isolated to half of one side of the prostate; usually smaller (can be larger if well-differentiated histology); PSA levels 6 to 10
   b. Stage IIB: Palpable tumor; isolated to one side of the prostate; moderately to poorly differentiated; PSA levels 6 to 10
   c. Stage IIC: Palpable tumor; isolated to the inside of the prostate; moderately to poorly differentiated; PSA levels 6 to 10

III. **Stage III:** High-grade tumors that invade the outer portion of the prostate and surrounding tissue; PSA levels are 10 to 20
   a. Stage IIIA: All components above plus spread to the seminal vesicle
   b. Stage IIIB: All components above plus spread to the bladder or rectum
   c. Stage IIIC: All components above plus poorly differentiated

IV. **Stage IV**: Tumors spread outside of the prostate
   a. Stage IVA: Involvement of the lymph nodes
   b. Stage IVB: Involvement of other organs (e.g., bone)

▶ EXAM TIP

Review the AJCC TNM Staging System for prostate cancer: https://www.cancer.org/cancer/prostate-cancer/detection-diagnosis-staging/staging.html.

● TREATMENT

▶ ACTIVE SURVEILLANCE

Active surveillance is a method to closely monitor prostate cancer. After the identification of abnormal prostate cells or slow-growing prostate cancer, the patient will have PSA levels drawn every 3 to 6 months, a follow-up biopsy within the first 6 to 12 months, an annual DRE, and a prostate biopsy every 2 to 5 years. The best candidates for active surveillance are asymptomatic patients at an advanced age (with no impact on the quality of life), low-grade lesions that are isolated to the prostate, and small and nonaggressive tumors. Active surveillance needs to be carefully discussed with provider and patient, particularly the possible quality-of-life issues related to complications of treatment versus the chance of missing the opportunity of cure.

Watchful waiting/observation may be an option for patients who have a significantly slow-growing lesion and no symptoms. The patient and family members are educated to understand any changes of symptoms related to the prostate.

▶ SURGICAL PROCEDURES

Surgery is the treatment of choice for prostate cancer to remove cancer and obtain a cure. Surgical options include:

- **Radical Prostatectomy**: Removal of the prostate gland, surrounding tissue, and seminal vesicles via an incision in the lower abdomen (pubic or perineal approach). The large incision requires increased healing time and has increased side effects and risk for complications such as infection.
- **Open/Laparoscopic Prostatectomy:** Removal of the prostate gland via several small incisions instead of one large incision. This is a more common procedure with fewer side effects and complications. In robotic-assisted laparoscopic prostatectomies, a surgeon physician uses a control panel to remove the prostate via small incisions.
- **Transurethral Resection of the Prostate (TURP):** Performed to identify if the prostate is enlarged. A resectoscope is inserted through the penis to visualize the prostate gland; the tissue is then shaved or removed.

▶ RADIATION THERAPY

Radiation can be an effective treatment option for prostate cancer; options include:

- External beam radiation therapy (EBRT)
- Brachytherapy
- Three-dimensional conformal radiation (3D-CRT)
- Intensity-modulated radiation therapy (IMRT)
- Stereotactic body radiation therapy
  - Gamma Knife
  - X-Knife
  - CyberKnife
  - Clinac
- Proton beam radiation
- Image guided radiation therapy (IGRT)
- Volumetric modulated arc therapy (VMAT): Provides increased accuracy of the radiation and decreases side effects

Due to the location of the prostate within the body, both surgery and radiation pose significant risks and side effects (Table 15.2). A common side effect is an erectile dysfunction, which can be treated with the following medications and procedures:

- **Oral medications:** Phosphodiesterase-5 inhibitors help to sustain erections, provided that the nerves have not been removed or damaged during surgery or radiation. Options include sildenafil (Viagra), vardenafil (Levitra), tadalafil (Cialis), and avanafil (Stendra). Common side effects include facial flushing, dizziness, and prolonged erections.
- **Suppositories:** Alprostadil is a prostaglandin E1 that can be inserted into the penis 5 to 10 minutes prior to sexual intercourse. Common side effects include dizziness and prolonged erection.
- **Vacuum devices:** A mechanical pump connected to the base of the penis and placed over the penis is used to create an erection prior to sexual activity. The air is deflated out of the pump to increase blood flow to the penis, thus producing an erection. The pump is removed after sex.

■ **Penile implants:** Surgical implants are an inflatable tube or semi-rigid tube/rod made of silicone that is surgically implanted within the penis. These devices do not promote sexual desire or sensation. Not recommended for patients with uncontrolled diabetes because infections are a primary risk factor, as well as adhesions and/or pump failure.

Table 15.2 Potential Side Effects From Surgery and Radiation Therapy for Prostate Cancer

Side Effect	Surgery	Radiation
Urinary incontinence (stress, overflow, urge)	X	X (radiation cystitis)
Erectile dysfunction	X	X
Bowel issues (e.g., fistula)		X
Changes in organs	X	
Loss of fertility	X	
Lymphedema	X	X
Fatigue		X
Decrease in penis length	X	
Inguinal hernia	X	

CHEMOTHERAPY

Chemotherapy tends not to be as effective as other treatment modalities for prostate cancer. It is usually administered as a single agent for advanced disease, and the primary goal is for palliation. Table 15.3 describes the most common chemotherapy agents utilized to treat metastatic prostate cancer.

Table 15.3 Common Chemotherapy Agents Used to Treat Advanced Prostate Cancer

Agent	Monitoring Considerations
Cabazitaxel (Jevtana)	Myelosuppression, bleeding, peripheral neuropathy
Docetaxel (Taxotere)	Infusion reactions, myelosuppression
Estramustine (Emcyt)	Liver functions; decreased libido
Mitoxantrone (Novantrone)	Peripheral neuropathy Vesicant precautions

▶ IMMUNOTHERAPY

Immunotherapy has shown to be highly effective with prostate cancer, namely a prostate vaccine and use immune checkpoint inhibitors. Sipuleucel-T (Provenge) is a cancer vaccine that is used in advanced prostate cancer, which stimulates the immune system to destroy the prostate cancer cells. It uses the patient's own white blood cells to create the vaccine by process of apheresis. The patient's cells are harvested and sent to the pharmaceutical company's laboratory to be processed with prostatic acid phosphatase (PAP). The processed cells are administered to the patient every 2 weeks for a total of 3 doses. The most common side effects include fever, chills, nausea, back, and joint pain.

Immune checkpoint inhibitors (nivolumab [Opdivo] and Pembrolizumab [Keytruda]) target the proteins on T-cells that block PD-1, which accelerates the immune system to target and destroy cancer cells.

▶ HORMONAL THERAPY

Like breast cancer, prostate cancer responds to hormonal treatment. Testosterone, which is an androgen, is responsible for the normal and abnormal growth of prostate cancer cells. Therefore, the goal is to reduce the production of testosterone from the testicles and decrease the opportunity for prostate cancer cells to grow. Hormonal therapies include:

- **Testosterone suppression (surgical/medical castration):** Shuts down the production of testosterone from the testis. Achieved with orchiectomy, removal of the testicles, or luteinizing hormone-releasing hormone (LHRH) analogs including goserelin (Zoladex), leuprolide (Lupron, Eligard), triptorelin (Trelstar), histrelin (Vantas). All are administered intramuscularly and can cause a flare reaction, which can cause pain and sexual dysfunction. LHRH antagonists (degarelix [Firmagon]) also decrease testosterone levels, but it does not cause the tumor flare reaction. It can cause sexual dysfunction.
- **Medications to decrease androgen levels:** Abiraterone (Zytiga; oral) blocks the enzyme CYP17, which is essential for stopping the production of androgens. It is used for men with elevated Gleason scores and / or metastatic disease or both. Ketoconazole (Nizoral) blocks the production of androgens via the adrenal gland and decreases testosterone levels. Both require daily prednisone to prevent disruption in the normal corticosteroid production. Side effects include nausea/vomiting, gynecomastia, and elevated liver enzymes.
- **Anti-androgens:** Anti-androgens (oral agents) decrease testosterone, preventing cancer cells from growing. These agents include flutamide (Eulexin), bicalutamide (Casodex), and nilutamide (Nilandron), as well as new agents such as enzalutamide (Xtandi), apalutamide (Erleada), and darolutamide (Neega), which is used for metastatic disease. They are often combined with LHRH to have the maximum benefit of testosterone decline, which is known as combined androgen blockade. The newer anti-androgens can be used in advanced and local diseases and can be given after previous hormone therapy has failed, which is known as non-metastatic castrate-resistant prostate cancer (CRPC). Side effects include nausea/vomiting, sexual dysfunction, and fatigue. Newer agents can cause nervous system complications such as dizziness and increased fall risk.
- **Estrogens:** Decrease testosterone; administered in advanced prostate cancer and when other hormones have failed. They are used less frequently due to the increased side-effect profile, including blood clots and gynecomastia.

⬤ SURVIVAL INFORMATION

According to the ACS (2020), the 5-year relative survival rate is approximately 90%. The rate of cure is also approximately 90%, with a diagnosis of localized prostate cancer.

The bibliography and references for this chapter are available on ExamPrepConnect; see inside front cover for access instructions.

1. Which genetic screening test is useful in determining the risk of recurrence in prostate cancer?

   A. BRAC1
   B. BRAC2
   C. Prolaris
   D. CDK4 inhibitor

2. Which of the following treatment options can cause decreased libido?

   A. External beam radiation
   B. Watchful waiting
   C. Anti-androgen therapy
   D. Phosphodiesterase-5 inhibitors

3. Which of the following chemotherapy agents is used to treat advanced prostate cancer?

   A. Cyclophosphamide (Cytoxan)
   B. Mitoxantrone (Novantrone)
   C. Doxorubicin (Adriamycin)
   D. 5-Fluorouracil (5FU)

4. The nurse is reviewing treatment options with a 65-year-old male patient newly diagnosed with prostate cancer. The patient has a Gleason score of 4. The nurse anticipates reviewing which of the following treatment options:

   A. Chemotherapy alone
   B. Surgery and radiation
   C. Surgery and hormone therapy
   D. Watchful waiting

5. The nurse is caring for a 72-year-old male patient post brachytherapy. Which of the following findings indicate that the patient has a serious complication from treatment?

   A. Decreased blood counts
   B. Pain and bleeding from the rectum
   C. Erectile dysfunction
   D. Stress incontinence

1. C) Prolaris

Prolaris is a genetic test that measures the activity of specific prostate cancer genes to determine metastatic risk. This test is scored from 0 to 10; the higher the score, the greater the chance of spreading aggressive disease. BRAC1 and BRAC2 are genetic tests to identify the risk of prostate cancer, not recurrence. CDK4 inhibitor is a genetic test used in breast cancer patients.

2. C) Anti-androgen therapy

Anti-androgen therapy is a hormonal therapy that can cause decreased libido. External beam radiation can cause erectile dysfunction and urinary incontinence. Phosphodiesterase-5 inhibitors are used to treat erectile dysfunction; they do not cause decreased libido. Watchful waiting is the choice of no treatment.

3. B) Mitoxantrone (Novantrone)

Mitoxantrone (Novantrone) is a single agent chemotherapy that is used to treat advanced prostate cancer. Cyclophosphamide (Cytoxan), doxorubicin (Adriamycin), and 5-Fluorouracil (5FU) are used in combination to treatment multiple cancers, including breast, lung, and colon cancers.

4. C) Surgery and hormone therapy

A Gleason score of 4 indicates that the patient has stage I and II prostate cancer. Surgery and hormone therapy are the most common treatment options for stage 1 and 2 prostate cancer. Chemotherapy alone is used in advanced cancer only. Watchful waiting is used in the elderly with limited disease.

5. B) Pain and bleeding from the rectum

Brachytherapy is a form of radiation therapy used to treat prostate cancer. Radiation therapy can cause serious bowel issues such as rectal fistula, leading to pain and bleeding from the rectum. Brachytherapy does not affect blood counts. Erectile dysfunction and stress incontinence are expected side effects of treatment, not serious complications.

Head and Neck and Thyroid Cancers

Head and neck cancer (HNC) are identified as tumors that involve the mouth, throat, nose, sinuses, and larynx. HNC is responsible for approximately 4% of cancers within the United Stated (Cancer Net, 2021). The average age of diagnosis is 62 years; however, it may be seen in patients younger than 55 years. Men are more affected than women, and African American males tend to be at the highest risk for HNC and mortality due to socioeconomic status, lifestyle, and limited access to care (Moore et al., 2012). HNC is divided among the cavities of the head and neck region (Figure 16.1).

- Oral cavity
- Pharynx: Nasopharynx, oropharynx, hypopharynx
- Larynx
- Paranasal sinuses and nasal cavity
- Salvia gland cancers

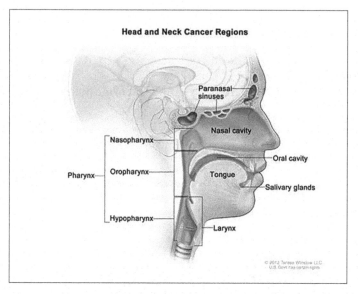

Figure 16.1 Head and neck cancer regions.
Source: Courtesy of Therese Winslow and the National Institutes for Health.

Squamous cell carcinoma is the most common type of cancer cell for HNC. Squamous cell cancer constitutes approximately 90% of all the forms of head and neck malignancies (Penn Medicine, 2021). Thyroid cancers are not identified as HNC; however, they will be addressed in this chapter.

The bibliography and references for this chapter are available on ExamPrepConnect; see inside front cover for access instructions.

RISK FACTORS

HNC risk factors include:

- Age
- Gender: More common in males than females
- Smoking and drinking alcohol: The combination causes a synergistic effect.
- Viruses: HPV and EBV
- Lichen Planus
- Sunlight exposure (specific to cancers of the lip)
- Suboptimal nutritional status
- Immunosuppressed patients: Graft versus host disease
- Genetic disorders: Fanconi Anemia and dyskeratosis congenita
- Occupational exposures:
  - Asbestos, wood, dust, nickel, and formaldehyde
  - Construction workers, textile workers, and laboratory workers
- Previous radiation exposure to the head and neck

SIGNS AND SYMPTOMS

The most common signs and symptoms of HNC include:

- Nonhealing lesions on the lips, nares, and tongue
- Continuous sore throat
- Voice changes, most notably hoarseness
- Pain
- Edema of face and neck
- Functional changes such as difficulty chewing and swallowing

DIAGNOSIS

Common diagnostic tests include:

- Biopsy of the affected area: Lips, tongue, nares, salivary glands, and larynx
- CT scan
- PET scans
- MRI

STAGING

As with other solid tumors, HNC uses the AJCC TNM (tumor, node, metastasis) Staging System. The TNM system is a cancer classification to identify whether the tumor has invaded other areas, such as the lymph nodes (NCBI, 2012). For complete staging information for the various HNC cancer regions, visit https://www.cancer.org/.

> ▶ **EXAM TIP**
>
> Review the AJCC TNM Staging System for HNC cancer regions: https://www.cancer.org/.

TREATMENT

▶ SURGICAL PROCEDURES

As with all solid malignancies, surgery is the first line of defense for HNC. The surgical procedure depends on the region that is involved (Table 16.1).

Table 16.1 Surgical Procedures for Head and Neck Cancers

Type of Cancer	Surgical Procedure
Oral cavity cancer/lips	Mohs surgery
Tongue	Glossectomy (partial or complete)
Nasopharyngeal	Maxillectomy
Ethmoid sinuses, frontal sinuses, and/or the sphenoid	Craniofacial resection
Larynx	Laryngectomy
Jaw/salivary glands	Mandibulectomy
Thyroid	Thyroidectomy

Note: Some of these surgeries require reconstructive surgery to enhance function and appearance.

▶ CHEMORADIATION

Radiation and chemotherapy combined, or chemoradiation, is used to treat HNC. Chemoradiation is the process of administering chemotherapy prior to the radiation therapy to sensitize the cancer cells, enhance the effectiveness of the radiation, and promote increased cell death. Radiation can be administered before or after surgery. The most common forms of radiation for HNC include:

- **Three-dimensional conformal radiation therapy (3D-CRT):** Allows the radiation treatment to be aimed more precisely and uses the same intensity throughout each beam, which enables safe use of higher doses and reduced damage to healthy tissue. It also helps to limit dry mouth and salivary gland damage.
- **Intensity-modulated radiation therapy (IMRT):** Targets the tumor, and radiation is varied within each field. Avoids more healthy tissue than the conventional 3D-CRT.

Due to the high toxicity profile of both chemotherapy and radiation therapy, there are several supportive procedures and therapies that can be recommended to combat the expected untoward side effects:

- **Feeding tube:** The use of a feeding tube is common practice when a patient with HNC cannot maintain nutritional intake. It is usually temporary and used only until the treatment regimen is complete.
  - Gastrostomy (G) tube
  - Percutaneous endoscopic gastrostomy (PEG) tube
  - Nasogastric feeding (NG) tube
- **Tracheostomy:** Post laryngectomy, permanent or temporary

▶ EXAM TIP

Radiation and chemotherapy are usually administered concomitantly to enhance cell-kill effect with head and neck malignancies (not thyroid cancers).

▶ CHEMOTHERAPY AND BIOTHERAPY

Common chemotherapy and biotherapy agents are described in Table 16.2.

Table 16.2 Common Chemotherapy and Biotherapy Agents Used to Treat Head and Neck Cancers

Agent	Treatment Modality	Monitoring Considerations
Albumin-bound paclitaxel (Abraxane)	Chemotherapy	Myelosuppression (can be dose-limiting), nausea/vomiting
Doxorubicin (Adriamycin)	Chemotherapy	Myelosuppression, mouth sores, nausea/vomiting Use of vesicant precautions during administration Potential to be cardiotoxic; requires a MUGA scan prior to administration of the first dose Lifetime max of drug: 550 mg/m^2; 450 mg/m^2 with commitment radiation Red urine 24–48 hr post infusion
Bleomycin (Blenoxane)	Chemotherapy (used infrequently)	Allergic reaction Test dose; PFT prior to administration; administer pre-medications if ordered Lifetime dose max: 400 units
Cyclophosphamide (Cytoxan; oral/IV)*	Chemotherapy	Myelosuppression, nausea/vomiting, hemorrhagic cystitis
Carboplatin (Paraplatin)	Chemotherapy	Kidney function, thrombocytopenia, nausea/vomiting Drug dosing based upon area under the curve (AUC)
Cetuximab (Erbitux)	Biotherapy	Acneiform rash, fatigue
Docetaxel (Taxotere)	Chemotherapy	Infusion reaction, neuropathy (peripheral)
5-Fluorouracil (5FU)	Chemotherapy	Diarrhea, skin and nail changes, myelosuppression
Hydroxyurea (Hydrea; oral)	Chemotherapy	Myelosuppression, cutaneous vasculitis
Methotrexate	Chemotherapy	Methotrexate levels, kidney functions, nausea/vomiting, use of Leucovorin
Nivolumab (Opdivo)	Biotherapy	Signs and symptoms of pneumonitis, colitis, hepatitis, nephritis; thyroid dysfunction
Paclitaxel (Taxol)	Chemotherapy	Anaphylaxis/infusion reaction, peripheral neuropathy (can be dose-limiting) Use of pre-medications; use of non-PVC tubing and 0.22-micron filter for administration
Pembrolizumab (Keytruda)	Biotherapy	Thyroid function, diarrhea, rash, neuropathy
Platinol (Cisplatin)	Chemotherapy	Kidney function, strict input and outputs, hydration and fluid replacement, nausea/vomiting, myelosuppression

*Used in combination with doxorubicin and plus or minus paclitaxel.
MUGA, multigated acquisition; PFT, pulmonary function tests.

● SURVIVAL INFORMATION

The 5-year survival rates are based upon the location and stage of the disease (ACS, 2020):

- Lips: Local 94%; regional 66%; metastatic 32%
- Tongue: Local 82%; regional 68%; metastatic 40%
- Oral cavity: Local 76%; regional 38%; metastatic 20%
- Average for other HNC regions: 60%

◐ THYROID CANCERS

Thyroid cancers are not identified as head and neck malignancies. The three most common types of thyroid cancers are papillary, medullary, and anaplastic.

▶ RISK FACTORS

- Gender: More common in women than men
- Age: Typically occurs between the ages of 25 and 55 years
- Race: Asian population has an increased risk
- Genetics: *RET* oncogene can be a risk factor
- Radiation exposure:
  - Previous radiation to the head and neck (e.g., treatment for Hodgkin's lymphoma)
  - Exposure from atomic weapons and nuclear power plant accidents (e.g., Chernobyl [1986], exposure to radioactive iodine (I-131)
- Low-iodine diets
- History of breast cancer

▶ SIGNS AND SYMPTOMS

The most common signs and symptoms of thyroid cancers include the following:

- Swelling of the neck and glands
- Lump in the anterior portion of the neck
- Hoarseness
- Difficulty swallowing
- Difficulty breathing
- Continuous cough
- Pain in the neck area

▶ TREATMENT

Treatment options include surgery, radiation, and chemotherapy.

SURGICAL PROCEDURES

Lobectomy or thyroidectomy (partial or total) are used for the treatment of thyroid cancers.

RADIATION

The use of I-131 is used to prevent micro-metastasis after surgical removal of either the thyroid gland or a portion of the thyroid gland. It is often recommended for patients with local invasion and positive lymph nodes. I-131 is a radioisotope, which is ingested. In order for the radioisotope to be most effective, there need to be elevated levels of thyroid-stimulating hormone to attach to I-131. Therefore, patient needs to stop taking levothyroxine (Synthroid) or take TSH (thyrotropin). The patient will experience signs and symptoms of hypothyroidism, which are temporary. In addition, the patient will need to have a low-iodine diet 1 to 2 weeks prior to the I-131. See Box 16.1 for pertinent patient education. External beam radiation can also be used in the advanced stages of the disease.

Box 16.1 Patient Education for the Use of I-131

- Drink water hourly during the first 8 hours
- Urination and use of bathroom
  - Sit while urinating (men and women)
  - Flush toilet twice
  - Use a private bathroom
- Maintain social distancing of at least 3 feet from family and friends
- Avoid public areas
- Do not share the following:
  - Eating utensils
  - Towels and washcloths
  - Bed linens
  - Clothing
- Sleep alone for 7 days
- Avoid contact with pregnant women and small children for 7 days

CHEMOTHERAPY

The most common chemotherapy agents used to treat thyroid cancers in advanced stages include:

- Carboplatin
- Cyclophosphamide
- Dacarbazine
- Doxorubicin
- Docetaxel
- Fluorouracil
- Paclitaxel
- Streptozocin
- Vincristine

BIOTHERAPY

Biotherapy agents can be added to chemotherapy regimens in advanced stages of the disease and when the patient is not responding to chemotherapy alone. The following agents can be used:

- Lenvatinib (Lenvima)
- Sorafenib (Nexavar)
- Selpercatinib (Retevmo)
- Larotrectinib (Vitrakvi)
- Entrectinib (Rozlytrek)
- Vandetanib (Caprelsa)
- Cabozantinib (Cometriq)
- Dabrafenib (Tafinlar)
- Trametinib (Mekinist)

▶ SURVIVAL INFORMATION

According to the ACS (2020), the 5-year survival rate for thyroid cancer is approximately 98%.

The bibliography and references for this chapter are available on ExamPrepConnect; see inside front cover for access instructions.

1. Which treatment will the nurse anticipate for a patient with stage I medullary thyroid cancer status post thyroidectomy?

   A. External beam radiation
   B. Chemoradiation
   C. I-131
   D. Chemotherapy with carboplatin

2. Which of the following statements regarding HNC is MOST accurate?

   A. HNC affects more women than men
   B. HNC affects more men than women
   C. HNC has an increased mortality rate
   D. HNC has a decreased mortality rate

3. Which oral chemotherapy agent can be used to treat HNC?

   A. Capecitabine (Xeloda)
   B. Bleomycin (Blenoxane)
   C. Docetaxel (Taxotere)
   D. Hydroxyurea (Hydrea)

4. The oncology nurse is assessing a 35-year-old patient with metastatic HNC who is receiving concurrent chemoradiation. Which of the following findings indicates that the patient is experiencing severe side effects?

   A. Abdominal pain, mucositis, and elevated temperature
   B. Increased white blood cell count, mucositis, and weight loss
   C. Decreased white blood cell count, mucositis, and weight loss
   D. Elevated temperature, increased white blood cell count, and abdominal pain

5. A patient is receiving nivolumab (Opdivo) for advanced HNC. The nurse recognizes that the patient should be monitored for which of the following complications?

   A. Myelosuppression
   B. Colitis
   C. Nausea/vomiting
   D. Fatigue

1. C) I-131
I-131 is the most common treatment following a thyroidectomy. Chemotherapy, radiation, and carboplatin are used in advanced stages.

2. B) HNC affects more men than women
HNC typically affects more men than women. The mortality rate is dependent upon the stage of disease at diagnosis.

3. D) Hydroxyurea (Hydrea)
Hydroxyurea is an oral agent used to treat HNC. Bleomycin and Docetaxel are IV chemotherapy agents used to treat HNC. Xeloda is not recommended for the treatment of HNC.

4. C) Decreased white blood cell count, mucositis, and weight loss
Chemotherapy can cause an increased white blood cell count. Side effects of radiation to the head and neck include mucositis and weight loss.

5. B) Colitis
The nurse should monitor for inflammatory responses such as colitis, pneumonitis, hepatitis, and thyroiditis in patients receiving treatment with nivolumab (Opdivo). Myelosuppression, nausea/vomiting, and fatigue are associated with a range of other chemotherapy agents, not nivolumab.

Section II: Liquid Tumors
Leukemia

● INTRODUCTION

Leukemia is a cancer of the blood and bone marrow, which causes the overgrowth of white blood cells either from the lymphoid or myeloid cell lines. The primary function of the bone marrow is to produce healthy blood, cells, white blood cells, red blood, cells, and platelets. Although there are different subtypes of leukemia, each of which is treated differently— all leukemia arises from a mutated cell. Leukemia cells (white blood cells) do not evolve into healthy functioning cells; they divide in order to produce more leukemia cells and ultimately crowd the bone marrow.

Leukemias are divided into two primary categories: acute or chronic. Acute leukemia is rapidly progressing in nature and usually requires urgent treatment with chemotherapy. The chemotherapy is administered in three phases: (i) induction, (ii) consolidation, and (iii) maintenance. Acute leukemia is sudden onset with symptoms appearing early and intensely, and without treatment, acute leukemia is fatal.

Chronic leukemia tends to follow a more indolent course, occurring in older individuals, slow to progress and often with fewer symptoms. Chronic leukemia is often easily treated with oral chemotherapy and biotherapy agents.

The four subtypes of leukemia are:

1. Acute myeloid leukemia (AML): Abnormal cells developed from the myeloid cell line
2. Acute lymphoblastic leukemia (ALL): Abnormal cells developed from the lymphoid cell line
3. Chronic myeloid leukemia (CML): Abnormal cells developed from the myeloid cell line
4. Chronic lymphocytic leukemia (CLL): Abnormal cells developed from the lymphoid cell line

▶ EXAM TIP

Understand the differences among the four subtypes of leukemia.

● RISK FACTORS FOR LEUKEMIAS

Unfortunately, the specific cause of leukemia development is unknown. It is believed that there is a genetic/hereditary component. Risk factors include:

- Gender: Men tend to have a higher risk than females
- Age: Typically occurs in individuals over the age of 55
- Family history: Direct first-degree relative
- Genetic disorders: Inherited disorders such as Down syndrome, neurofibromatosis, and several other genetic mutations.
- Previous exposure to chemotherapy or radiation therapy
- Exposure to viruses such as human T cell leukemia (HTLV-1)

The bibliography and references for this chapter are available on ExamPrepConnect; see inside front cover for access instructions.

- Exposure to chemicals:
  - Smoking
  - Herbicide
  - Agent Orange (linked to CLL and CML)
  - Benzene (linked to ALL and AML)

ACUTE MYELOID LEUKEMIA

▶ RISK FACTORS

Most commonly, it is unclear what causes AML; however, the following factors have been identified as putting a person at a higher risk for developing AML:

- Male gender
- Older adults
- Prior chemotherapy/radiation exposure
- Benzene exposure (industrial workers)
- Smoking history

▶ SIGNS AND SYMPTOMS

The signs and symptoms of AML are like those of many other illnesses. They are often nonspecific and, if present, require additional workup and testing. The signs and symptoms of AML are mainly attributed to abnormal blood counts and their sequelae. Generally, the abnormalities appear suddenly, evolving in a matter of days to weeks. An abnormal CBC is often the first signal of bone marrow dysfunction. Newly diagnosed AML patients usually have either extremely high or extremely low white blood cell counts (either >10 or <4), decreased hemoglobin (<12), and decreased platelet count (<150,000). Common symptoms include:

- Fever
- Abnormal bleeding/easy bruising
- Infections
- Bone pain
- Unexplained weight loss

▶ DIAGNOSIS

A diagnosis of AML is established when 20% of leukemia cells or "immature blasts" of myeloid cell line origin are identified either in the peripheral blood or a bone marrow sample. In the bone marrow of a healthy person, stem cells mature and differentiate into functional blood cells. In a person with AML, mutations in their DNA forces the stem cell to "get stuck" in an immature phase which does not allow them to differentiate into functional blood cells. These immature blast cells replicate and crowd the bone marrow, not allowing room for healthy functional cells to develop. The gold standard diagnostic tool for AML is a bone marrow biopsy. A bone marrow biopsy is often prompted by abnormal bloodwork.

▶ STAGING INFORMATION

CYTOGENETIC TESTING

Cytogenetic testing examines the chromosomes under a microscope. A normal human cell has 23 pairs of chromosomes, whereas, in certain cases of AML, changes on the chromosomes are detectable (deletions, translocations, and/or extra chromosomes). These cytogenetic changes can help risk stratify the disease, which can guide treatment planning and can suggest overall prognosis. Table 17.1 describes the risk category for cytogenetic abnormalities.

Table 17.1 Risk Category for Cytogenetic Changes in Acute Myeloid Leukemia

Risk Category	Cytogenetic Abnormality
Low risk	Inversion of chromosome 16, translocation between chromosome 8 and 21
Intermediate risk	Trisomy 8, translocation between chromosomes 9 and 11
High risk	Deletion of chromosome 5 or 7, more than three abnormalities, inversion of chromosome 3

MOLECULAR TESTING

Molecular tests can be obtained from either the peripheral blood or from a bone marrow sample. It is highly sensitive DNA testing that examines mutations in genes. Molecular testing is frequently used in hematologic malignancies to identify mutations that are targetable. Targeting the mutations can aid which targeted immune therapy can be utilized. Once identified, these gene mutations can also help predict the prognosis and potential outcomes. The following are commonly occurring examples of mutations and their risk category:

- *CEBPA* mutation → Low risk
- *NPM1* → Moderate risk
- *TP53, RUNX1, ASXL1* → High risk

▶ TREATMENT

The standard approach to treating AML in otherwise healthy adults is with chemotherapy. To make an accurate treatment plan, several factors must be considered:

- Age
- Comorbid conditions
- Previous chemotherapy exposure
- Performance status
- Cytogenetic and molecular abnormalities

The first phase of treatment is referred to as *induction therapy*. The goal is to control the disease burden and destroy as many leukemia cells as possible. Induction therapy is typically administered in the hospital setting as patients require close monitoring and supportive care. If remission is achieved with induction therapy, the patient proceeds to the next phase of treatment: consolidation therapy. Induction therapy (at least a month of therapy) includes:

- **Cytarabine + daunorubicin or idarubicin**
  - Commonly referred to as "7+3" because 7 consecutive days of cytarabine are administered and 3 days of either daunorubicin or idarubicin.
  - Most commonly used therapy for adults with newly diagnosed leukemia who can tolerate intensive chemotherapy
- **Vyxeos** (combination of daunorubicin and cytarabine)
  - This therapy is approved for adults with treatment-related leukemia; it can be administered in a hospital or office setting.
- **Stem cell transplant**
  - The purpose of a stem cell transplant is to give the recipient a new immune system so that it can recognize and fight cancer cells. It is a treatment option for patients with higher risk AML in combination with chemotherapy. Stem cell transplants have a high mortality rate, and several factors must be considered before proceeding with this option.

ACUTE LYMPHOBLASTIC LEUKEMIA

ALL, also called acute lymphocytic leukemia, is leukemia that arises from DNA mutations in the lymphoid cell line. It more commonly occurs in children; however, ALL has a much higher mortality rate when it occurs in adults.

▶ RISK FACTORS

It is largely unknown what causes ALL; however, certain factors have been identified that place individuals at higher risk for developing the disease:

- Genetic disorders such as Down syndrome
- Age: commonly affects young children (1–4 years of age) and older adults (>70 years of age)
- Male gender
- Race: Hispanic and Caucasian individuals
- Prior chemotherapy/radiation exposure

▶ SIGNS AND SYMPTOMS

- Night sweats
- Fatigue and weakness
- Abnormal bleeding/bruising
- Bone pain
- Splenomegaly
- Unintentional weight loss

▶ DIAGNOSIS

ALL is diagnosed via a bone marrow biopsy. A bone marrow biopsy entails taking a liquid sample of the bone marrow and removing a small chip of bone for evaluation. To diagnose ALL, blast cells (of lymphoid origin) must be present in the bone marrow. Once ALL is identified in the bone marrow, further testing is indicated to determine the subtype of ALL and the presence or absence of the Philadelphia chromosome (a translocation of chromosomes 9 and 22).

▶ STAGING INFORMATION

ALL is further subdivided into either B-cell or T-cell involvement. This subdivision yields differing treatment and prognostic outcomes.

1. B-cell leukemia is more commonly occurring and generally associated with better outcomes.
2. T-cell leukemia accounts for approximately 25% of ALL cases and has fewer treatment options, particularly in the setting of relapse.

▶ TREATMENT

Similar to AML, the standard first-line treatment for ALL is chemotherapy. Chemotherapy regimens for ALL patients are comprised of a combination of multiple drugs. In addition to chemotherapy, ALL patients require central nervous system prophylaxis to prevent leukemia cells from traveling to the brain and spinal fluid. The method of delivering CNS prophylaxis is injecting chemotherapy directly into spinal fluid; this procedure is called a "lumbar puncture."

Following an initial diagnosis of ALL, patients receive induction chemotherapy in the hospital. Once remission is achieved, they proceed with consolidation chemotherapy and ultimately maintenance therapy. Bone marrow transplant is indicated for certain ALL patients and is often a consideration. For patients with relapsed or refractory disease. Table 17.2 reviews the chemotherapy agents used to treat ALL.

Table 17.2 Chemotherapy Agents Used to Treat Acute Lymphoblastic Leukemia

Chemotherapy Agent	Monitoring Considerations	Induction or Maintenance
Doxorubicin (Adriamycin)	Use of vesicant precautions during the administration Potential to be cardiotoxic; requires a MUGA scan prior to administration of the first dose Lifetime max of drug: 550 mg/m²; 450 mg/m² with commitment radiation Creates red urine 24–48 hours post infusion Monitor for myelosuppression, mouth sores, N/V	Induction
Cytarabine (Ara-C)	Administer eye drops as ordered Liver functions Monitor for cerebellar ataxia (check handwriting)	Induction

(continued)

Table 17.2 Chemotherapy Agents Used to Treat Acute Lymphoblastic Leukemia (*continued*)

Chemotherapy Agent	Monitoring Considerations	Induction or Maintenance
Cyclophosphamide (Cytoxan)	Monitor for myelosuppression, N/V, hemorrhagic cystitis	Induction
Methotrexate	Methotrexate levels, kidney functions; use of leucovorin Monitor for N/V	Induction/oral route for maintenance
Mercaptopurine	Liver and kidney functions	Maintenance
Pegaspargase (Oncaspar® PEG-L-asparaginase)	Monitor for acute allergic reaction, diarrhea, pancreatitis (rare cases)	Maintenance
Vincristine (Vincasar Marqibo, PFS)	Vesicant Monitor for severe constipation	Induction/maintenance

MUGA, multigated acquisition; N/V, nausea/vomiting.

In the event of the presence of the Philadelphia chromosome in an ALL patient, an oral tyrosine kinase inhibitor (TKI) agent is added to the treatment plan. This class of medications works by blocking an overactive enzyme (tyrosine kinase) which affects the growth and functional development of cells. TKI therapy may be continued for many years after maintenance treatment has been completed.

IMMUNOTHERAPY

■ **Blinatumomab**
  ● Indicated for relapsed/refractory B-cell ALL or B-cell ALL with minimal residual disease detected, often used as a bridge to bone marrow transplant
  ● Administered through an IV over the course of 28 days, requires close neurological monitoring, may cause seizure, confusion, balance disturbances.
■ **Intotuzumab ozogamicin**
  ● Indicated for relapsed/refractory B-cell ALL
  ● Administered through an IV
  ● Targets a protein (CD22) expressed on the surface of B-cells; can be administered in the outpatient setting
  ● Side effects: Bleeding, fatigue, cytopenia, and liver toxicity

CHRONIC MYELOID LEUKEMIA

CML is a chronic form of leukemia that involves the myeloid white blood cells. It is characterized by the presence of the gene *BCR-ABL1*. This gene is caused by a translocation of chromosomes 9 and 22. The resulting abnormal chromosome 22 is referred to as the Philadelphia chromosome. The vast majority of CML patients have the *BCR-ABL1* gene; <5% of CML cases are Philadelphia chromosome negative.

▶ RISK FACTORS

It is largely unknown what causes CML; however, certain factors have been identified that place individuals at higher risk for developing the disease:

- Advanced age; primarily affects older adults
- Slightly more common in men

▶ SIGNS AND SYMPTOMS

CML is a chronic or slow-growing disease; therefore, patients often experience no signs or symptoms to indicate an illness. However, those with symptoms often report the following:

- Weakness
- Fatigue
- Shortness of breath
- Unexplained weight loss
- Night sweats
- Pain/fullness on the left side (enlarged spleen)

▶ DIAGNOSIS

CML, like most forms of leukemia, is diagnosed with a bone marrow biopsy. However, CBC testing can be useful to first identify an abnormality. A patient with CML often has an extremely high white blood cell count and decreased red blood cells and platelets. Additionally, FISH testing, PCR, and cytogenetic analysis are used to diagnose CML.

FISH (fluorescence in situ hybridization)
- Lab test that can identify the *BCR-ABL1* gene using color probes.
- Shows the translocation between chromosomes 9 and 22.

PCR (polymerase chain reaction)
- Most sensitive to quantify the *BCR-ABL1* gene
- The *BCR-ABL1* gene blood test is used to track treatment response and should be performed every 3 months for CML patients.
  - Cytogenetic response → No cells with *BCR-ABL1* gene detected.
  - Molecular response → Decrease in cells with *BCR-ABL1* gene
  - Early molecular response → *BCR-ABL1* gene is 10% or less at approximately 3–6 months of treatment with TKI therapy
  - Major molecular response → *BCR-ABL1* gene 0.1%

▶ TREATMENT

The standard treatment for adults with CML is the use of a tyrosine kinase inhibitor (TKI), an oral agent taken either once or twice per day. Treatment with TKI therapy is highly effective and can control the disease for decades. Choosing an appropriate TKI is based on age, comorbidities, and phase of CML at diagnosis. For the majority of patients, TKI therapy can yield disease control. Compliance is extremely important for successful disease control. It is important for patients to notify their providers of any and all side effects associated with TKI therapy so they can be appropriately managed.

TARGETED THERAPY: TKI INHIBITORS

- Gleevec (imatinib)
  - Taken daily with food.
  - Side effects: nausea/vomiting, diarrhea, swelling, muscle cramps, fatigue, rash, periorbital edema
- Sprycell (dasatinib)
  - Taken daily with or without food
  - Side effects: nausea, diarrhea, headache, fatigue, shortness of breath, rash
    - Fluid retentions surrounding the lungs and heart can occur; must inform prescribing physician immediately.
- Tasigna (nilotinib)
  - Taken twice per day on an empty stomach.
  - Separate from H2 blockers, avoid antacids.
  - Side effects: arrhythmias, nausea, diarrhea, headache, fatigue, joint pain, night sweats
    - Serious side effects can include blood clots, pancreatic irritation, QT prolongation.
- In the event of resistance to one or more of the above TKI agents
  - Bosutinib (Bosulif)
    - Taken daily with or without food.
    - Side effects: fluid retention, rash, fatigue, fluid retention, diarrhea, nausea, and vomiting
  - Ponatinib (Iclusig)
    - Indicated for patients with a *T3151* mutation or those who have failed all other therapies
    - Taken daily with or without food
    - Side effects: rash, abdominal pain, hypertension, blood clots, fluid retention, blurry vision, heart failure

● SURVIVAL INFORMATION FOR LEUKEMIA

According to the Lymphoma and Leukemia Society (2021) overall survival data, the approximate 5-year survival rates are as follows:

- ALL: 71.7% in adults; 91.9% in children
- AML: 29.4% in adults; 94.1% in children
- CLL: 88.2% overall
- CML: 69.7% overall

The bibliography and references for this chapter are available on ExamPrepConnect; see inside front cover for access instructions.

1. A 65-year-old female patient is being evaluated for suspected AML. The MOST concerning risk factor in the patient's medical history is:

    A. Prior chemotherapy and radiation for breast cancer 15 years ago
    B. 0.5 pack-per-day smoking history for 5 years; quit 2 years ago
    C. Patient's sister had ALL as a child
    D. History of type 2 diabetes mellitus

2. Which of the following agents should be added to the treatment plan for a 45-year-old male patient newly diagnosed B-cell ALL who was found to be Philadelphia chromosome positive?

    A. Vyxeos
    B. Inotuzumab
    C. Dasatinib
    D. Blinatumomab

3. A 55-year-old female patient with recently diagnosed ALL is experiencing new-onset headaches and blurry vision. The last cycle of chemotherapy was 3 weeks ago. The nurse will perform which intervention first?

    A. Lumbar puncture with intrathecal chemotherapy
    B. PET scan
    C. Bone marrow biopsy
    D. Additional chemo cycle

4. Which of the following CBC results MOST LIKELY depicts an acute myeloid leukemia?

    A. WBC 4.9, Hgb 11.9, Plt 149
    B. WBC 10.9, Hgb 17.4, Plt 680
    C. WBC 1.1, Hgb 8.8, Plt 95
    D. WBC 11.5, Hgb 9.0, Plt 265

5. Which of the following patients is MOST LIKELY to require a bone marrow transplant?

    A. An 80-year-old male with ALL in remission
    B. A 35-year-old female with AML, normal cytogenetics
    C. A 60-year-old female with AML, *TP53* mutation
    D. A 45-year-old male with CML in remission

1. A) Prior chemotherapy and radiation for breast cancer 15 years ago
Having received chemotherapy or radiation for another malignancy is a risk factor for AML. This is referred to as a "treatment-related AML" and is often associated with a poor prognosis. Smoking is also a risk factor, but previous chemotherapy is more likely the cause. A sister with malignancy is also a risk factor, but the chemotherapy is a direct link to leukemia. Diabetes has no effect on developing leukemia; it just complicates the care of the leukemic patient.

2. C) Dasatinib
Philadelphia chromosome positivity in an ALL patient calls for the addition of a TKI agent. The following agents are approved to treat Ph+ (Philadelphia chromosome positive) ALL: imatinib, dasatinib, and ponatinib. Vyxeos is approved for adults with treatment-related AML. Inotuzumab is indicated for relapsed/refractory B-ALL. Blinatumomab is indicated for relapsed/refractory B-cell ALL or B-cell ALL with minimal residual disease detected.

3. A) Lumbar puncture with intrathecal chemotherapy
Invasion of leukemia into the central nervous system occurs more frequently in ALL than AML. Prophylaxis with intrathecal chemotherapy is a standard part of treatment even without the presence of CNS symptoms.

4. C) WBC 1.1, Hgb 8.8, Plt 95
CBC testing is useful in identifying abnormalities in the blood so that further workup can be investigated. AML is often characterized by cytopenia—that is, low white blood cells, low red blood cells, and low platelets. CBC results of WBC 1.1, Hgb 8.8, Plt 95 indicate AML.

5. C) A 60-year-old female with AML, *TP53* mutation
TP53 mutated leukemia is considered a high-risk or unfavorable molecular abnormality. Patients with high-risk diseases should be evaluated for bone marrow transplants as a potentially curative treatment option.

Lymphoma

INTRODUCTION

The immune system is a complex mechanism that uses numerous cell types and various signaling pathways to identify and combat unhealthy cells, bacteria, and viruses. All immune cells come from precursor cells that originate in the bone marrow. Each cell type has different functionality. The immune cells can identify unhealthy cells as well as communicate with other cells to prevent, limit, and/or kill foreign bodies. One mechanism that is regulated by the immune system is to recognize danger cues within the body, also referred to as danger-associated molecular patterns (DAMPs). This occurs when cells in the body are unhealthy due to infection, cancer, and genetic malformation, and are targeted to be removed and/or eliminated. Figure 18.1 depicts the lymphatic organs.

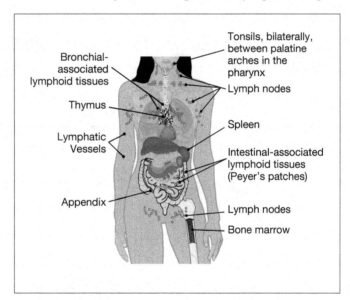

Figure 18.1 Lymphatic organs.
Source: From Gawlik, K. S., Melnyk, B. M., & Teal, A. M. (2021). *Evidence-based physical examination: Best practice for health and well-being assessment.* Springer Publishing Company.

LYMPHATIC SYSTEM

The lymphatic system is a key element of the immune system. The lymphatic vessels are responsible for transporting lymph which is a colorless liquid throughout the body. Lymph nodes are bean-shaped structures that act as a filter for the lymph fluid. The lymph fluid

---

The bibliography and references for this chapter are available on ExamPrepConnect; see inside front cover for access instructions.

and lymph nodes contain white blood cells, which are further divided into B and T cells, and aim to fight infection and destroy abnormal cells. In addition, the immune system utilizes cytokines, which act as the messengers to signal the immune system. Lymphocytes, which aid in the adaptive immune response, have the ability to remember the foreign agent and attack when it becomes present. However, in many patients with cancer, the immune system fails to recognize the foreign agent; in this case, cancer cells that have abnormal DNA pass through the immune system and the cells continue to grow.

▶ OVERVIEW OF B AND T CELLS

The white blood cells, B and T, are responsible for the adaptive immune response (Figure 18.2). These cells are created in the bone marrow; B cells originate and grow in the bone marrow while T cells mature in the thymus.

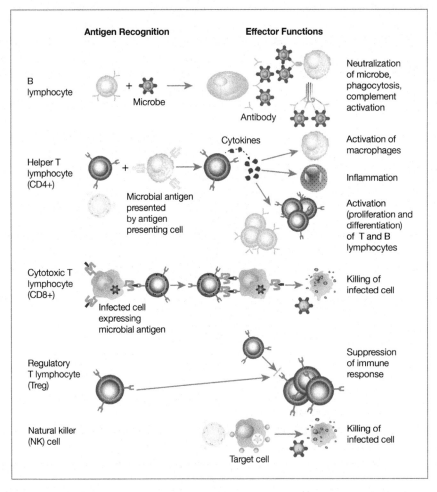

Figure 18.2 Lymphocytes.
Source: From Gawlik, K. S., Melnyk, B. M., & Teal, A. M. (2021). *Evidence-based physical examination: Best practice for health and well-being assessment.* Springer Publishing Company.

1. B cells are responsible for the protection from infections and other invaders. B cells are known to create antibodies in response to an antigen.

2. T cells are also responsible for protection; however, they function differently. T cells interact with specific foreign bodies. T cells do not attack all antigens but rather circulate within the body until they meet their specific antigen. T cells are subdivided into:

a. T-helper cells: Responsible for stimulating the immune system to produce natural T-killer cells as well as increase the B-cell antibody production.

b. T-natural killer cells: Responsible for directly attacking and killing the infection and/or abnormal cells within the body.

⬤ LYMPHOMAS

Lymphomas are liquid malignancies of the lymphatic system arising from white blood cells. There are over 70 different subtypes ranging from slow growing to extremely aggressive life-threatening cancers. Lymphomas are divided into two categories: Hodgkin's and non-Hodgkin's.

▶ HODGKIN'S LYMPHOMA

Hodgkin's lymphoma (HL) arises from abnormal B-lymphocytes known as Reed-Sternberg cells. Unlike other malignancies, there are no useful screening tests or exams to identify the disease. There are four subtypes of Hodgkin's lymphoma:

1. **Nodular sclerosis Hodgkin's lymphoma** is the most common sub-type accounting for about 70% of cases. It is the most common type found in young adults and has a higher incidence with women.
2. **Mixed cellularity Hodgkin's lymphoma** is the second most common type accounting for 20% to 25% of cases. It is more prevalent in males, older adults, and patients with HIV infections. Lymph nodes involved have Reed-Sternberg cells.
3. **Lymphocyte-rich Hodgkin's lymphoma** accounts for about 5% of all cases. It is usually diagnosed at early stages and is more common in males. The lymph nodes involved contain numerous normal-appearing lymphocytes among Reed-Sternberg cells.
4. **Lymphocyte-depleted Hodgkin's lymphoma** is a rare form of HL. Median age ranges between 30 and 37 years old and is more prevalent in those with HIV infection. This form of HL tends to be more aggressive and is usually diagnosed with an advanced stage. Lymph nodes involved generally contain few normal lymphocytes and numerous Reed-Sternberg cells.

RISK FACTORS

There are several risk factors that are associated with HL:

- **Age:** Usually diagnosed between the ages of 20 and 40 and over the age of 55.
- **Gender:** Tends to affect more males; however, the subtype of nodular sclerosis HL is more commonly seen in the female population.
- **Epstein-Barr virus (EBV) infection/mononucleosis:** EBV, which causes infectious mononucleosis, is associated with HL. The virus also has been identified in the Reed-Sternberg cells.
- **Family history:** There is a link between family members and HL, specifically siblings. If a sibling (e.g., brother) has the disease, there is an increased risk for the other siblings (e.g., sister or brother) to develop HL. In addition, there is a significantly higher risk for an identical twin if the other has HL.
- **Immunocompromised status:**
  - HIV infection
  - Immunosuppressive medications: Post-organ transplant patients
  - Autoimmune disorders

Nodular lymphocyte-predominant Hodgkin's lymphoma, which is characterized by the presence of lymphocyte-predominant cells, is sometimes termed "popcorn cells," which are a variant of Reed-Sternberg cells. It accounts for about 5% of Hodgkin's lymphoma cases and is most common in those who are 30 to 50 years old. This subtype is more common in males and is highly curable; however, it can be slow-growing and relapse many years later. In about 7% of cases, nodular lymphocyte-predominant Hodgkin's lymphoma can transform to aggressive non-Hodgkin's lymphoma.

▶ SIGNS AND SYMPTOMS

Common signs and symptoms include:

- Painless enlarged lymph nodes
- Persistent fatigue
- Pruritus
- Cough
- Shortness of breath
- Chest pain
- Other symptoms:
  - Fever (which can come and go over several weeks) without an infection.
  - Drenching night sweats
  - Unintentional weight loss (at least 10% of your body weight <6 months)

◗ NON-HODGKIN'S LYMPHOMA

Non-Hodgkin's lymphoma (NHL) is one of the most common cancers in the United States; NHL is not a single disease but rather a global term that refers to several cancers called lymphoid neoplasms. There are over 80 different subtypes of NHL. The different subtypes of NHL are related to the pathological appearance, molecular features, growth patterns, and response to treatment.

▶ SUBTYPES OF NON-HODGKIN'S LYMPHOMA

The subtypes of lymphoma are divided by the type of cell involved, including B-cell or T-cells, and the growth rate of the disease. Table 18.1 describes the most common subtypes of NHL.

Table 18.1 Common Subtypes of Non-Hodgkin's Lymphoma

Subtype	Cell Type	Growth Rate	Recommended Treatment
Diffuse large B-cell lymphoma (DLBCL) *Can spread to cerebrospinal spinal fluid*	B cell	Aggressive	Chemotherapy, biotherapy, and radiation; CNS chemotherapy may be recommended
Follicular lymphoma *Has the potential to transform to DLBCL*	B cell	Slow growing; indolent at times	Watchful waiting until symptoms occur Chemotherapy, targeted therapy, and radiation

(continued)

Table 18.1 Common Subtypes of Non-Hodgkin's Lymphoma (*continued*)

Subtype	Cell Type	Growth Rate	Recommended Treatment
Mantle Cell *Involves chromosomes 11 and 14*	B cell	Slow growing	Watchful waiting if slow-growing non-active disease Chemotherapy, monoclonal antibodies, stem cell transplant
Small lymphocytic lymphoma	B cell	Indolent	Watchful waiting until symptoms occur Chemotherapy and biotherapy
Double hit lymphoma *Involves older adults; gene mutations of MYC and either BCL2 or BCL6* Triple Hit Lymphoma *Involves all three gene mutations: MYC, BCL2, and BCL6*	B cell	Highly aggressive	Chemotherapy and biotherapy
Primary mediastinal large B-cell lymphoma *(Presents with a large mass in the mediastinal)*	B cell	Aggressive	Chemotherapy, biotherapy, and radiation to the chest mass are often recommended; CART therapy and stem cell transplant can also be recommended for unresponsive disease
Extranodal marginal zone B-cell lymphoma (MALT) *Involves the stomach and can be correlated to an autoimmune disease*	B cell	Aggressive	Biotherapy (Rituxan) with or without chemotherapy
Splenic marginal zone B-cell lymphoma *Involves the spleen*	B cell	Slow growing	Removal of the spleen, watchful waiting, and rituxan and chemotherapy in some cases
Burkitt lymphoma/Burkitt cell leukemia (Rare) *May be associated with EBV and HIV infections*	B cell	Aggressive	Chemotherapy biotherapy; some cases, stem cell transplant
Anaplastic large cell lymphoma primary cutaneous type *Involves the skin*	T cell	Indolent to aggressive	Radiation for local disease; chemotherapy with systematic disease
Peripheral T-cell lymphoma *Involves CD4 or CD8*	T cell	Aggressive	Chemotherapy and stem cell transplantation
Adult T-cell lymphoma/ leukemia	T cell	Aggressive	Allo transplant and biotherapy are beneficial; chemotherapy is not responsive
Mycosis fungoides (Rare) *Involves the skin; not a curable disease*	T cell	Indolent at first; has the potential to be aggressive	Topical agents, radiation therapy, chemotherapy, and biotherapy

▶ RISK FACTORS

- ■ Age: Older than age 60 years is a strong risk factor in lymphoma.
- ■ Gender: Men tend to have an increased risk than women.
- ■ Race/ethnicity: Whites are more likely to develop NHL than African Americans or Asian Americans.
- ■ Family history: Increased risk with a first-degree relative
- ■ Chemical exposure: Benzenes, herbicides, and insecticides (research still ongoing)
- ■ Drug exposure: Chemotherapy drugs; drugs used to treat autoimmune diseases such as methotrexate and tumor necrosis factor inhibitors.
- ■ Radiation: Survivors of atomic bombs, nuclear reactor accidents, or patients treated with radiation therapy for other cancers.
- ■ Immunocompromised population:
  - ● Patients taking immunosuppressive medications
  - ● HIV infections
  - ● Genetically inherited syndrome: Ataxia-telangiectasia and Wiskott-Aldrich syndrome
- ■ Autoimmune diseases:
  - ● Rheumatoid arthritis
  - ● Systemic lupus erythematosus (SLE or lupus)
  - ● Sjogren disease
  - ● Celiac disease (gluten-sensitive enteropathy)
- ■ Viral and bacterial infections
  - ● Human T-cell lymphotropic virus (HTLV-1)
  - ● Epstein-Barr virus (EBV)
  - ● Human herpes virus 8 (HHV-8)
  - ● Human immunodeficiency virus (HIV)
  - ● Hepatitis C
  - ● *Helicobacter pylori*
  - ● *Chlamydophila psittaci*

▶ SIGNS AND SYMPTOMS

Common signs and symptoms that fluctuate over the course of days to weeks:

- ■ Fever
- ■ Night sweats
- ■ Weight loss >10% of body within 6 months
- ■ Enlarged lymph nodes
- ■ Weight loss
- ■ Chills
- ■ Fatigue (feeling very tired)
- ■ Swollen abdomen (belly)
- ■ Feeling full after only a small amount of food
- ■ Chest pain or pressure
- ■ Shortness of breath or cough
- ■ Severe or frequent infections
- ■ Easy bruising or bleeding

DIAGNOSIS OF LYMPHOMA

1. History and physical
2. Blood work:
   - CBC with differential, platelets, erythrocyte sedimentation rate
   - Comprehensive metabolic panel, lactate dehydrogenase (LDH), liver function tests
   - Pregnancy test for women of childbearing age
   - HIV and hepatitis B
3. PET/CT scan (orbits to mid-thigh or head to toe in certain cases)
4. Diagnostic contrast-enhanced CT scans
5. Bone marrow biopsy
6. Pre-treatment:
   - Pulmonary function tests (PFTs) to assess lung function
   - Echocardiogram to evaluate ejection fraction (MUGA scan)

SURGICAL BIOPSY OF LYMPH NODES

A diagnosis of lymphoma is best obtained by taking a biopsy of the lymph node or nodes. There are several biopsies options:

1. Fine needle aspiration (FNA) biopsy
2. Core needle biopsy
3. Excisional or incisional biopsy: Removal of the lymph node and surrounding tissue

MOLECULAR INFORMATION

- Immunohistochemistry—used to identify the specific protein the lymphoma is expressing
- Flow cytometry
- Fluorescence in situ hybridization (FISH)—test often used to determine the genomic changes of the lymphoma tissue

▶ STAGING OF LYMPHOMA

Lymphoma staging is not based on the TNM (tumor, nodes, metastases) staging, as this is considered a liquid malignancy. It is staged using the Lugano Classification, which was based upon the Ann Arbor System. The Lugano Classification has four stages.

- **Stage I:** Either of the following:
  - Lymphoma is found in only one lymph node area.
  - Lymphoma is found only in one part or one organ outside the lymph system (IE).
- **Stage II:** Either of the following:
  - Two or more lymph node areas on the same side of (above or below) the diaphragm (II).
  - Lymphoma extends locally from one lymph node area into a nearby organ (IIE).

- **Stage III:** Either of the following:
  - Lymphoma found in lymph node areas on both sides of (above and below) the diaphragm (III).
  - Lymph nodes above the diaphragm and in the spleen.
- **Stage IV:**
  - Lymphoma has spread widely into at least one organ outside of the lymph system, such as the liver, bone marrow, or lungs.

Other modifiers may also be used to describe the lymphoma stage, which includes the size of the lesions, also referred to as bulky disease. The letter A or B may also be added as the identification of B symptoms.

▶ TREATMENT OF LYMPHOMA

RADIATION THERAPY

Due to the advances with biotherapy agents, radiation is used less frequently with lymphoma treatments. However, external beam radiation therapy can be used to treat HD patients as well as lymphoma patients with advanced disease. Lastly, radiation therapy can be used in the palliative setting for advanced uncontrolled lymphoma patients.

CHEMOTHERAPY AND BIOTHERAPY

Treatment options do not include surgery as primary option with lymphomas. The most common first-line treatment includes a combination of chemotherapy plus immunotherapy. Table 18.2 provides the treatment options for B-cell non-Hodgkin's lymphomas, Hodgkin's lymphoma, and T-cell lymphomas.

Table 18.2 Common Treatment Options for Lymphomas

Lymphoma Diagnosis	Treatment Regimen
Classic Hodgkin's lymphoma	**Primary Treatment:** ■ ABVD (adriamycin, bleomycin, vinblastine, and dacarbazine) ■ BEACOPP (bleomycin, etoposide, doxorubicin, cyclophosphamide, vincristine, procarbazine, prednisone) ■ Brentuximab Vedotin + AVD (adriamycin, bleomycin, dacarbazine) **Second-Line Therapy:** ■ Brentuximab Vedotin (BV) ■ BV + Bendamustine ■ BV+ Nivolumab ■ ICE (ifosphamide, carboplatin, etoposide) ■ GVD (gemcitabine, vinorelbine, doxorubicin) ■ IGEV (ifosfamide, gemcitabine, vinorelbine) ■ DHAP (dexamethasone, cytarabine, cisplatin) Once a good response is achieved after second-line therapy, then consolidation with high dose chemotherapy followed by autologous stem cell transplant (+/– Brentuximab Vedotin maintenance) is performed.

(continued)

Table 18.2 Common Treatment Options for Lymphomas (*continued*)

Lymphoma Diagnosis	Treatment Regimen
Diffuse large B-cell lymphoma	■ Rituxan + CHOP (cyclophosphamide, doxorubicin, vincristine, prednisone) ■ Dose-adjusted EPOCH (cyclophosphamide, doxorubicin, vincristine, etoposide, prednisone) was given as continuous IV infusion. **High Grade Lymphomas:** ■ R-Hyper CVAD (cyclophosphamide, doxorubicin, vincristine, dexamethasone, methotrexate, and cytarabine) ■ R-CODOX-M/R-IVAC: (cyclophosphamide, doxorubicin, vincristine, dexamethasone, methotrexate and ifosfamide, cytarabine, etoposide)
Follicular lymphoma	Bendamustine + Rituxan or Obinutuzamab CHOP (cyclophosphamide, doxorubicin, vincristine, prednisone) + rituxan or obinutuzamab CVP (cyclophosphamide, vincristine, prednisone) + rituxan or obinutuzamab Lenalidomide + rituxan or obinutuzamab
Peripheral T-cell lymphoma (PTCL), anaplastic large cell lymphoma (ALCL), and angioimmunoblastic T-cell lymphoma (AITL)	Brentuximab vedotin + CHP (cyclophosphamide, doxorubicin, prednisone) CHOP (cyclophosphamide, doxorubicin, vincristine, prednisone) CHOEP (cyclophosphamide, doxorubicin, vincristine, etoposide, prednisone) Dose-adjusted EPOCH (cyclophosphamide, doxorubicin, vincristine, etoposide, prednisone) given as continuous IV infusion Consider consolidation with high dose therapy and autologous stem cell rescue as consolidation
Cutaneous T-cell lymphoma (CTCL)	Brentuximab vedotin (anti-CD30 antibody-drug conjugate) Romidepsin HDAC (histone deacetylase inhibitor) Alemtuzumab (anti-CD52 antibody therapy)

▶ **EXAM TIPS**

■ Oncology nurses should always check PFTs before the first dose of Bleomycin and have a test dose.

■ MUGA scan should always be checked prior to the first dose of Adriamycin.

TARGETED THERAPIES

In lymphoma, the most valuable checkpoints are the anti-programmed death receptor PD-1 antibody and antibody directed against cytotoxic T-lymphocyte-associate protein-4 CTLA-4. Treatment response has been seen with Nivolumab and pembrolizumab, which inhibit PD-1, and Ipilimumab, which inhibit CTLA-4.

CHIMERIC ANTIGEN RECEPTOR T-CELL THERAPY

One of the newer immuno-oncology/cellular therapy treatments for lymphoma and other malignancies is Chimeric antigen receptor (CAR) T-cell therapy. CAR T-cell therapy removes the T cells and is genetically altered to have specific chimeric antigen receptors on their surface that can attach to proteins on the surface of lymphoma cells. The genetically modified T cells are multiplied in a lab and then infused back into the patient. The CAR T-cells then expand within the person's body and launch an immune attack on the lymphoma cells. CAR T-cell therapy can cause cytokine release syndrome (CRS), in which immune cells in the body release large amounts of cytokines into the blood, causing a cytokine-mediated systemic inflammatory response. Symptoms of this life-threatening syndrome can present with fevers, myalgias, hypotension, and hypoxia. CRS can be mild and self-limiting, or progress into a severe life-altering situation.

STEM CELL TRANSPLANT

Autologous stem cell transplantation is often used following high-dose chemotherapy for patients with aggressive lymphoma, which has relapsed. Allogeneic stem cell transplant is also a treatment option for certain subtypes of lymphoma, particularly T-cell lymphomas.

SURVIVAL INFORMATION FOR LYMPHOMA

According to the ACS (2020), the 5-year survival rate for HL is 87%; however, it is 92% if diagnostic in the early stages, 94% in regional disease, and 78% in metastatic disease. According to the ACS (2020), The 5-year survival rate for NHL is 72%; however, in regional disease, it is 90% and 85% in metastatic disease (ACS, 2020).

The bibliography and references for this chapter are available on ExamPrepConnect; see inside front cover for access instructions.

1. Which treatment options are commonly used with a diagnosis of non-Hodgkin's lymphoma?

   A. Surgery, chemotherapy, biotherapy, and radiation therapy

   B. Watchful waiting, chemotherapy, biotherapy, radiation therapy, and stem cell transplantation

   C. Watchful waiting, surgery, chemotherapy, biotherapy, and radiation therapy

   D. Watchful waiting, surgery, chemotherapy, and stem cell transplantation

2. A patient is receiving their first dose of R-CHOP for a diagnosis of diffuse large cell lymphoma. The nurse should check all the following before administering the medications, EXCEPT:

   A. Allergies

   B. MUGA scan

   C. Venous access

   D. PFTs

3. The nurse is planning care for a patient who has been diagnosed with follicular lymphoma and is 5 days post treatment with Bendamustine and Rituxan. The nurse's priority intervention is to:

   A. Assess for nausea and vomiting

   B. Monitor neutrophil count

   C. Monitor BUN levels

   D. Assess for constipation

4. Common risk factors for both HL and NHL include:

   A. Age, gender, family history, and genetic mutations

   B. Age, infections, and chemical exposures

   C. Age, gender, autoimmune disorders, and family history

   D. Age, family history, and EBV exposure

5. Which system is used to stage lymphomas?

   A. Ann Arbor System

   B. TNM Staging System

   C. Lugano Classification

   D. Grading System

(See answers next page.)   **227**

1. B) Watchful waiting, chemotherapy, biotherapy, radiation therapy, stem cell transplantation

Watchful waiting is recommended for some indolent lymphomas, as is chemotherapy, biotherapy, and radiation therapy. In some cases with advanced disease, stem cell transplantation may be recommended. Surgery is not a recommended treatment option.

2. D) PFTs

The nurse should review the patient's allergy for risk of hypersensitivity reaction to the Rituxan, MUGA scan for Doxorubicin, and venous access due to the vesicants in the regimen. PFTs is not required because bleomycin is not part of the regimen.

3. B) Monitor neutrophil count

The nurse's priority intervention is to monitor neutrophil count. Depending on how much treatment the patient has had, the neutrophil count can be affected, and the patient is at risk for infection. Nausea and vomiting are not expected 5 days post-chemotherapy. BUN levels should be assessed prior to administration of chemotherapy and biotherapy, not after. Bendamustine and Rituxan do not cause constipation.

4. A) Age, gender, family history, and genetic mutations

Age, gender, family history, and genetic mutations are risk factors for both HD and NHL. Chemical exposure and EBV exposure are risk factors for NHL.

5. C) Lugano Classification

The Lugano Classification is used to stage lymphomas. It is based on the Ann Arbor system. TNM is used to stage solid cancers, and grading is a pathology system.

Multiple Myeloma

INTRODUCTION

Multiple myeloma (MM) is a plasma cell dyscrasia disorder that accounts for 1% to 2% of all cancers and approximately 17% of the hematological malignancies. Multiple myeloma occurs in all races; however, it occurs in about twice as many African Americans than Caucasians and is more common in men than in women. Unfortunately, it is an incurable disease, with a 5-year relative survival rate for patients living with multiple myeloma of approximately 54% (https://seer.cancer.gov/statfacts/html/mulmy.html).

Multiple myeloma is a bone marrow disease where abnormal plasma cells interfere with normal organ function. Plasma cells account for <5% of the cells in the bone marrow, and their function is to produce antibodies (immunoglobulins [Igs]/proteins) in response to infection or other immune-triggering events. They develop from stem cells in the bone marrow, mature into B lymphocytes, and circulate in the body. Multiple myeloma occurs when there is an insult to the plasma cell either by genetics or changes in the bone marrow microenvironment, which results in the normal plasma cell becoming malignant. The malignant plasma cell then starts reproducing a clone of itself which results in an excess of a single type of unnecessary and ineffective immunoglobulin called the myeloma or M protein and reduced amounts of normal functional immunoglobulins. The single unwarranted type and amount of immunoglobulin/protein produced varies among patients and is measured in the blood serum or urine.

▶ IMMUNOGLOBULINS

Immunoglobulin or antibodies are produced by plasma cells and are responsible for humoral immunity. They are glycoproteins that bind to antigens on infectious agents such as bacteria, viruses, fungi, and parasites resulting in the deactivation of the microorganism. Approximately 20% of the protein in plasma is made up of immunoglobulin (https://www.ncbi.nlm.nih.gov/books/NBK513460/).

INTACT IMMUNOGLOBULIN

Immunoglobulins/proteins contain two types of smaller molecules: heavy chains and light chains. There are five heavy chain immunoglobulins called subtypes: IgG, IgA, IgM, IgD and IgE. IgG and IgA are the most common types of M protein, accounting for 80% of all cases. There are two types of light chains—kappa and lambda (Figure 19.1).

The bibliography and references for this chapter are available on ExamPrepConnect; see inside front cover for access instructions.

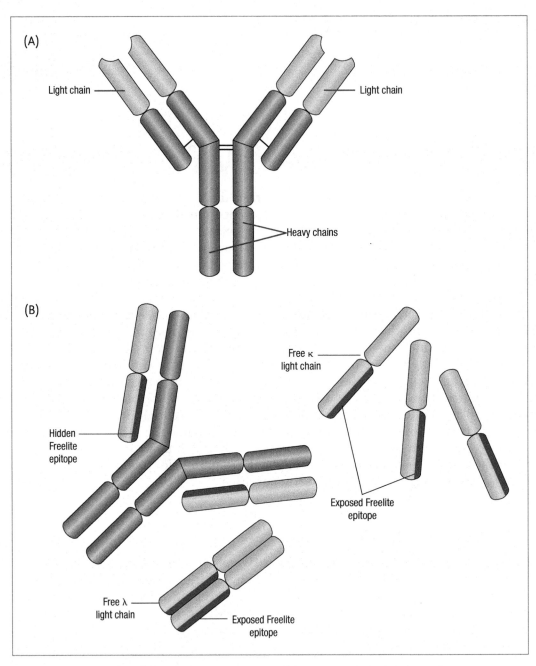

Figure 19.1 Light chains. (A) Light and heavy chains. (B) Kappa and Lambda light chains.

▶ MYELOMA PROTEINS: PATHOLOGIC FEATURES

There are four types of myeloma (Figure 19.2):

■ **Intact immunoglobulin myeloma:** Intact immunoglobulins are composed of 2 heavy chains and two light chains attached to the heavy chains. They can be secreted in the serum or urine. For example, a patient may produce IgG kappa multiple myeloma, IgG lambda multiple myeloma, IgA kappa multiple myeloma, and IgA lambda multiple myeloma.

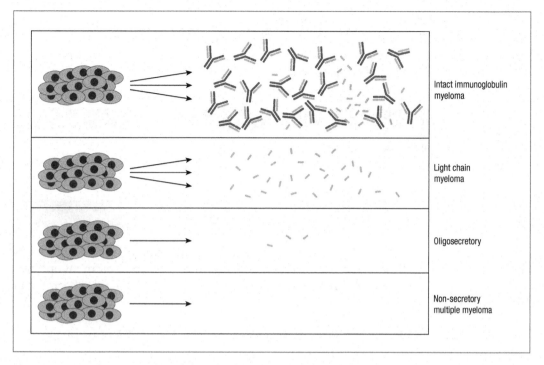

Figure 19.2 Myeloma proteins.

- **Light chain multiple myeloma:** The abnormal protein produced are either kappa or lambda light chains that have broken off the heavy chains. They can be secreted in the serum or urine. When they are secreted in the urine, they are called Bence Jones protein. For example, a patient may produce free kappa light chain or free lambda light chain multiple myeloma.
- **Oligo-secretory myeloma:** A rare form of myeloma and is defined as the absence of measurable disease in serum or urine.
- **Non-secretory multiple myeloma:** The patient does not secrete an abnormal protein that is detectable in the blood or urine.

▶ CRAB CRITERIA

The unrestrained growth of myeloma/clonal plasma cells and the immunoglobulin/ protein it produces is associated with many clinical manifestations and symptoms. These are often referred to as the CRAB criteria. The CRAB criteria are four features or events of specific end-organ damage that have been established by the International Myeloma Working Group as determinants of progression from a benign state MGUS to the active cancer form of the disease multiple myeloma. The attributable CRAB features include hypercalcemia, renal failure, anemia, and bone lesions. CRAB is an acronym for:

- **C**alcium elevation from bone disease due to increase osteolytic activity of osteoclasts and suppression of osteoblasts resulting hypercalcemia.
- **R**enal dysfunction caused by hypercalcemia and accumulation of immunoglobulin light chains.

- **A**nemia caused by inhibition of erythropoiesis.
- **B**one pain occurs due to the stimulation of osteoclast-activating growth factors, cytokine release, and suppression of osteoblasts and may result in pathological fractures, vertebral collapse, and spinal cord compressions.

> ▶ **EXAM TIP**
>
> Understand and memorize the CRAB criteria for MM.

⬤ RISK FACTORS

Most risk factors for MM are unclear. Ongoing research into the potential risk factors has enabled insight into the disease process and to development of targeted treatment options. The risk factors for developing MM include (Atul, 2015; Kyle et al. 2003; Lauby-Secretan et al. 2016; Lynch et al., 2005):

- Age: It is a disease of older age; the median age at diagnosis is 65 to 74 years of age.
- Sex: It is more prevalent in men than women.
- Obesity: The risk increases with body mass.
- Ethnicity: Occurs in all races but affects twice as many African Americans than Caucasians.
- Environmental exposure: Exposure to ionizing radiation and toxins such as pesticides, herbicides, dioxin, and petroleum products has been shown to increase risk.
- Genetics: The risk of developing MM is approximately four times higher for persons with a first-degree relative with MM. Monoclonal gammopathy of undetermined significance (MGUS), a condition that precedes MM, is an important factor associated with the development of MM.

⬤ SIGNS AND SYMPTOMS

At the time of diagnosis, approximately 73% of patients present with symptoms of anemia, 67% present with symptoms of bone pain, 48% present with renal issues, 32% present with fatigue or generalized weakness, 28% with hypercalcemia, and 24 % with weight loss (Kyle et al., 2003). While most patients present with subacute signs and symptoms, a small number of patients will present with acute signs that require immediate intervention. These include spinal cord compression, kidney failure, and hyperviscosity (Kyle et al., 2003).

⬤ DIAGNOSIS

▶ INTERNATIONAL MYELOMA WORK GROUP CRITERIA

To diagnose MM, the criteria established by the International Myeloma Work Group (IMWG) must be met (Box 19.1).

Box 19.1 International Myeloma Work Group Criteria for Multiple Myeloma

Clonal bone marrow (BM) plasma cells of ≥10%

OR

Biopsy-proven bony or extramedullary plasmacytoma

AND

One or more myeloma-defining events:≥1 CRAB feature(s)

OR

≥1 SLIM CRAB feature(s)

Plasmacytoma is a cluster of MM that can grow inside or outside the bone. A solitary plasmacytoma is referred to as extramedullary when it grows outside the bone. An isolated plasmacytoma grows within the bone.

▶ SLIM CRAB CRITERIA

Myeloma-defining events are evidence of end-organ damage that can be attributed to the underlying plasma cell proliferative disorder. Table 19.1 defines the SLIM CRAB criteria.

Table 19.1 Slim Crab Criteria

S	Clonal BM plaSma cell %	≥60%
LI	Free LIght chain ratio (FLC)	FLC ratio involved/uninvolved ≥100
M	MRI	>1 focal lesion (≥5 mm each)
C	Calcium elevation	>11 mg/dL or >1 mg/dL higher than upper limit of normal
R	Renal insufficiency	Creatinine clearance <40 mL/min or serum creatinine >2 mg/dL
A	Anemia	Hbg <10 g/dL or 2 g/dL <normal
B	Bone lesion	≥1 lytic lesion on skeletal radiography, CT, or PET-CT
		If the BM has less than 10% clonal plasma cells, more than one bone lesion is required to distinguish it from a solitary plasmacytoma with minimal marrow involvement.

BM, bone marrow.

▶ EXAM TIP

Understand and memorize the SLIM CRAB criteria for defining MM.

▶ CLASSIFICATION

There are several differential diagnoses for B-cell plasma cell dyscrasias and each has a different treatment recommendation. MM is usually preceded by a premalignant condition called monoclonal gammopathy of undetermined significance (MGUS) in nearly all cases and occurs in about 1% of the general population. The risk of progression from MGUS to MM is approximately 1% to 2% per year. Box 19.2 includes the IMWG criteria for MGUS.

Smoldering Myeloma

Smoldering myeloma is defined as asymptomatic myeloma. See Box 19.3 for the IMWG criteria for smoldering myeloma.

The risk of progression to symptomatic multiple myeloma is approximately 10% each year for the first 5 years from diagnosis, 3% between years 5 and 10 and about 1% in succeeding years. MGUS and SMM are generally found on routine examination when a monoclonal (M) protein is detected during laboratory workup of patients with multiple comorbidities.

Box 19.2 IMWG Criteria for Monoclonal Gammopathy of Undetermined

---

Significance

Serum monoclonal protein (IgG or IgA or IgM) <3g/dL

AND

Clonal BM plasma cells <10%

AND

No myeloma-defining events

OR

Light chain MGUS (all criteria must be met)

Abnormal sFLC ratio <0.26 or >1.65

AND

Increased level of the appropriate involved light chain (increased Kappa sFLC in patients with ratio >1.65 and increased Lambda sFLC patients with A.26)

AND

No immunoglobulin heavy chain on immunofixation

AND

Clonal BM plasma cells <10%

AND

Urinary monoclonal protein >500 mg/24 hr

No myeloma-defining events

IMWG, International Myeloma Work Group Criteria for Multiple Myeloma.

Box 19.3 IMWG Criteria for Smoldering Myeloma

Serum monoclonal protein (IgG or IgA) ≥3 g/dL

OR

Urinary monoclonal protein ≥500mg/24

AND/OR

Clonal BM plasma 10% to 60%

AND

No myeloma-defining events or amyloidosis

IMWG, International Myeloma Work Group Criteria for Multiple Myeloma.

▶ DIAGNOSTIC TESTING

See Table 19.2 for the recommended (IMWG) initial diagnostic workup and expected findings for MM.

Table 19.2 Diagnostic Work Up and Expected Findings for Multiple Myeloma

Diagnostic Workup	Expected Findings
History and physical	Focus on the CRAB symptoms
CBC with differential	Decreased Hgb, WBC, platelets
BUN/creatinine, electrolytes imbalances	Increased BUN, creatinine, uric acid
Calcium/albumin	Elevated Ca+/decreased albumin prognostic indicator
Lactate dehydrogenase (LDH)	Elevated lactate dehydrogenase prognostic indicator
Beta-2 microglobulin	Elevated levels/measures/tumor burden
Serum Free Light Chain FLC assay	Increased free light chains/measures the level of free Kappa and Lambda in the blood
Serum quantitates immunoglobulins	Measures the type of protein produced
Serum protein electrophoresis (SPEPS)	Elevated/M spike establishes presence of a monoclonal band
Serum immunofixation electrophoresis (SIFE)	Confirms the presence and type of the protein light/heavy chain type of M protein
24-hour urine for total protein	Elevated monoclonal protein (Bence Jones)
Urine protein electrophoresis (UPEP)	Confirms the presence of protein of urine/elevated
Imaging: Skeletal survey	Reveals osteolytic lesions/osteoporosis/compression fractures
Imaging: MRI	Reveals focal lesions bone marrow involvement
Imaging: PET scan	Reveals sites of localized extramedullary disease
Bone marrow aspirate and biopsy	>10% plasma cells no translocations
Bone marrow immunohisto-chemistry and bone marrow flow cytometry	Flow cytometry/examines the percentage of PC in the S phase mitosis and abnormalities
Fluorescence in situ hybridization (FISH)	FISH examines genes and chromosomes and how they deviate from the normal structure

Sources: From Faiman, B. Clinical Updates and Nursing Considerations for Patients with Multiple Myeloma. Clin J Oncol Nurs. 2007; 11:831–840; https://www.myeloma.org/international-myeloma-working-group-imwg-criteria-diagnosis-multiple-myeloma.

⬤ STAGING

Once a diagnosis of MM has been confirmed, patients undergo disease staging. Staging is used to verify the extent of the disease, to determine prognosis, the best treatment options, and clinical trials that are appropriate for each patient. Two staging systems were developed to stage MM: the Durie Salmon and the ISS-RISS.

The Durie Salmon Staging System was established in 1975. It measures the myeloma cell mass, hemoglobin, calcium, bone health, M protein, and Bence-Jones protein (Table 19.3). The purpose of this staging system is to associate the amount of myeloma with the damage it has caused. For example, the amount of cell mass with the level of Hgb, stage of renal function, and if bone disease is present. It does not predict prognosis and survival.

Table 19.3 Durie Salmon Staging System

Stage	Durie Salmon Criteria	Measured Myeloma Cell Mass (myeloma cells in billions/m²)

I (low cell mass)	All the following:
	■ Hemoglobin value >10 g/dL
	■ Serum calcium value normal or ≤12 mg/dL
	■ Bone x-ray, normal bone structure or solitary bone plasmacytoma only
	■ Low M-component production rate
	  ● IgG value <5 g/dL
	  ● IgA value <3 g/dL
	  ● Bence Jones protein <4 g/24 hr
		600 billion

II (intermediatecell mass)	Neither stage I nor stage III	600 to 1,200 billion

III (high cell mass)	One or more of the following:
	■ Hemoglobin value <8.5 g/dL
	■ Serum calcium value >12 mg/dL
	■ Advanced lytic bone lesions
	■ High M-component production rate
	  ● IgG value >7 g/dL
	  ● IgA value >5 g/dL
	  ● Bence Jones protein >12 g/24 hr
		>1,200 billion

Subclassification Criteria		
A	Normal renal function (serum creatinine level <2.0 mg/dL)	
B	Abnormal renal function (serum creatinine level ≥2.0 mg/dL)	

The International Staging System (ISS) was developed in 2005 to provide a dependable, simple staging system that could be applied internationally for classification and stratification. It integrates two disease parameters—the Serum Beta-2 Microglobulin (B2M) and Serum Albumin levels—by separating disease burden into three stages with prognostic implications (Box 19.4). Serum Beta-2 Microglobulin reflects tumor mass and renal function, and Serum Albumin is an alternative marker for IL-6 activity. Decreased albumin is the result of the inflammatory cytokines such as interleukin-6 secreted caused by the myeloma microenvironment (Greipp et al., 2005).

Box 19.4 International Staging System for Multiple Myeloma

Stage I: B2M <3.5 mg/L and serum albumin ≥3.5 g/dL

Stage II: Neither stage I nor stage III

Stage III: B2M ≥5.5 mg/L

B2M, serum beta-2 microglobulin.

The ISS was revised in 2015. The Revised International Staging System includes the prognostic indicators of serum lactate dehydrogenase (LDH) and high-risk chromosomal abnormalities acquired from the bone marrow biopsy—interphase fluorescence in situ hybridization (FISH). See Box 19.5.

Box 19.5 Revised International Staging System

R-ISS I (n = 871) – ISS stage I (B2M <3.5 mg/L and serum albumin ≥3.5 g/dL) and normal LDH and not del (17p), t (4;14), or t (14;16) by FISH.
R-ISS II (n = 1894) – Neither stage I nor stage III.
R-ISS III (n = 295) – ISS stage III (B2M ≥5.5 mg/L) plus LDH above normal limits and/or detection of one of the following by FISH: del(17p), t (4;14), or t (14;16).

Source: Palumbo, A., et al 2015.

TREATMENT

The diagnostic evaluation establishes a diagnosis, identifies the subtype and stage, estimates prognosis, and determines the need to initiate treatment (Kurtin et al., 2016):

- **Differential diagnosis:** MGUS, smoldering myeloma, or multiple myeloma
- **Subtype:** Heavy chain, light chain, oligo-secretory, non-secretory, solitary plasmacytoma
- **Staging:** Durie Salmon, ISS, and R-ISS
- **Prognosis:** Cytogenetics, FISH, ploidy, LHD, albumin, B2M, %BMPC
- **Treatment:** Urgent intervention and treatment based on risk
  (Kurtin et al., 2016)

Figure 19.3 depicts the treatment options for the different staging of MM.

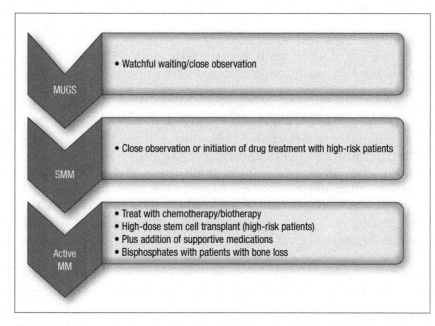

Figure 19.3 Treatment options for the different stages of multiple myeloma.

▶ TREATMENT IN NEWLY DIAGNOSED

Patients who present with newly diagnosed multiple myeloma and subacute symptoms will be considered for one of two initial treatment pathways: transplant or nontransplant. The risk stratification and comprehensive assessment obtained from the focused diagnostic workup help in determining the initial treatment pathway.

The comprehensive assessment provides a guide as to how the patient may tolerate cancer treatment by recognizing comorbidities and age-related organ-specific physiologic changes which can impede tolerance to cancer therapy. The assessment should include functional status, comorbid medical conditions, cognitive status, psychological state, social support, nutritional status, and a review of the medication list (Mohile et al., 2018).

Risk stratification is also considered when determining initial treatment as it provides prognostic information. Patients who express at least one of the following clinical or pathologic criteria are considered to have high-risk MM: t (4;14), t (14;16), t (14;20), del17p13, or gain 1q by FISH and/or lactate dehydrogenase (LDH) levels ≥2 times the institutional upper limit of normal. Patients with standard risk MM have the following pathologic features t (11;14), and t (6;14) (Palumbo, 2015).

It has been shown that autologous stem cell transplant (ASCT) when compared with chemotherapy alone appears to prolong time to relapse and overall survival. Stem cells should be collected early in the initial course of treatment regardless of whether ASCT will immediately follow the initial course of treatment or occurs at time of first relapse. Patients who are eligible for transplant should have minimal exposure to treatment agents that may impair stem cell collection or damage stem cells during the initial course of treatment (Nishimura, 2020). There is no consensus of preferred initial/induction therapy, the regimens used differ among providers and are influenced by availability of medication and provider level of expertise.

Generally, patients who are transplant eligible will receive a three-drug regimen for approximately 3 to 4 months to decrease symptoms, alleviate end-organ damage and diminish the number of cells found in the bone marrow. After 3 to 4 cycles of treatment the patient will complete stem cell collection. Patients who choose not to go to ASCT immediately following stem cell collection will complete several more cycles of pretreatment therapy before being placed on maintenance therapy and will remain on maintenance until disease progression or adverse treatment toxicity.

Patients who are not eligible for transplant will receive 8 to 12 cycles of a three-drug regimen followed by maintenance therapy and will remain on maintenance until progression of disease or adverse treatment toxicity. Patients who cannot tolerate a three-drug regimen will be placed on a two-drug regimen. These patients may also have their stem cells collected for future use with other treatments.

While on therapy, patients are evaluated monthly until best response and then every 3 months. Work up includes CBC with differential, CMP, heavy and light chains, SPEP and other labs as dictated by pathological features of the disease and individual considerations.

During all phases of multiple myeloma treatment decisions are guided by National Comprehensive Cancer Network (NCCN) guidelines. The NCCN puts forth updated evidence-based practice guidelines regarding treatments and supportive services to assist providers in achieving optimal outcomes.

When relapse or progression of disease is suspected restaging is completed. Workup includes repeat bone marrow, repeat imaging, monitoring of end organ damage, serum protein electrophoresis, serum quantitate immunoglobulins, SIFE, serum free light chains, LDH and reassessing comorbidities.

When choosing a treatment regimen for patients who are relapsed and refractory the following factors must be considered: Quality and duration of previous response, aggressiveness of the disease, age, pre-existing toxicities from previous treatment regimens, performance status, bone marrow reserve, and renal function.

▶ CHEMOTHERAPY AND BIOTHERAPY

Over the past two decades the MM treatment landscape has changed dramatically. Clinical trials have resulted in the development of novel agents and advances in diagnostic and prognostic procedures have led to risk modified therapies. These advances have resulted in improved patient outcomes. Currently, the FDA has approved nine therapeutic classes of drugs to treatment MM. These include immunomodulatory imide drugs (IMiDs), proteasome inhibitors, monoclonal antibodies, histone deacetylase inhibitors (HDACs), corticosteroids, chemotherapy, alkylating agents, nuclear export inhibitor, and anti-BCMA; antineoplastic agent, antibody drug conjugate. See Table 19.4 for chemotherapy/biotherapy agents used to treat MM.

Table 19.4 Chemotherapy/Biotherapy Agents Used to Treat Multiple Myeloma

Chemotherapy/Biotherapy	Indications	Route of Administration and Treatment Combinations
Immunomodulatory Imide Drugs		
Lenalidomide (Revlimid)	Newly diagnosed, relapsed, refractory	Oral VRD KRD
Pomalidomide (Pomalyst)	Relapsed, refractory	Oral Elo/Pom Dara/Pom
Thalidomide (Thalomid)	Newly diagnosed, relapsed, refractory	Oral VTD KTD
Proteasome Inhibitors		
Bortezomib (Velcade)	Newly diagnosed, relapsed, refractory	IV Sub Q VRD Velcacde +Panobinastat
Carfilzomib (Kyprolis)	Newly diagnosed, relapsed, refractory	IV KRD KCD
Ixazomib (Ninlaro)	Relapsed	Oral IRD
Monoclonal Antibodies		
Daratumumab (Darazelex) Daratumumab Hyaluronidase (Darzalex Faspro)	Newly diagnosed in transplant ineligible patients, relapsed, refractory	IV Sub Q Dara/Rev Dara/Pom
Elotuzumab (Empliciti)	Relapsed, refractory	IV Elo/Rev Elo/Pom
Isatuximab (Sarclisa)	Relapsed, refractory	IV Isa/Rev Isa/Pom
Belantamab Mafodotin Blen Rep	Relapsed, Refractory MM	IV Single Agent
Histone Deacetylase Inhibitors		
Panobinostat (Farydak)	Relapsed, refractory	Oral Velcade/Panobinistat

(continued)

Table 19.4 Chemotherapy/Biotherapy Agents Used to Treat Multiple Myeloma (*continued*)

Chemotherapy/Biotherapy	Indications	Route of Administration and Treatment Combinations
Chemotherapy		
Doxorubicin	In combination with ortezomib for patients who have not received Bortezomib and have received at least 1 prior line of therapy	IV VRDD
Alkylators		
Melphalan (Alkeran, Alphalan)	Newly diagnosed, relapsed, refractory	IV High Dose conditioning prior to stem cell transplant Oral for palliative treatment
Cyclophosphamide (Cytoxan)	Newly diagnosed, relapsed, refractory	IV and Oral VCD KCD

Source: https://www.cancer.gov/about-cancer/treatment/drugs

TARGETED THERAPY

Immunomodulators

Immunomodulators inhibit proliferation and induce apoptosis of certain hematopoietic tumor cells including multiple myeloma. Available through the FDA Risk Evaluation and Mitigation Strategy (REMS) program to prevent fetal exposure. REMS is a drug safety program that helps ensure the benefits of the medication outweigh the risks. Black box warnings for lenalidomide, pomalidomide, thalidomide include:

- Risk of venous thrombosis treat with anticoagulation therapy prophylactically
- Embryo-fetal toxicity; pregnancy test monthly for women of childbearing age
- Hematologic toxicity associated with Lenalidomide and Pomalidomide, monitor CBC

Proteasome Inhibitors

Proteasome Inhibitors block the action of proteasomes, which are cellular complexes that break down proteins. Key drug-specific considerations include:

- Bortezomib, Carfilzomib, Ixazomib: Acyclovir or Valacyclovir prophylaxis for the prevention of herpes zoster
- Bortezomib:
  - Monitor for peripheral neuropathy on every visit
  - Subcutaneous administration decreases the risk of developing peripheral neuropathy
  - Myelosuppression, particularly thrombocytopenia
- Carfilzomib
  - Monitor for cardiac and pulmonary toxicities especially in the elderly
  - Hydration prior to each dose of cycle 1
  - Monitor for tumor lysis syndrome during treatment
- IIxazomib
  - GI toxicity: Nausea, vomiting, diarrhea treat with antiemetic therapy
  - Rash

Monoclonal Antibodies

Monoclonal antibody therapy is a type of immunotherapy that targets plasma cell antigens. Elotuzamab is a humanized IgG1 immunostimulatory monoclonal antibody that targets signaling lymphocytic activation molecule family member 7 (SLAMF7) on myeloma cells and mediates antibody-dependent cellular cytotoxicity. Infusion reactions include chills, fatigue, fever, and cough; treat accordingly. Pre-medicate patients with antihistamines, antipyretics, and corticosteroids.

Daratumumab is an IgG1κ human monoclonal antibody that binds to CD38, a cell surface glycoprotein expressed on myeloma cells, inhibiting the growth of CD38-expressing tumor cells by inducing apoptosis. Infusion reactions also include chills, fatigue, fever, and cough; treat accordingly. Pre-medicate patients with antihistamines, antipyretics, and corticosteroids. Other key considerations:

- Myelosuppression: particularly neutropenia, monitor CBC.
- Interferes with serological testing resulting in false positive direct Coombs test.
- Re-activation of hepatitis B: test for hepatitis B before initiating treatment.
- Interferes with cross-matching and red blood cell antibody and red blood cell antibody screening. Draw type and screen prior to starting treatment.
- Interference with determination of complete response: It is a human IgG kappa monoclonal antibody and can be detected on both the serum protein electrophoresis (SPE) and immunofixation (IFE) assays used for the clinical monitoring of endogenous M-protein.

Isatuximab is an IgG1-derived human monoclonal antibody that binds to CD38, a cell surface glycoprotein expressed on myeloma cells, inhibiting the growth of CD38-expressing tumor cells by inducing apoptosis.

Infusion-related reactions include dyspnea, cough, chills, and nausea; treat accordingly. Pre-medicate patients prior to infusion with acetaminophen, H2 antagonists, diphenhydramine, or equivalent and dexamethasone. Most common severe signs and symptoms included hypertension and dyspnea. It interferes with cross-matching and red blood cell antibody and red blood cell antibody screening. Draw type and screen prior to starting treatment.

Histone Deacetylase Inhibitors

Histone deacetylase inhibitors inhibit enzymatic activity of HDACs resulting in increased acetylation of histone proteins which results in an accumulation of acetylated histones and other proteins inducing cell cycle arrest and apoptosis. Panobinostat carries the following boxed warnings:

- **Gastrointestinal events:** Severe diarrhea occurred in 25% of panobinostat-treated patients. Monitor for symptoms, institute antidiarrheal treatment, interrupt panobinostat, and then reduce dose or discontinue panobinostat.
- **Cardiovascular events:** Severe and fatal cardiac ischemic events, severe arrhythmias, and EKG changes have occurred in patients receiving panobinostat. Arrhythmias may be exacerbated by electrolyte abnormalities. Obtain EKG and electrolytes at baseline and periodically during treatment as clinically indicated.

Alkylators

Cyclophosphamide is an alkylating agent that prevents cell division by cross-linking DNA strands and decreasing DNA synthesis. It has the following boxed warnings:

- Carcinogenesis, mutagenesis, and impairment of fertility
- Second malignancies; most frequently, urinary bladder
- Myeloproliferative or lymphoproliferative malignancies
- Potential for fetal harm when administered to a pregnant woman
- Cyclophosphamide interferes with oogenesis and spermatogenesis

Anti-BCMA; Antineoplastic Agent; Antibody Drug Conjugate

Belantamab mafodotin is an anti-BCMA; antineoplastic agent, antibody drug conjugate. It has the following boxed warnings:

- Restricted access: Available only through the REMS program due to the risk of ocular toxicity. Corneal epithelium changes resulting in changes in vision, including severe vision loss and corneal ulcer, and symptoms, such as blurred vision and dry eyes.
- Conduct ophthalmic exams at baseline, prior to each dose, and promptly for worsening symptoms.
- Withhold belantamab mafodotin until improvement and resume, or permanently discontinue, based on severity.

COMMON COMPLICATIONS

▶ BONE DISEASE

Patients with lytic bone disease should receive bisphosphate therapy to reduce the risk of skeletal fractures. Obtaining baseline dental examination is strongly recommended prior to initiating therapy. While on therapy, patients should be assessed for osteonecrosis of the jaw and closely monitored for renal function. Patients who present with symptomatic vertebral compression fractures should be evaluated for kyphoplasty or vertebroplasty. Patients with bone disease should be monitored for hypercalcemia throughout all phases of therapy.

Diagnostic workup may include ionized calcium, an elevated creatinine from baseline, albumin, potassium, sodium, magnesium, complete blood count, echocardiogram, and multiple myeloma workup. Treatment options include calcitonin, hydration, and bisphosphonate therapy zoledronic acid or pomidronate, and denosumab.

▶ ANEMIA

There are several reasons why myeloma patients develop anemia; they include:

- Myeloma plasma cells suppress the microenvironment of the bone marrow
- Myeloma treatment
- Renal impairment
- Nutritional deficiencies (Niesvizky & Badros 2010).

Signs and symptoms of anemia include fatigue, shortness of breath, lightheadedness, dizziness or syncope, tachycardia, chest pain and pale skin. Treatments include erythropoiesis-stimulating agents (ESAs) and packed red blood cell transfusions.

▶ NEUTROPENIA

Patients with decreased neutrophils need to be monitored for fever, infection, and sepsis. Neutropenia in myeloma patients may be a result of the disease itself or treatment. Febrile neutropenia is defined as a single temperature of 38.3°C over 1 hour, neutropenia <500 mcL or <1000 neutrophils and a predicted decline to <500 neutrophils/mcL over the next 48 hours. Treatment may include colony stimulating growth factors such as filgrastim and pegfligrastim and anti-infectives including viral fungal and bacterial (https://www.nccn.org/professionals/physician_gls/pdf/growthfactors.pdf).

▶ INFECTION

MM patients have compromised immune systems which place them at greater risk for recurrent infections. To help prevent and decrease the frequency of infections NCCN guidelines recommend:

- Intravenous immunoglobulin therapy in the setting of recurrent infections
- Pneumococcal conjugate vaccine and polysaccharide vaccine one year later
- Herpes zoster to prevent shingles
- Antifungal prophylaxis in high dose dexamethasone regimens

▶ RENAL DISEASE AND VENOUS THROMBOSIS

National Comprehensive Cancer Network (NCCN) guidelines recommend supportive care measures for patients experiencing a decline in renal function including hydration, discontinuation of nephrotoxic medications, treatment of hypercalcemia, hyperuricemia other metabolic abnormalities, dialysis, and renal dosing of all medications.

Anticoagulation therapy is recommended by the NCCN for all patients treated with immunomodulatory-based therapy and for those at high risk for thrombosis.

▶ SUPPORTIVE CARE

MM patients from the time of diagnosis and throughout their disease course will require supportive care measures for bone disease, hypercalcemia, myelosuppression, renal disease, infections, and venous thrombosis.

⬤ ONCOLOGICAL EMERGENCIES

Patients presenting with acute signs and symptoms need immediate attention to prevent these events from becoming life-threatening; these include spinal cord compression, hypercalcemia, and renal failure. Multiple myeloma patients with bone disease are at risk for developing two significant oncological emergencies spinal cord compression (SCC) and hypercalcemia of malignancy (HOM). These emergencies can occur at diagnosis and at times of relapse.

● SURVIVORSHIP

Multiple myeloma is an incurable disease with a disease trajectory of multiple responses, remissions, and relapses. The plasma cell clone which emerges at each relapse will be different from the clonal plasma cell identified at diagnosis. With each relapse the remission duration becomes shorter until the disease becomes refractory. Patients receive continuous therapy until disease progression or unacceptable toxicities, and over time will be exposed to multiple lines of therapy. The use of novel agents in MM have improved overall survival rates in both newly diagnosed and relapsed myeloma patients transforming myeloma into a chronic disease.

These factors make survivorship and supportitve care both unique and challenging in myeloma patients. Survivorship starts at time of diagnosis with the goal of achieving a deep response with initial therapy, managing treatment toxicites and complications while maintaining quality of life. The evolution of myeloma into a chronic disease requires a intergrated approach with the hematologist/medical oncologist managing the disease and related complications and the primary care physician and subspecialities overseeing noncancer comorbidities. All disciplinces must partner with the patient in order to execute a seamless plan of care (Chakraborty, 2020).

The bibliography and references for this chapter are available on ExamPrepConnect; see inside front cover for access instructions.

1. The myeloma/clonal plasma cells produce an immunoglobulin/protein associated with the CRAB symptoms. CRAB stands for:

   A. Decrease in calcium and increase in phosphorous, decrease in renal function (renal insufficiency) increase in hemoglobin, and bone pain/lesion.

   B. Increase in calcium and decrease in phosphorous, increase in hemoglobin, and bone pain/lesion.

   C. Increase in calcium, decrease in renal function (renal insufficiency), decrease hemoglobin, and bone pain/lesion.

   D. Calcium within normal limits, renal function within normal limits, hemoglobin within normal limits and bone pain/lesion.

2. The International Staging System was revised in 2015 to include which two prognostic indicators?

   A. Myeloma mass and bone health

   B. M spike or M protein and hemoglobin

   C. Calcium and hemoglobin

   D. Serum lactate dehydrogenase (LDH) and high-risk chromosomal abnormalities acquired from the bone marrow biopsy

3. The International Myeloma Working Group revised the diagnostic criteria to include the SLIM biomarkers of malignancy for a diagnosis of MM. Which biomarker is required for the diagnosis of multiple myeloma?

   A. Uninvolved:involved serum free light chain ratio ≥60

   B. Clonal bone marrow plasma cell percentage ≥60%

   C. Magnetic resonance imaging studies >5 focal lesions

   D. Involved:uninvolved serum free light chain ratio ≥60

4. Which treatment medications interfere with cross-matching and red blood cell antibody and red blood cell antibody screening and require a type and screen drawn prior to initiating treatment?

   A. Elotuzumab and daratumumab

   B. Daratumumab and isatuximab-Irfc

   C. Elotuzumab and isatuximab-Irfc

   D. Daratumumab and ixazomib

5. Which of the following CRAB symptoms is the most common symptom present when multiple myeloma is diagnosed?

   A. Bone pain

   B. Fatigue

   C. Neuropathy

   D. Anemia

(See answers next page.)
  245

1. C) Increase in calcium, decrease in renal function (renal insufficiency), decrease hemoglobin, and bone pain/lesion

CRAB is an acronym for: **C**alcium elevation from bone disease, **R**enaldysfunction, **A**nemia, and **B**one pain/lesion.

2. D) Serum lactate dehydrogenase (LDH) and high-risk chromosomal abnormalities acquired from the bone marrow biopsy

The ISS Revised Staging System is a simple and reliable prognostic staging system that stratifies MM patients using LDH and high-risk chromosomal abnormalities which helps guide risk adapted treatment. It was revised in 2015 to include serum lactate dehydrogenase (LDH) and high-risk chromosomal abnormalities acquired from the bone marrow biopsy.

3. B) Clonal bone marrow plasma cell percentage ≥60%

According to the International Myeloma Working Group revised criteria, clonal bone marrow plasma cell percentage ≥60% is required for the diagnosis of MM.

4. B) Daratumumb and isatuximab

Daratumumb and isatuximab monoclonal antibodies that interfere with cross-matching and red blood cell antibody and red blood cell antibody screening and require a type and screen drawn prior to initiating treatment.

5. D) Anemia

At time of diagnosis, approximately 73% of patients present with symptoms of anemia, 67% present with symptoms of bone pain, and 32% present with fatigue or generalized weakness. Neuropathy is not a common presenting symptom.

Part IV
Symptom Management and Oncologic Emergencies

Integumentary Side Effects

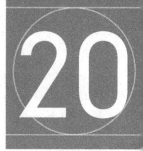

INTRODUCTION

Integumentary side-effect profiles can vary greatly due to the variety of treatment options. Chemotherapy and biotherapy agents cause systemic reactions, while radiation side effects are localized to the area irradiated and the surrounding tissue. This chapter discusses the most common integumentary side effects from chemotherapy/biotherapy and radiation, as well as recommended treatment options.

> **EXAM TIP**
>
> To reduce the chance of missing a potential skin side effect, think about side effects from the head-to-toe assessment perspective.

ALOPECIA

Alopecia is hair loss related to chemotherapy and radiation therapy. Chemotherapy targets rapidly growing cells; hair follicles are rapidly growing cells, so they are usually the first to be damaged. Hair loss occurs within 7 to 14 days after receiving or being exposed to the causative agent. Total body irradiation can also contribute to hair loss, as well as radiation for primary brain tumors. Regrowth of hair typically occurs 3 to 6 months after chemotherapy and radiation are completed.

There are no treatment options for alopecia; however, breast cancer patients can use scalp hypothermia (scalp cooling or cold caps) to reduce or prevent hair loss from chemotherapy agents. Keeping the scalp cold reduces damage to the hair follicles during chemotherapy administration. Scalp hypothermia is not recommended with liquid malignancies as it increases the risk for scalp metastasis. Patients should be educated about this potential risk.

▶ NURSING CARE RECOMMENDATIONS

Nursing care recommendations include:

- Instruct patients to keep their heads covered to retain warmth during the winter months.
- Instruct patients to keep their heads covered to protect the scalp from the sun.
- Promote good body hygiene and avoid micro-organisms.
- Provide emotional support, active listening, and resources on how to cope with hair loss.

The bibliography and references for this chapter are available on ExamPrepConnect; see inside front cover for access instructions.

GINGIVAL HYPERPLASIA

Gingival hyperplasia is a condition that is manifested by the overgrowth of the gum tissue over and around the teeth. It is a side effect of acute myeloid leukemia (AML) and chemotherapy agents. There are two methods to surgical remove excessive gum tissue: laser surgery and gingivectomy. Treatment includes:

- Dental treatments: Deep cleaning to remove plaque and bacteria scaling and planing, ultrasonic treatments, medicated mouthwashes
- Systematic antibiotics: Azithromycin or erythromycin

NAIL CHANGES

Chemotherapy-related nail and toenail changes can be unsightly, cause pain, inhibit activities of daily living, and be a vehicle for infection. The nail changes are related to the alteration in the nail matrix. Like hair regrowth, once the causative agent is stopped, the nails will return to normal. Table 20.1 identifies the chemotherapy and biotherapy agents that can cause common nail changes. Treatment for nail changes includes topical and oral antibiotics for infections, topical and oral antifungals, and pain medications when indicated.

▶ NURSING CARE RECOMMENDATIONS

Nursing care recommendations include:

- Avoid visiting a manicurist while receiving cancer treatment.
- Examine nails and toenails daily.
- Keep nails and toenails clean and short.
- Use a water-soluble nail lacquer to protect and strengthen nails.

Table 20.1 Chemotherapy and Biotherapy Agents That Cause Nail Changes

Nail Changes	Causative Chemotherapy and Biotherapy Agents
Beau's lines: Transverse lines and indents of the nail	Cyclophosphamide, doxorubicin, docetaxel, hydroxyurea, idarubicin, ifosfamide, 5-fluorouracil
Hyperpigmentation: Change in the color/pigment of the nail bed	Cetuximab and panitumumab, bleomycin, capecitabine, cyclophosphamide, dacarbazine, daunorubicin, doxorubicin, erlotinib and gefitinib, idarubicin, melphalan, methotrexate
Onycholysis: Detachment of the nail from the nail bed; usually does not cause pain	Dacarbazine, daunorubicin, everolimus and temsirolimus, mitoxantrone
Paronychia: Inflammation of the nail bed that can lead to infection of the nail and nail bed	Cetuximab, dacomitinib, doxorubicin, docetaxel, erlotinib, everolimu and temsirolimus, gefitinib, nab-paclitaxel, necitumumab, paclitaxel, panitumumab
Splinter hemorrhage: Tiny red lines that represent bleeding under the nail	Docetaxel, doxorubicin, nab-paclitaxel, paclitaxel
Fissures: Breaks in the nail and nail bed; extremely painful and lead to an infectious process	Targeted therapy or immunotherapy monoclonal antibodies (cetuximab, panitumumab)

⬤ SKIN REACTIONS

Biotherapy, chemotherapy, and radiation therapies can cause a variety of skin reactions, which can be localized or acute systemic episodes. Occasionally, the reactions can be associated with a life-threatening event such as anaphylactic reactions. Common reactions include hyperpigmentation and photosensitivity.

A patient with **hyperpigmentation** will present with darkening of the gums, skin, and/or nails. It is commonly caused by chemotherapy agents and typically occurs within 2 to 3 weeks of initiation of chemotherapy and dissipates between 10 and 12 weeks after stopping the chemotherapy agent. There is no treatment for the skin reaction except to educate the patient that darkening of the skin may occur and that it will resolve when agents are completed. Causative agents include busulfan, cyclophosphamide, cisplatin, 5FU (can also cause darkening of the veins), ifosfamide, thiotepa, docetaxel, and etoposide.

▶ CHEMOTHERAPY-INDUCED SKIN REACTIONS

Photosensitivity is an increased response of the skin when it is exposed to sunlight. **Phototoxic reactions** can occur when a patient is exposed to sunlight after chemotherapy administration. They will present with a severe sunburn with redness, edema, blistering, peeling, and pain. A **photoallergic reaction** is similar to a phototoxic reaction; however, it extends beyond the skin that was directly exposed to the sunlight. A **UV recall reaction** occurs in skin that was previously damaged by sunburn within a week of chemotherapy or administration. When chemotherapy is administered, the sunburn is reactivated in the area that was originally exposed. Depending on the severity, it would be treated as a burn: topical steroids, nonsteroid creams such as silver sulfadiazine, barrier protectors in some cases, pain medications in severe cases.

NURSING CARE RECOMMENDATIONS

Prevention is a key factor that requires detailed patient education:

- Avoid sunlight when receiving chemotherapy.
- Wear protective clothing while outside, especially during the summer months.
- Use daily sunscreen, especially on exposed skin.
- Avoid tanning salons.

▶ RADIATION-INDUCED SKIN REACTIONS

Radiation-induced skin reactions (RISR), or radiation dermatitis, are localized reactions isolated to irradiated areas. They occur days to weeks post radiation therapy. Risk factors include inadequate nutritional status, history of skin disorders, use of skin creams prior to radiation therapy, obesity, history of repeated radiation exposure, and doses of radiation therapy greater than 55 Gy (total dose). RISR is subcategorized as acute or chronic. Acute RISR occurs post radiation and causes redness, tenderness, pain, and, in severe cases, tissue necrosis. Chronic RISR causes long-term damage to the skin, including thinning, scarring, sensitivity, telangiectasia, and pain. There are four grades of acute RISR:

- **Grade 1:** Initial redness and/or desquamation
- **Grade 2:** Increased swelling, erythema, and sometimes patches found in skin folds with moist desquamation
- **Grade 3:** Significant swelling (including pitting edema) and moist desquamation not limited to skin folds
- **Grade 4:** Development of skin necrosis

Treatment, which is based on the grade of dermatitis, includes topical steroids, nonsteroid creams such as silver sulfadiazine, barrier protectors in some cases, and pain medications in severe cases.

Radiation recall reactions are localized skin reactions that occur post radiation and is manifested by the use of chemotherapy agents. Patients present with redness that resembles a sunburn and can progress to necrosis, ulceration, and/or bleeding. The most common treatment is topical steroids.

NURSING CARE RECOMMENDATIONS

Nursing care recommendations include:

1. Practice excellent hygiene.
2. Wash the affected area with soap and water.
3. Avoid perfumes and scented lotions.
4. Avoid sunlight and tanning salons.

▶ RASHES

HAND AND FOOT SYNDROME

Hand and foot syndrome, or palmer-plantar erythrodysesthesia, is the capillary leakage of a drug, which leads to an inflammatory response. Signs and symptoms include red swollen palms and soles of the feet, dryness, sloughing, and blistering of the skin, and pain, numbness, and tingling. Causative chemotherapy agents include cytarabine, doxorubicin, 5FU, and capecitabine. Causative biotherapy agents include axitinib, cabozantinib, sorafenib, pazopanib, and regorafenib.

Treatment includes the application of ice packs to hands and feet for 15- to 20-minute intervals; emollients such as Aveeno, Lubriderm, Udder Cream, Bag Balm, steroids in severe cases, antibiotics with secondary infection of skin, and pain medications as needed.

Nursing Care Recommendations

Prevention is highly recommended to avoid complications such as the inability to perform daily activities. Patients should be encouraged to:

- Keep the skin clean, moist, and intact.
- Reduce friction and heat exposure.
- Avoid hot showers and baths, washing dishes in hot water, aerobics and aggressive exercise, and the use of gardening tools, screwdrivers, or any other tools or tasks that require the squeezing motion of the hands on a hard surface. In addition, avoid chopping foods with a knife that can increase pressure.

- Wear comfortable cotton socks, supportive cushions in shoes, and cotton gloves for shopping, gardening, and activities of daily living.
- Apply daily moisturizer.
- Avoid scratching affected areas.

ACNEIFORM RASH

Acneiform rash, or epidermal dermal growth factor (EFRGI) rash, occurs in the majority of patients who receive targeted therapy with epidermal growth factor medications. Several weeks after therapy, patients will present with pruritic, acne-like nodules, papules, pustules, and/or cysts in the head, face, and trunk. Causative agents include cetuximab, panitumumab, erlotinib, and gefitinib. It is treated with antibiotics (tetracycline, minocycline, or doxycycline) and topical steroids.

Nursing Care Recommendations

Patients should be educated regarding the risk for rash and be encouraged to follow the following recommendations:

- Keep skin clean and avoid harsh soaps.
- Do not scratch or pick at pustules, nodules, or cysts.
- Avoid contact with harsh cleaning chemicals.
- Use daily fragrance-free moisturizers.
- Avoid long hot showers or baths.

HYPERSENSITIVITY REACTIONS

A hypersensitivity reaction, or allergic reaction, results from an overactive immune response to the foreign agent. There are four types of hypersensitivity reactions:

1. **Type 1 reaction:** Acute-onset allergic reaction that can manifest within minutes. Anaphylaxis is a potentially life-threatening type 1 reaction. Signs and symptoms include facial flushing, hives, itching, shortness of breath, chest pain, and swelling (angioedema). Reactions can be caused by chemotherapy (Taxanes, L-Asparaginas, Bleomycin) and biotherapy agents (monoclonal antibodies).
2. **Type 2 reaction:** Acute immune response caused by a reaction to an antibody. Examples include hemolytic anemia and blood and platelet transfusion reactions.
3. **Type 3 reaction:** A systemic reaction that occurs hours to days after the immune system has been triggered. Examples include serum sickness, systemic lupus erythematosus, and immune-complex glomerulonephritis.
4. **Type 4 reaction:** Delayed responses that occur several days after the exposure. Examples include contact dermatitis and organ-transplant rejection.

Pre-medications may be ordered to reduce the immune response, including antihistamines, such as Benadryl, Claritin, and Pepcid (to target the GI receptors); steroids, such as hydrocortisone (systemic), solumedrol (systemic), and beclovent (inhaled); and bronchodilators, such as albuterol and epinephrine, which can be used in life-threatening events.

EXTRAVASATIONS

Extravasations are a complication of chemotherapy administration, specifically vesicants, which are highly caustic to the vein and can cause damage to the surrounding tissue, leading to decreased function and potentially necrosis. The risk of extravasations is increased when agents are administered via the peripheral route (PIV); however, central line (CIV) extravasations can also occur. Signs and symptoms include loss of blood return, pain, redness, swelling, burning, and any visible changes at the injection site (PIV or CVC). If extravasation is suspected, the following steps should be taken:

1. Stop infusion immediately and leave the needle (either Huber needle or Angio catheter) in place.
2. Aspirate residual agent.
3. Administer antidote to the causative agent if appropriate.
4. Remove needle.
5. Apply a cold or warm compress, depending on the causative agent.
6. Notify healthcare providers and follow organizational policy and procedure.
7. Provide patient education.

Treatment is dependent upon the causative agent. See Table 20.2 for recommended treatment for extravasations.

Table 20.2 Recommended Treatment for Extravasations

Causative Chemotherapy Agents	Warm or Cold Compress	Antidote
Alkylating Agents* Nitrogen mustards: Chlorambucil, cyclophosphamide, ifosfamide, melphalan Nitrosoureas: Carmustine, lomustine, streptozocin Alkyl sulfonates: Busulfan Triazines: Dacarbazine Ethylenimines: Thiotepa	Cold compress	Sodium thiosulfate
Antitumor Antibiotics (Vesicants) Anthracycline: Doxorubicin, daunorubicin, epirubicin Miscellaneous: Mitoxantrone, bleomycin	Cold compress	Dexrazoxane for 3 days (anthracyclines)
Taxanes (Plant Alkaloids) Paclitaxel, docetaxel	Cold compress	Hyaluronidase
Vinca Alkaloids (Vesicants) Vinblastine, vinorelbine, vincristine	Warm compress	Hyaluronidase

*First chemotherapy agents developed.

The bibliography and references for this chapter are available on ExamPrepConnect; see inside front cover for access instructions.

1. The nurse suspects that a patient has an extravasation. The nurse's INITIAL action is to:

   A. Immediately stop the infusion and remove the needle
   B. Administer an antidote
   C. Immediately stop the infusion and keep the needle
   D. Apply warm compresses

2. Paclitaxel can cause which type of hypersensitivity reaction?

   A. Type 1
   B. Type 2
   C. Type 3
   D. Type 4

3. All of the following nursing care considerations should be included in the patient education package for a patient receiving concomitant chemotherapy and radiation therapy, EXCEPT:

   A. Restrict fluid intake
   B. Avoid sunlight
   C. Wear daily sunscreen
   D. Wear protective clothing

4. Which of the following agents has the highest risk of causing hand and foot syndrome?

   A. Cisplatin
   B. Cyclophosphamide
   C. Capecitabine
   D. Cetuximab

5. The first-line treatment for a patient experiencing photoallergic reactions is:

   A. Systemic antibiotics
   B. Systemic steroids
   C. Topical steroids
   D. Topical antibiotics

1. C) Immediately stop the infusion and keep the needle

When extravasation is suspected, the nurse should immediately stop the infusion and keep the needle. Administering antidote depends on the agent being administered. Not all agents require warm compresses; the majority require cold compresses.

2. A) Type 1

Paclitaxel cau type 1 allergic/hypersensitivity reaction. It is an acute-onset allergic reaction that can manifest within minutes. Signs and symptoms include facial flushing, hives, itching, shortness of breath, chest pain, and swelling (angioedema). Reactions can be caused by chemotherapy (taxanes such as paclitaxel, L-Asparaginas, Bleomycin) and biotherapy agents (monoclonal antibodies).

3. A) Restrict fluid intake

A patient receiving concomitant chemotherapy and radiation therapy should be advised to avoid sunlight and wear daily sunscreen and protective clothing. A patient receiving chemotherapy and radiation therapy should increase fluid intake (not restrict) to flush the chemotherapy from the system and improve kidney function.

4. C) Capecitabine

Capecitabine causes hand and foot syndrome. Cisplatin causes kidney toxicity, cyclophosphamide causes hemorrhagic cystitis, and cetuximab causes acneiform rashes.

5. C) Topical steroids

Topical steroids are the first-line treatment for photoallergic reactions. Systematic therapy is used for other skin reactions, such as hypersensitivity reactions.

Hematologic Side Effects

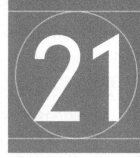

INTRODUCTION

Cancer treatments can cause a variety of significant side effects. One of the most serious and common effects is hematologic dysfunction. This chapter discusses the expected side effects from chemotherapy, radiation, and biotherapy agents, which include myelosuppression, neutropenia, anemia, and thrombocytopenia.

MYELOSUPPRESSION

Myelosuppression, also known as bone marrow suppression, is a condition where there is a significant decrease in activity in the bone marrow, which results in fewer blood cells being produced. Cytopenia is a condition in which the number of blood cells is lower than normal. Myelosuppression and cytopenia are side effects of cancer treatments, such as chemotherapy and radiation therapy. These agents are responsible for causing direct damage to the stem cells. Myelosuppression can also be due to crowding in the bone marrow, which is a result of the growth of the tumor in relationship to cancers that involve the bone marrow, such as leukemia and lymphomas. Bone marrow failure is another reason for myelosuppression, which is driven by the inability of the bone marrow to adequately recover from extensive doses of chemotherapy, radiation, and/or from bone marrow or stem cell transplantation.

NEUTROPENIA

Neutropenia is defined as the decreased level of neutrophils in circulation. Neutrophils are a type of WBCs that form from the stem cells in the bone marrow and act as the first line of defense against infections, ingesting microorganisms, bacteria, and other organisms. When a patient receives cancer treatment, the neutrophils can become depleted, and the ability to fight inflammation or infections can be significantly compromised.

The best method to determine if the body is producing an adequate number of neutrophils is to monitor the absolute neutrophil count (ANC), which is the number of circulating neutrophils and is essential for assessing the patient's risk of infection and grading the level of neutropenia. In the clinical setting, there is a formula to calculate the patient's ANC. In some instances, specific laboratories and organizations will have the ANC already calculated; however, oncology nurses should not rely on these measures for safety.

The bibliography and references for this chapter are available on ExamPrepConnect; see inside front cover for access instructions.

> ▶ **EXAM TIP**
>
> Understanding how to calculate the ANC formula will be important when answering questions regarding neutropenic patients.
>
> Total WBC count × (% neutrophils + % bands) = ANC
>
> Example: Total WBC count of patient is 3.0 = 3,000; segs = 30%; bands = 10%
>
> 3,000 × (.30 + .10) = ANC
>
> 3,000 × .40 = 1,200
>
> ANC = 1,200 or read as 1.2

▶ GRADING OF NEUTROPENIA

The grading system for neutropenia is based upon the degree or severity of the risk of an infection process. Neutropenia can be gauged depending on the nadir, the time point at which the white blood count falls to its lowest level after chemotherapy treatment. The nadir depends on the specific cytotoxic agents and the dosages administered to the patient. For example, carmustine has a delayed nadir up to 6 weeks after administration, while doxorubicin causes a nadir within 10 to 14 days after administration. Neutropenia usually occurs approximately 8 to 12 days after having received a chemotherapy treatment and resolves about 21 to 28 days after completion of treatment. The lower the ANC, the higher the risk for infection:

- ANC 1,500/mcL to lower level of normal: No risk (Grade 1)
- ANC 1,000–1,500/mcL: Mild risk (Grade 2)
- ANC 500–1,000/mcL: Moderate risk (Grade 3)
- ANC <500mcL: High risk (Grade 4)

▶ CAUSES OF NEUTROPENIA

Neutropenia can be caused by chemotherapy, radiation therapy, and immunotherapy, as well as bone marrow or stem cell transplantation. Certain chemotherapy agents can cause damage to the bone marrow resulting in decreased production of neutrophils as well as obliterating existing mature neutrophils in the circulation. Chemotherapy-induced neutropenia (CIN) is associated with systemic chemotherapy treatments and is a dose-limiting toxicity that may be life-threatening and result in delays in treatment, affecting survival rates. Radiation therapy to areas such as the pelvis, ribs, sternum, spine, and legs can also suppress bone marrow function and cause neutropenia. Blood malignancies such as leukemias and lymphomas can crowd the bone marrow with malignant cells and impede normal function.

▶ RISK FACTORS

There are many risk factors that are related to neutropenia, including age >65 years, cancer in advanced stages, poor performance or nutritional status, gastrointestinal mucosal compromise, prolonged or high-dose corticosteroid therapy, history of neutropenia, dose-intensive chemotherapy with cell cycle-specific agents (e.g., antimetabolites), dose-dense chemotherapy, chemotherapy regimens that include cell cycle-nonspecific agents (e.g., alkylating agents, nitrosoureas), and hematologic malignancies (e.g., leukemia, lymphoma, multiple myeloma, myelodysplastic syndrome).

▶ SIGNS AND SYMPTOMS

Neutropenia, per se, does not present with any specific set of signs or symptoms. It can only be detected via a CBC. A neutropenic patient will be more susceptible to developing an infection that can quickly become profoundly serious or life-threatening, leading to sepsis, septic shock, and death. Signs of infection that should be identified and immediately acted upon include fever greater than 100.5°F, chills, sweats, cough or difficulty breathing, sore throat, new-onset pain, and unexplained redness, swelling, or pain at the site of a wound or catheter.

▶ TREATMENT

Neutropenia can be prevented by including the use of granulocyte-colony stimulating factors (G-CSF) in the patient's treatment plan as supportive therapy. G-CSF is used when a patient has experienced febrile neutropenia, is at high risk for developing febrile neutropenia (FN), or is receiving dose-dense chemotherapy (Marrs, 2006). G-CSF such as filgrastim (Neupogen) or pegfilgrastim (Neulasta) are biologic response modifiers used to stimulate the production of granulocytes and stem cells. Both filgrastim and pegfilgrastim bind to receptors on the surface of stem cells, thus stimulating the hematopoiesis of neutrophils. These cells are then released into the bloodstream, where they mature even further and become active. Because the potential sensitivity of rapidly dividing myeloid cells to cytotoxic agents and the simultaneous use of G-CSF has not been established, G-CSF should not be administered within 24 hours before the start of chemotherapy treatment or within 24 hours after completing chemotherapy (AMGEN, 2016).

Filgrastim is administered via intravenous infusion or subcutaneous injection daily for multiple days because of its half-life of 3.5 hours, whereas pegfilgrastim has a much longer half-life of 15 to 80 hours due to the polyethylene glycol (PEG) molecule attached, thus eliminating the need for daily dosing (Quirion, 2009).

Pegfilgrastim is administered only subcutaneously by manual injection or via a delivery system called an on-body injector (Neulasta Onpro). The device is applied to the patient's arm or abdomen on the day of chemotherapy treatment and set by an automatic timer to release the pegfilgrastim 27 hours after application onto the patient. The device is then removed by the patient after the 28th hour upon completed delivery of the pegfilgrastim. This novel delivery system eliminates the need for the patient to return to the clinic the day after treatment for pegfilgrastim via manual injection by the nurse.

Various biosimilars are now available on the market that can be prescribed to treat or prevent neutropenia. Biosimilars are biologic products similar to an already existing and approved biologic medication. Overall, biosimilars have a similar structure, size, and function as the reference drug. They can also be a more affordable alternative. They are all administered by subcutaneous injection.

G-CSF are extremely helpful in combating neutropenia. However, all medications have side effect profiles which are important to include in patient eduation. The most common side effects of G-CSF include bone pain due to increased activity within the bone marrow (sternal bone pain may feel like chest pain), low-grade, arthralgia, myalgia, nausea, rash, headache, irritation at the injection site, cough, and shortness of breath. Severe reactions include splenomegaly or splenic rupture, acute respiratory distress syndrome (ARDS), severe sickle cell crisis in sickle cell patients, capillary leak syndrome, and allergic reaction/hypersensitivity/anaphylaxis.

Granulocyte macrophage-colony-stimulating factor (GM-CSF) such as sargramostim (Leukine) may also be used and is administered intravenously or subcutaneously. GM-CSF should also not be administered within 24 hours before the start of chemotherapy treatment or within 24 hours after completing chemotherapy. The most common side effects of GM-CSF include fever, bone pain, myalgia, arthralgia, headache, alteration in blood pressure, tachycardia, facial flushing, lightheadedness, irritation at the injection site, fatigue, rash, nausea, and diarrhea. Severe reactions include hypersensitivity/anaphylaxis, infusion-related reactions, effusions including pleural or pericardial, edema, capillary leak syndrome, supraventricular arrhythmias, and leukocytosis.

FEBRILE NEUTROPENIA

Febrile neutropenia (FN) is defined as a fever associated with a temperature higher than 101°F and lasting longer than 1 hour in the presence of grade 3 or higher neutropenia (ANC of <1000/mcL). FN is the main cause of hospital admissions for chemotherapy patients and can result in treatment delays and/or dose reductions of chemotherapy, thus compromising the efficacy of the treatment.

FN places the patient at an extreme risk for systemic infection, which can easily progress to sepsis, septic shock, and even death. Therefore, it is imperative that the severely neutropenic patient receives treatment with broad-spectrum antibiotics immediately, within 1 hour of spiking a temperature, to reduce their risk for septic shock. A review of the patient's allergies to antibiotics must be performed prior to administration. Patients who are at high risk for complications of FN may be placed on prophylactic antibiotics and antifungals. Occasionally, the neutropenic patient may not manifest the most common signs and symptoms of infection (such as redness, swelling, pus) due to the low neutrophil count not triggering a normal inflammatory response by the body.

▶ NURSING INTERVENTIONS

Hand hygiene is paramount in caring for the oncology patient and is the most effective measure in infection control and prevention, especially before eating and after using the bathroom. This should always be emphasized to patients and caregivers. The nurse should also provide the patient and caregiver education on FN and on all interventions being performed. In addition, the nurse should:

1. Review the patient's allergies, past medical history, and medications.
2. Perform a rapid and full physical assessment, including all catheter sites. Report immediately if the patient has rigors, chills, clammy or sweaty skin, altered mental status, redness, swelling, pain, pus at catheter sites, wounds, or in any area.
3. Monitor vital signs and report immediately if the patient is hypotensive, febrile, tachycardic, tachypneic.
4. Establish IV access and obtain blood work as ordered, including CBC with differential, comprehensive metabolic panel (CMP), and C-reactive protein (CRP) (an elevated level may indicate the presence of infection or inflammation).
5. Obtain two sets of blood cultures from different sites.
   a. If the patient does not have a central venous access device (VAD), then the patient should be venipunctured twice, once for each set of blood cultures.

    b. If the patient has a central VAD, then one set should be drawn from the device without initially flushing the VAD to prevent further entry of possible colonized bacteria in the VAD. The other set should be collected peripherally via venipuncture.

    *The presence of a central VAD or other foreign body always places the patient at risk for infection.

  6. Collect a urine sample for analysis and culture to rule out a urinary tract infection.

  7. Collect a stool sample if diarrhea is present to rule out gastrointestinal pathogens and *Clostridium difficile.*

  8. Collect a nasal or throat swab, sputum for culture if respiratory symptoms are present.

  9. Collect viral cultures from ulcerated skin lesions if present.

10. Swab the VAD site for culture if inflammation is present.

11. Obtain a chest x-ray to rule out any respiratory infection.

12. Admit the patient to the hospital or transfer the patient to the intensive care unit if indicated (Wilson, 2019).

▶ TREATMENT

After all cultures have been collected, promptly administer intravenous empiric broad-spectrum antibiotics, antipyretics, and CSFs if ordered. Oncology nurses play a key role in educating oncology patients and their caregivers on how to minimize their risk for infection. The nurse should educate that patient on the signs and symptoms of infection; the importance of effective hygiene including handwashing, oral, personal (bathing daily), and perineal (wiping from front to back after toileting); and side effects of CSFs. The nurse should instruct the patient to (Marrs, 2006):

- Avoid crowded places and people who may have a cold or flu
- Maintain a bowel regimen with stool softeners to avoid constipation
- Avoid suppositories and enemas
- Wash fruits and vegetables thoroughly
- Eat meat that is thoroughly cooked
- Avoid handling pet excrement
- Avoid fresh flowers or plants

Neutropenia must be managed properly to prevent delays in treatment, negative patient outcomes, as well as reduced quality of life. Nurses need to understand that FN can increase the morbidity and mortality rate and requires prompt treatment. Nurses have the responsibility to educate patients and their caregivers not only on the side effects of the cancer treatment but also the risks, signs, and symptoms of infection, as well as neutropenic precautions.

● ANEMIA

Anemia is defined as the decreased level of red blood cells (RBCs or erythrocytes) or the hemoglobin (Hgb). RBCs are the most common type of blood cell in the human body and are the primary means by which oxygen is delivered to all the organs and tissues via the circulatory system. There are several components to the RBC, which serve important functions and include:

■ **Hemoglobin (Hgb):** The iron-containing protein within the RBC responsible for transporting oxygen from the lungs to organs and tissues within the body and transporting carbon dioxide from the organs and tissues back to the lungs. Iron is necessary to produce hemoglobin.

■ **Hematocrit (hct):** The proportion of RBCs to plasma in the blood and is expressed in percentage. The hematocrit value is usually three times greater than the hemoglobin value.

■ **Reticulocytes (retic):** Circulating immature RBCs newly released from the bone marrow. The reticulocyte count may be ordered when working up or treating a patient for certain types of anemia, such as iron deficiency anemia or hemolytic anemia. Normal levels for the reticulocyte count are 0.5% to 1.5%.

■ **Mean corpuscular volume (MCV):** Measurement of the average size of RBCs. The larger the RBC size, the higher the MCV value will be and vice versa.

■ **Mean corpuscular hemoglobin (MCH):** The amount of hemoglobin in a typical RBC. RBCs that contain more hemoglobin will have a higher MCH and vice versa.

■ **Mean corpuscular hemoglobin concentration (MCHC):** The concentration of hemoglobin per RBC (or MCH) as compared to the average size of the RBC (or MCV).

■ **Red cell distribution width (RDW):** This measurement reflects the size of the smallest RBC as well as the size of the largest RBC.

See Table 21.1 for the reference ranges of the components of the RBC in a CBC.

Table 21.1 References Ranges for Red Blood Cells, Hemoglobin, and Hematocrit in a CBC

CBC Component	Reference Ranges
Red blood cell (RBC) count	Male: 4.7–6.1 trillion cells/L (4.7–6.1 million cells/mcL) Female: 4.2–5.4 trillion cells/L (4.2–5.4 million cells/mcL)
Hemoglobin (Hgb)	Male: 14.0–18.0 g/dL (140–180 g/L) Female: 12.0–16.0 g/dL (120–160 g/L)
Hematocrit (Hct)	Male: 42.0–52.0% Female: 37.0–47.0%
Mean corpuscular volume (MCV)	80.0–90.0 fL
Mean corpuscular hemoglobin (MCH)	27.0–31.0 pg
Mean corpuscular hemoglobin concentration (MCHC)	32.0–36.0 g/dL
Red cell distribution width (RDW)	11.5–15.5%

▶ **KEY FACT**

All of these values in the CBC may be low in the patient with anemia and increased in the patient with dehydration.

▶ CAUSES OF ANEMIA

Anemia in adults is defined as a hemoglobin level <11 g/dL. There are numerous causes of anemia which include decreased RBC production (e.g., bone marrow suppression, renal failure), increased RBC destruction (e.g., chemotherapy), inadequate levels of EPO from compromised EPO production and stimulation, kidney disease/kidney dysfunction due to nephrotoxic chemotherapy agents or radiation therapy, loss of blood or hemorrhaging, genetic disorders (e.g., thalassemia, sickle cell anemia), deficiencies in iron, vitamin B12, or folate, and hypothyroidism. Grading and assessing the risk of anemia is essential for treatment planning of this patient population:

- Grade 1: Mild anemia: Hgb 10 g/dL to lower level of normal
- Grade 2: Moderate anemia: Hgb 8–10 g/dL
- Grade 3: Severe anemia: Hgb 8 g/dL or lower
- Grade 4: Life-threatening anemia: Requires immediate medical attention

▶ TYPES OF ANEMIA

The types of anemia include:

1. Vitamin deficiency anemia: It is caused by low levels of folic acid, vitamin B12, and vitamin C needed for RBC production. Pernicious anemia may occur when vitamin B12 is not absorbed by the gastrointestinal tract. Macrocytic anemia is most often caused by vitamin B12 and/or folate deficiency.
2. Aplastic anemia (AA): Disorder of the bone marrow in which the bone marrow is unable to produce RBCs due to insufficient stem cells.
3. Hemolytic anemia: It may be genetic or caused by autoimmune disorders, infection, hypersplenism, or heart valvular dysfunction.
4. Sickle-cell anemia: Hereditary disease in which the RBCs are sickle-shaped due to abnormal hemoglobin, which leads to vascular obstruction, decreased blood flow throughout the body causing swelling, and episodes of excruciating pain called sickle cell crises.
5. Thalassemia: A hereditary blood disorder in which there are mutations in the DNA of cells that produce hemoglobin, causing the body to produce abnormal forms or insufficient amounts of hemoglobin.
6. Iron-deficiency anemia: The reticulocyte count may be low (hypoproliferative state) due to inadequate amounts of iron, B12, or folate available in the body to produce RBCs, or there may be bone marrow disease such as leukemia or aplastic anemia or high (hyperproliferative state) caused by hemolytic anemia, hemorrhaging, blood transfusions.

Anemia is confirmed with an iron panel; see Table 21.2 for components and normal reference ranges:

Table 21.2 Iron Panel Components and Their Reference Ranges

Iron Panel Component	Reference Ranges
Serum iron (SI)	Adult male: 59–158 mcg/dL Adult female: 37–145 mcg/dL
Ferritin	Adult male: 12–300 ng/mL Adult female: 12–150 ng/mL
Transferrin	200–360 mg/dL
Total iron-binding capacity (TIBC)	45–72 µmol/L TIBC = UIBC + SI
% saturation (transferrin saturation)	Males: 20–50% Females: 15–50%
Unsaturated iron-binding capacity (UIBC)	Males: 12–43 µmol/L Females: 13–56 µmol/L

▶ IRON-DEFICIENCY ANEMIA

Iron deficiency occurs when the body slowly depletes its iron stores resulting in inadequate amounts of hemoglobin which in turn leads to insufficient oxygen being transported throughout the body. The body then compensates by accelerating transferrin production to increase the transport of iron. This leads to the production of fewer and smaller RBCs which can eventually result in iron deficiency anemia. In this case, the serum iron, ferritin, % saturation levels will decrease, while the transferrin, TIBC, and UIBC levels increase. This may also be present during pregnancy.

Iron deficiency anemia signs and symptoms are due to tissue hypoxia from low hemoglobin levels, thus compromising their oxygen-carrying ability. The most common signs and symptoms include fatigue, weakness, pallor, and headaches. Patients may have dry hair and skin, brittle nails, and soreness and swelling of the oral mucosa.

TREATMENT

Treatment interventions directed toward the underlying cause of anemia can include:

- Iron, vitamin B12, and folate supplementation
- Nutritional counseling
- PRBC transfusions for Hgb <8 g/dL or if patient is symptomatic
- Administering erythropoiesis-stimulating agents (ESAs) such as Epoetin alfa (Procrit, Epogen), darbepoetin alfa (Aranesp), which is a long-acting ESA and allows for less frequent dosing, and epoetin alfa-epbx (Retacrit), which is a biosimilar.

Nursing interventions for managing anemia include:

- Review the patient's allergies, past medical history, and medications.
- Assess for signs and symptoms of anemia.
- Monitor vital signs.
- Obtain and monitor blood work. Maintain current type and screen.
- Administer ESAs or biosimilar as ordered.
- Administer PRBC transfusions. Monitor for reactions as previously discussed.
- Provide oxygen therapy as needed.

Educate the patient and caregiver on signs and symptoms of anemia and side effects of EPO, blood transfusion procedure and associated risks, and how to manage fatigue:

- Conserving energy with frequent rest periods
- Scheduling activities during the time of the day when the energy level is at its peak.
- Exercising as energy level allows
- Incorporating complementary therapies (e.g., massage, yoga, relaxation)
- Maintaining a well-balanced diet and adequate hydration

Severe anemia can lead to a reduction of doses or delay with chemotherapy treatments, delay of surgical procedures, and cause suboptimal results from radiation therapy. Anemia is a main contributing factor for fatigue which can greatly impact a patient's ability to perform activities of daily living. When effectively treated, it can greatly improve the patient's quality of life, physical and psychosocial well-being, and survival.

THROMBOCYTOPENIA

Thrombocytopenia is the decrease in circulating platelets which can result in bleeding. Platelets are identified as thrombocytes and are responsible for thrombosis production and maintaining hemostasis. Hemostasis is the opposite of hemorrhage and is defined as the process of preventing bleeding by keeping blood within damaged blood vessel walls to promote wound healing. Platelets generally circulate in the blood in an inactive and nonadhesive state and are activated in response to a vascular injury or an alteration in normal blood flow.

The body maintains a normal level of platelets (150,000 to 400,000/mcL) circulating throughout at any given time. The spleen serves as storage for approximately one-third of the reserve platelets, which are released when stimulated by the sympathetic nervous system. Old platelets that are cleared from the circulation are phagocytosed in the liver and spleen. Platelets have a life span of 8 to 10 days. Effective control in bleeding involves adequate platelet count (which is the number of platelets as shown in the CBC) as well as platelet function. The normal range is 150 to 400 billion/L (150,000 to 400,000/mcL). Thrombocytopenia is graded as follows:

- Grade 1: Minimal risk: Platelets 75,000/mcL to lower level of normal
- Grade 2: Mild risk: Platelets 50,000–75,000/mcL
- Grade 3: Moderate risk: Platelets 25,000–50,000/mcL
- Grade 4: Severe risk: Platelets <25, 000/mcL

The mean platelet volume (MPV) in the CBC indicates the average size of the platelets in the blood (normal range is 7.4–10.4 fL). An examination of a peripheral blood smear under the microscope may be employed to study the appearance of a patient's platelets. A bone marrow aspiration may be used to diagnose the reason for the decreased production of platelets (e.g., tumor invasion in the bone marrow, leukemia).

Thrombosis (intravascular clot) occurs when platelets respond to an abnormality on the vessel wall instead of a bleeding injury leading to inappropriate platelet adhesion and activation. In other words, thrombosis is when a clot is formed in an undesired location and is the opposite of hemostasis. Thromboembolism is part of a thrombus that breaks off and travels through the circulation and lodges somewhere. Venous thrombosis can result in congestion of the affected area. Venous thromboembolism lodged in the lung is a pulmonary embolism. Arterial thrombosis will result in tissue ischemia, necrosis, infarction if cardiac in origin, stroke if in the brain or carotid artery.

▶ ADDITIONAL COAGULATION STUDIES RELATED TO PLATELET FUNCTION

In addition to the platelet count, coagulation studies may also be ordered to see how quickly a patient's blood clots and may include the following. See Table 21.3 for normal reference ranges.

- Prothrombin time (PT): Evaluates the blood's ability to clot and can be affected by warfarin therapy, deficiency or high intake of vitamin K, hormone replacements, oral contraceptives, disseminated intravascular coagulation (DIC), and liver disease
- International normalized ratio (INR): Created to standardize PT results; ensures that PT results are the same between two different laboratories.
- Partial thromboplastin time (PTT): Helps to determine if there is a clotting disorder and if heparin therapy is effective. PTT can be affected by heparin therapy, liver disease, and systemic lupus erythematosus (SLE).
- Thrombin time (TT): Measures the activity of fibrinogen. Thrombin is an enzyme formed from prothrombin that acts on fibrinogen to form fibrin needed to form a blood clot.
- Fibrin degradation products (FDP): Products from the dissolved clot and fibrin net that are released into the bloodstream. FDP levels help determine the presence of DIC, deep vein thrombosis (DVT), pulmonary embolism (PE), leukemia, kidney disease, and stroke.
- D-dimer: A protein produced by a blood clot after it dissolves in the body. This assay is helpful in diagnosing and monitoring for conditions such as DIC, DVT, PE, and stroke.

See Table 21.3 for the normal reference ranges for coagulation studies for a patient who is not on anticoagulant therapy.

Table 21.3 Normal Reference Ranges for Coagulation Studies
for a Patient *Not* on Anticoagulant Therapy

Coagulation Study	Reference Range
Prothrombin time (PT)	10 to 12 s
INR	1 to 2
Partial thromboplastin time (PTT)	30 to 45 s
Thrombin time (TT)	12 to 14 s
Fibrinogen	200 to 400 mg/dL
Fibrin degradation products (FDP)	<10mg/L
D-dimer assay	0 to 0.50

▶ CAUSES OF THROMBOCYTOPENIA

Examples of thrombocytopenia related to decreased platelet production include bone marrow disease (e.g., leukemia, lymphoma, multiple myeloma, aplastic anemia, myelodysplastic syndrome), viral infections (e.g., rubella, Epstein-Barr, mumps, varicella, HIV, CMV, hepatitis C), cancer therapy (e.g., systemic chemotherapy, radiation therapy), medications (anticonvulsants and estrogen therapy), chronic alcohol abuse, and deficiency in vitamin B12 and folic acid.

Examples of thrombocytopenia related to increased platelet destruction include idiopathic thrombocytopenic purpura (ITP), thrombotic thrombocytopenic purpura (TTP), DIC, chronic lymphocytic leukemia (CLL), SLE, post bone marrow or stem cell transplantation, medications such as sulfa antibiotics, heparin, anticonvulsants, and sepsis.

▶ SIGNS AND SYMPTOMS

Mild bleeding may occur when the platelet count falls below 50,000/mcL. Signs and symptoms of thrombocytopenia usually appear when the platelet count falls below 20,000/mcL and would be manifested by signs of bleeding, prolonged bleeding, and bruising.

Common signs and symptoms include bleeding (including from gums or oral mucosa), epistaxis, hematemesis, hemoptysis, melena, hematuria, prolonged/heavy menstrual periods, and petechiae.

▶ TREATMENT

Treatment for thrombocytopenia depends on the cause and severity of signs and symptoms and may include:

- Corticosteroids to abate platelet destruction
- Immunoglobulin therapy
- Rho (D) immune globulin
- Rituximab therapy for ITP
- Platelet transfusions which may be from random donors or single donors
- Thrombopoietic growth factors such as oprelvekin
- Thrombopoietin receptor agonist for thrombocytopenia related to ITP with little or no response to corticosteroids, immunoglobulins, or splenectomy such as Romiplostim or Eltrombopag
- Splenectomy

Nursing interventions include:

- Review the patient's allergies, past medical history, and medications.
- Obtain and monitor CBC and other blood tests.
- Assess for signs and symptoms of thrombocytopenia. Monitor for signs of bleeding or bruising (e.g., GI or GU bleeding, intracranial bleeding).
- Monitor vital signs, which can indicate signs of occult bleeding.
- Monitor for fever and signs of sepsis which can contribute to platelet destruction.
- Institute bleeding precautions in the plan of care.
- Administer glucocorticoids if ordered.
- Administer thrombopoietic agents if ordered.
- Administer platelet or PRBC transfusions. Monitor for reactions. Obtain post-platelet count at least 30 minutes after transfusion to evaluate response if ordered.
- Administer plasma to replenish clotting factors.
- Administer immunoglobulin if ordered. Monitor for reactions.

Patient and caregiver education includes:

- Signs and symptoms of thrombocytopenia, fever, infection, and when to call the provider
- Bleeding precautions and safety measures to prevent injury and trauma, including safety measures in the home (e.g., removing area rugs)
- Gently blowing the nose and how to treat bleeds such as nosebleeds by applying pressure, ice, and hemostatic agents
- Applying pressure to venipuncture or fingerstick sites
- Using electric razors rather than straight-edge blades and soft bristle toothbrushes; avoiding flossing
- Avoiding the use of enemas, suppositories, and tampons

■ Bowel regimens to avoid constipation.
■ Use of lubricants during sexual intercourse
■ Reasons for withholding anticoagulant therapy

The oncology nurse has the responsibility to assess, monitor, and evaluate responses to treatment when caring for a patient with thrombocytopenia. Thorough education of the patient and caregiver on thrombocytopenia, treatments and interventions, and necessary follow-up can greatly impact the abilities of these patients to care for themselves in hopes of improving or maintaining their quality of life.

The bibliography and references for this chapter are available on ExamPrepConnect; see inside front cover for access instructions.

1. Which of the following is a risk factor for infection?

    A. Frequent handwashing
    B. Bathing daily
    C. Poor oral hygiene
    D. Cooking meats thoroughly

2. A patient's WBC count is 4,000 cells/mcL, segmented neutrophils are 35%, and bands are 15%. What is the calculated ANC?

    A. 200
    B. 20,000
    C. 20
    D. 2,000

3. All of the following are contributing factors for anemia, EXCEPT:

    A. Vitamin B12 deficiency
    B. Decreased thyroid function
    C. Impaired kidney function
    D. Sickle-cell disease

4. All of the following interventions would be appropriate for a patient admitted to hospital for chemotherapy-induced anemia, EXCEPT:

    A. Administering erythropoiesis-stimulating agents
    B. Iron supplementation
    C. Single-donor platelet transfusion
    D. Monitoring of vital signs

5. Which of the following assessments should the nurse expect when a patient is diagnosed with thrombocytopenia?

    A. A platelet count of 150,000/mcL
    B. A platelet count of 50,000/mcL
    C. Administration of Epogen
    D. Administration of Filgrastim

1. C) Poor oral hygiene
Poor oral hygiene will lead to halitosis, dental cavities, periodontal disease, and gum disease, all of which can place the patient at risk for infection. Frequent handwashing, bathing daily, and cooking meats thoroughly minimize the risk of introducing microbes into the body.

2. D) 2,000
The patient's ANC would be calculated as follows:

Total WBC count of patient is 4,000 (or read as 4.0)

segs = 35%; bands = 15%

$4,000 \times (.35 + .15) = ANC$

$4,000 \times .50 = 2,000$

$ANC = 2,000$ (or read as 2.0)

3. B) Decreased thyroid function
Thyroid function is unrelated to RBC production and anemia. Vitamin B12 is necessary for RBC production. Therefore, vitamin B12 deficiency can cause anemia. Impaired kidney function can compromise erythropoietin production necessary for RBC production in the bone marrow. Sickle cell disease causes the sickle-shaped RBCs to break apart and die, resulting in a decreased RBC count.

4. C) Single-donor platelet transfusion
A single-donor platelet transfusion would be ordered for a thrombocytopenic patient with alloimmunization concerns. Interventions and treatments for the patient with anemia include administering erythropoiesis-stimulating agents, iron supplementation, and monitoring of vital signs.

5. B) A platelet count of 50,000/mcL
A platelet count of 50,000/mcL is expected with thrombocytopenia. A platelet count of 150,000/mcL is a normal platelet range and would not place a patient at risk for bleeding. Epogen is used for patients with anemia, and filgrastim is used to treat neutropenia.

Pulmonary Side Effects

INTRODUCTION

Cancer treatment regimens are comprised of drugs with varying mechanisms of action that can lead to numerous side effects. Combining chemotherapy and biotherapy with or without radiation therapy will increase the toxicity profile. Pulmonary toxicities are often interrelated and occur in stages. Signs and symptoms of pulmonary side effects can be difficult to diagnosis because they can resemble many other side effects and disease profiles. For example, infections, lung tumor recurrence, and lung cancer progression can share similar symptoms to pulmonary side effects.

Cancer treatments cause pulmonary toxicities by forming free radicals, which directly damage healthy cells. Free radicals are unstable molecules with an unpaired electron and are produced during normal cellular metabolism. They seek stability by binding with other electrons, thereby causing damage to cells, proteins, and DNA. Free radicals can also be produced as a result of exposure to environmental carcinogens such as tobacco, UV radiation, and asbestos.

The most common types of cancer treatments that can cause injury and/or damage the pulmonary system include systemic chemotherapy, particularly alkylating agents, antimetabolites, and antitumor antibiotics; targeted therapy agents such as checkpoint inhibitors, *HER2* inhibitors, and (e.g., trastuzumab), and tyrosine kinase inhibitors (TKI); and radiation therapy for cancers of the lung, breast, esophageal, thymus, mesothelioma, and lymphoma. The combination of treatment modalities significantly increases the risk for pulmonary complications.

The interrelated pulmonary toxicities that will be discussed in this chapter include interstitial lung disease (ILD), pulmonary edema, pleural effusion, pulmonary embolism, and treatment-related pneumonitis.

INTERSTITIAL LUNG DISEASE

Interstitial lung disease (ILD) is a group of approximately 100 respiratory conditions that affect the interstitium of the lungs. Various pathological processes of ILD involve inflammation (pneumonitis) and thickening. Alveolar damage can progress to scarring of lung tissue (fibrosis). Scarring inhibits adequate oxygenation of the blood and is usually irreversible. Once symptoms occur, the goal of treatment is to prevent further lung damage and pulmonary fibrosis. ILD can lead to complications that are life-threatening, such as pulmonary hypertension, cor pulmonale (right-sided heart failure), and respiratory failure. ILD can be caused by chemotherapy or radiation. Risk factors include chemotherapy (bleomycin), chest radiation therapy, interstitial pneumonia, exposure to environmental carcinogens, autoimmune disorders, smoking.

The bibliography and references for this chapter are available on ExamPrepConnect; see inside front cover for access instructions.

The signs and symptoms of ILD are common among other pulmonary conditions making it difficult to diagnose. The most common symptoms include dyspnea, nonproductive cough, decreased tolerance to exercise, fatigue, and weight loss. Diagnostic tests include chest x-ray, CT scan, PFTs, and lung biopsy via bronchoscopy, video-assisted thoracoscopic surgery (VATS), or thoracotomy (open lung biopsy).

▶ TREATMENT

Treatment for ILD includes:

1. Medications:
   a. Antibiotics: to treat interstitial pneumonia (e.g., antifungal, antibacterial)
   b. Corticosteroids: to reduce inflammation in the lungs (e.g., prednisone)
   c. Immunosuppressants: (e.g., azathioprine, cyclosporine, cyclophosphamide, methotrexate)
2. Oxygen therapy
3. Pulmonary rehabilitation
4. Lung transplant (in advanced cases): Oncology patients may not be candidates for this type of treatment due to the cancer diagnosis.

⬤ PULMONARY FIBROSIS

Pulmonary fibrosis is a restrictive lung disease involving the development of fibrous scar tissue causing stiffness of the lungs. Pulmonary fibrosis can also be a secondary condition of other diseases such as interstitial lung diseases. The scarring reduces elasticity of the lungs resulting in inadequate intake of oxygen and impaired gas exchange. Fibrosis may or may not accompany inflammation (pneumonitis) and can lead to further complications including respiratory failure. Pulmonary fibrosis is permanent and irreversible. Progression of pulmonary fibrosis can lead to complications such as pulmonary hypertension, respiratory failure, pneumothorax, cor pulmonale, and pulmonary emboli. Risk factors for pulmonary fibrosis include chemotherapy (Bleomycin, Busulfan, Mitomycin), chest radiation therapy, medications such as amiodarone and nitrofurantoin, exposure to environmental carcinogens, smoking, autoimmune disorders, and respiratory infections.

Signs and symptoms of pulmonary fibrosis include dyspnea, nonproductive cough, rales, pleuritic chest pain, fever, nail clubbing of fingers or toes, fatigue, weight loss, arthralgias, and myalgias. Diagnostic tests for pulmonary fibrosis include chest x-ray, CT scan, ultrasound, MRI, and lung biopsy.

▶ TREATMENT

There is currently no cure for pulmonary fibrosis. The goal of treatment is to slow the progression of the lung scarring, reduce inflammation, and maintain pulmonary function. Treatment includes:

1. Medications: Corticosteroids, immunosuppressants, antifibrotics (pirfenidone, nintedanib), and opioid analgesics

2. Oxygen therapy
3. Pulmonary rehabilitation
4. Lung transplant

▶ PULMONARY FIBROSIS FROM BLEOMYCIN

Bleomycin is an antitumor antibiotic chemotherapy agent commonly used to treat Hodgkin's lymphoma and testicular cancer. Pulmonary side effects can occur in up to 20% of patients treated with bleomycin. Bleomycin is known to cause alveolar damage resulting in ILD and fibrosis. The patient receiving bleomycin can also develop chest pain which usually resolves with discontinuation of the infusion.

It is recommended that bleomycin be discontinued if the patient's pulmonary diffusion capacity for carbon monoxide (as noted in PFT studies) falls below 35% of the pretreatment value. The risk of bleomycin-related lung complications can be compounded by combining treatment with chest radiation.

Clinical Pearls

- A baseline PFT may be obtained prior to administration of the first dose.
- The incidence of pulmonary toxicity tends to be dose related (total dose >400 units).
- Lifetime cumulative dose should be recorded and tracked before administering each dose. Total lifetime dose should not be >400 units.
- Hypersensitivity or anaphylactoid reactions can occur. A test dose of 2 units may be administered for the first two doses prior to administering the remaining dose.
- Patients symptomatic of pulmonary side effects usually respond to corticosteroids.

● PULMONARY HYPERTENSION

Pulmonary hypertension primarily refers to the arteries of the lungs. It is a condition in which the blood pressure within the pulmonary arteries of the lungs is increased. Over time, the affected blood vessels become stiff and thick (fibrosis). This vascular narrowing leads to vasoconstriction, thrombosis, and inflammation with dysfunctional apoptosis in the walls of the vessels. These alterations cause impaired blood flow out of the heart, resulting in an increase in workload for the right ventricle. Eventually, the right ventricle becomes unable to compensate with the increased demand and gradually results in reduced cardiac output and right-sided heart failure. This leads to decreased blood flow to the lungs and less oxygenated blood returning to the left heart.

Pulmonary hypertension can become life-threatening. Complications include systemic congestion from right-sided heart hypertrophy and failure (cor pulmonale), exhibiting the following signs: jugular vein distension, pitting lower extremity edema, ascites, anasarca, hepatomegaly, splenomegaly, hepatojugular reflex, and parasternal heave. It can also lead to thromboembolism, arrhythmias, hemoptysis from pulmonary hemorrhaging, and complications during pregnancy.

▶ RISK FACTORS FOR PULMONARY HYPERTENSION

Many other conditions and agents can contribute to the incidence of pulmonary hypertension. See Box 22.1 for the risk factors for pulmonary hypertension.

Box 22.1 Risk Factors for Pulmonary Hypertension

- Proteasome inhibitors (bortezomib, carfilzomib)
- TKI (dasatinib)
- Chest radiation therapy
- Direct compression of tumor on pulmonary arteries
- Tumor invasion of pulmonary arteries
- Pulmonary embolism
- COPD
- ILD
- Cardiac conditions: Mitral valve disease, congenital heart disease
- Polycythemia vera
- HIV/AIDS
- Chronic hemolytic anemia: Sickle-cell disease
- Inflammatory disorders: Sarcoidosis, vasculitis
- Cocaine
- Amphetamines
- Exposure to high altitudes
- Female sex

Pulmonary hypertension can develop gradually without any signs or symptoms. Early signs and symptoms include dyspnea, palpitations, fatigue, chest discomfort or pain, upper right quadrant abdominal pain, and decreased appetite. Late signs and symptoms include lightheadedness, syncope, cyanosis, cool extremities, and pitting lower extremity edema.

Diagnostic tests for pulmonary hypertension include a physical exam to assess for signs of right-sided heart failure, EKG, Doppler echocardiogram, right heart catheterization to measure pulmonary arterial pressure (PAP) via Swan-Ganz catheter to assess the severity and confirm the diagnosis, chest x-ray and CT, ventilation/perfusion (V/Q) scan, PFTs, and ABG.

▶ TREATMENT

Currently, there is no cure for pulmonary hypertension. The goal of treatment is to provide supportive measures to ameliorate symptoms.

1. Medications
   a. Vasodilators: Epoprostenol, treprostinil, iloprost
   b. Calcium channel blockers: Amlodipine, diltiazem, nifedipine
   c. Anticoagulants: Warfarin
   d. Prostacyclins
   e. Digoxin
   f. Diuretics
   g. Endothelin receptor antagonists: Bosentan, ambrisentan, macitentan, and sitaxentan

2. Oxygen therapy

3. Lung transplant for severe cases

▶ PULMONARY VENO-OCCLUSIVE DISEASE (PVOD)

Pulmonary veno-occlusive disease (PVOD) is a rare form of pulmonary hypertension involving narrowing of the pulmonary veins. This results in elevated arterial blood pressure within the lungs and eventually heart failure. There is also dilation of alveolar capillaries leading to pulmonary edema. PVOD can be progressive and has a poor prognosis with a life expectancy of 2 years after being diagnosed. Risk factors include alkylating chemotherapy agents (cyclophosphamide, procarbazine, carmustine, cisplatin), antitumor antibiotics (bleomycin, mitomycin), chest irradiation, viral infections, genetic mutations, HIV/AIDS, and bone marrow/stem cell transplantation.

Signs and symptoms of PVOD include dyspnea (also when supine), fatigue, syncope, hemoptysis, chest pain, cyanosis, and hepatosplenic congestion. Lung biopsy, chest X-ray, and CT scan are used for diagnosis.

TREATMENT

The prognosis for PVOD is worse than pulmonary hypertension. Administering medications used to treat primary pulmonary hypertension, such as prostacyclins and endothelin receptor antagonists, can worsen symptoms and cause pulmonary edema. Currently, there is no medical treatment for PVOD. Supportive therapy includes oxygen therapy and diuretics. Lung transplant is the only definitive therapy that can provide a potential for long-term survival.

⬤ PULMONARY EDEMA

Pulmonary edema is an accumulation of excess fluid in the alveolar sacs causing impaired gas exchange and poor oxygenation of the blood. This condition can result in respiratory failure. The origin of pulmonary edema can be classified as either cardiogenic or noncardiogenic. Cardiogenic pulmonary edema is usually associated with left-sided heart failure or left ventricular failure. The reduced cardiac output by the left ventricle causes increased pressure in the pulmonary veins and forces fluid into the alveolar sacs. Noncardiogenic pulmonary edema occurs as a result of increased capillary permeability leading to accumulations of fluid and protein in the alveoli. Causes can include injury to the pulmonary tissue or pulmonary vessels. Progressive pulmonary edema can result in pulmonary hypertension.

Pulmonary edema can be caused by chemotherapy (e.g., anthracyclines, cyclophosphamide), radiation therapy (e.g., high-dose external beam radiation therapy), immunotherapy (e.g., IL-2), and all-trans retinoic acid (ATRA).

Acute pulmonary edema can have a sudden onset, and emergency care is crucial in order to avoid respiratory failure or cardiac arrest. Signs of chronic pulmonary edema usually manifest gradually over time. See Box 22.2 for the acute and chronic symptoms of pulmonary edema.

Box 22.2 Signs and Symptoms of Pulmonary Edema

Acute (call 911 for these symptoms):

- Dyspnea: Orthopnea, with or without diaphoresis
- Cough with frothy, blood-tinged, or pink sputum
- Feeling like drowning
- Wheezing
- Cold, clammy skin
- Anxiety, restlessness
- Cyanosis
- Palpitations
- Lightheadedness
- Dizziness
- Weakness

Chronic:

- Dyspnea even when lying down: Orthopnea, paroxysmal nocturnal dyspnea
- Worsening cough
- Wheezing
- Fatigue
- Rapid weight gain
- Lower extremity edema

Imaging tests used for pulmonary edema include chest x-ray and CT, EKG, echocardiogram, and lung ultrasound. In addition, diagnostic tests include pulse oximetry, ABG, chemistry panel, BNP, C-reactive protein, coagulation panel, cardiac catheterization, and coronary angiogram.

▶ TREATMENT

Prompt treatment leads to better patient outcomes. The focus of treatment is to improve respiratory function, treat the underlying cause, and prevent further lung damage.

1. Medications: Diuretics, morphine to alleviate respiratory distress, antihypertensives, inotropes to increase cardiac output
2. Oxygen therapy
3. Positive airway pressure to avoid the need for mechanical ventilation: BIPAP (bilevel positive airway pressure), CPAP (continuous positive airway pressure)
4. Limit dietary sodium intake

● PLEURAL EFFUSION

Pleural effusion is an abnormal accumulation of fluid within the pleural cavity that can be as much as 300 mL or more. This amount of excess fluid limits lung expansion, thus impairing respiration. Pleural effusion occurs when there is a disruption in homeostasis, and the rate of pleural fluid production exceeds the rate of fluid absorption. Pleural effusion is a complication often associated with lung cancer, breast cancer, mesothelioma, and lymphoma; medications such as methotrexate, dasatinib, amiodarone, and phenytoin; or the pleura as a site of metastasis as with ovarian or GI cancer. It can occur as a result of inflammation in the pleura from chest irradiation and may be seen up to 6 months after completing treatment. It can also be a result of chemotherapy treatment.

▶ MALIGNANT PLEURAL EFFUSION

If a pleural effusion is suspected to be caused by cancer, a thoracentesis is performed to collect pleural fluid for purposes of analysis and cytology. Cancer cells in malignant pleural effusion will cause an increase in pleural fluid production and a decrease in pleural fluid absorption. Malignant cells metastasize to the pleura via the bloodstream and by invading the visceral pleura. Malignant pleural fluid usually contains proteins, cancer cells, and lymphoid and myeloid immune cells. The presence of a malignant pleural effusion is usually indicative of cancer in advanced stages. Generally, the prognosis for the patient with malignant pleural effusion is poor and depends on various other factors such as age, performance status, type of cancer and stage, comorbidities, cytology of pleural fluid, and responsiveness of cancer to treatment.

▶ RADIATION-INDUCED PLEURAL EFFUSION

Chest radiation therapy for cancers of the lung, breast, esophagus, and lymphoma is a risk factor for developing pleural effusion. The incidence of radiation-induced pleural effusion depends on the dose of radiation and the volume of lung tissue exposed during treatment. Symptoms can manifest much later after radiation treatments have been completed.

▶ IMMUNOTHERAPY-INDUCED PLEURAL EFFUSION

Immunotherapy agents can cause an alteration in capillary permeability, leading to pleural effusions. These usually resolve without intervention once treatment is discontinued.

▶ CHEMOTHERAPY-INDUCED PLEURAL EFFUSION

Methotrexate elimination has been noted to be reduced in patients with ascites, renal insufficiency, and pleural effusions. Methotrexate is known to slowly clear from third space compartments (such as pleural effusions and ascites), leading to prolonged exposure and toxicity. It is recommended that third space fluid be removed prior to initiating treatment with methotrexate.

For docetaxel, it is recommended that patients be premedicated with corticosteroids such as dexamethasone 8 mg twice daily for 3 days, beginning 1 day prior to treatment to reduce fluid retention and hypersensitivity reactions. This is especially pertinent to lung cancer patients as they are already at risk for developing pleural effusion. Fluid retention also pertains to the development of peripheral edema.

▶ SIGNS AND SYMPTOMS

Patients can have asymptomatic pleural effusions. These effusions may be of small volume and may not require therapeutic drainage. As symptoms develop, dyspnea is usually the first complaint, followed by chest discomfort and cough. Signs and symptoms appear depending on the rate of pleural fluid reaccumulation.

▶ DIAGNOSTIC TESTS

Diminished breath sounds and pleural friction rub may be noted on physical exam. A pleural friction rub is an adventitious breath sound produced when the inflamed pleurae rub against each other during respiration. It is usually accompanied by pleuritic chest pain upon inspiration. Chest x-ray should be used to confirm a pleural effusion and may show tracheal deviation. It should also be done after a thoracentesis to determine the presence of any residual fluid or a pneumothorax. Other diagnostic tests include chest CT and ultrasound, thoracentesis with or without a sampling of fluid for cytology, and thoracoscopy with biopsy (may or may not include pleurodesis).

▶ TREATMENT

The goal of treatment for pleural effusion is to manage the underlying cause, provide symptom relief, and improve the patient's quality of life. For malignant pleural effusion, treatment may be for palliative reasons and to prevent a recurrence. Inadequate treatment for pleural effusion can lead to empyema, sepsis, and trapped lung (when the lung does not fully expand). Supportive measures include oxygen therapy, analgesics, and chest physical therapy. If congestive heart failure is the cause, treatment includes diuretics. If cancer is the cause, treatment includes chemotherapy, immunotherapy, radiation therapy, and intrapleural therapy.

For relief of respiratory symptoms:

1. Therapeutic thoracentesis for prompt relief of symptoms. The recommended amount of pleural fluid to be removed should be no more than 1500 mL to prevent re-expansion pulmonary edema (when a collapsed lung expands rapidly).
2. Chest tube placement via thoracostomy for drainage.
3. Pleurodesis (pleural sclerosis) via chest tube or indwelling pleural catheter (IPC) to obliterate the pleural space by fusing the parietal and visceral pleurae. The sclerosing agent instilled can promote an inflammatory response between the layers causing pleural fibrosis and fusion. The most commonly used agents include talc slurry, zinc sulfate, bleomycin, tetracycline, and silver nitrate.
4. Chemical pleurodesis via chest tube at the bedside or during a thoracostomy or thoracotomy.
5. Indwelling pleural catheter (IPC), which allows for repeated fluid drainage at home by the patient and/or caregiver.

Surgical procedures include:

1. Video-assisted thoracoscopic surgery (VATS): A camera is inserted to visually examine the pleurae and take samples for biopsy. Agents such as sterile talc or antibiotics may be instilled to prevent reaccumulation of fluid.
2. Complete or partial pleurectomy: A resection of the visceral and parietal pleura with or without decortication (removal of the fibrous pleural rind to allow for lung expansion).
3. Pleuroperitoneal shunt: Diverts pleural fluid into the peritoneum.
4. Thoracotomy: Performed to remove the fibrous tissue and evacuate possible infection from the pleural cavity. Chest tubes are usually placed to continue fluid drainage.

PULMONARY EMBOLISM

Pulmonary embolism (PE) is a blood clot in the lungs that can lead to respiratory distress and possibly death; thus, it requires emergency management. PE usually begins as a complication of a DVT with a blood clot forming in the vein of the lower extremities and traveling to the lungs via the vena cava and pulmonary blood vessels. Normal hemostasis involves the constant destruction of microscopic clots formed in the venous circulation. Tumors can cause hypercoagulability in the blood by releasing substances that promote clotting via the activation of factor X. Chemotherapy can cause vasculitis and alter the integrity of the blood. Risk factors for pulmonary embolism include immobility; cancer treatment with chemotherapy, radiation therapy, and immunomodulatory/anti-angiogenic agents; cancer (pelvic tumors, disease progression); surgery; and medications such as hormone replacement therapy/estrogen therapy, erythropoiesis-stimulating agents, or oral contraceptives.

The signs and symptoms of PE are usually vague, and most patients will not present with any classic complaints. For this reason, PE may lead to sudden death. Any sign of PE should be quickly worked up and treated in order to reduce further complications. The classic triad of symptoms are dyspnea with tachypnea, hemoptysis, and pleuritic chest pain.

The physical exam should include assessment for decreased oxygen saturation, Homan's sign, and swelling, pain, redness, palpable cord of a thrombosed vein in a lower extremity. Lab studies include D-dimer, PT/PTT/TT, CBC, chemistry panel, ESR, and troponin. Other diagnostic tests include ABGs, EKG, echocardiogram, chest x-ray, spiral CT, CT pulmonary angiography, and ventilation-perfusion (V/Q) scan.

▶ KEY FACTS

- D-dimer is a protein fragment of fibrin clot digestion. Blood clots usually break down after forming, which releases D-dimer into the blood. Therefore, D-dimer serves as a highly sensitive marker to indicate recent or current clot formation and lysis.
- A normal or negative D-dimer level can help rule out a PE (normal range is 0.0 to 0.5 mcg/mL).
- An elevated D-dimer level of >0.5 mcg/mL may indicate an abnormally high level of fibrin degradation products and can help confirm a PE.

▶ TREATMENT

Treatment for PE includes:

1. Oxygen therapy for hypoxemia
2. Medications
   a. Anticoagulant therapy: Unfractionated heparin, low-molecular-weight heparin (LMWH)
   b. Thrombolytics: Streptokinase, alteplase
3. Invasive procedures: IVC filter placement, pulmonary embolectomy
4. Preventive measures for pulmonary embolism
   a. Incorporate mobility and ambulation, especially following surgery and when seated for long periods of time.

b. Perform leg exercises.

c. Wear compression stockings.

d. Use a sequential compression device.

⬤ PNEUMONITIS

Combining immunotherapy agents with chemotherapy and radiation has been shown to significantly prolong survival, as seen with advanced stage III non-small cell lung cancer (NSCLC). This patient population often has pre-existing nonmalignant lung diseases with hypoxia. It is important to distinguish differential diagnoses of tumor progression, pulmonary infections, pulmonary embolism, and the category of pneumonitis. This can be accomplished by obtaining a high-resolution CT scan.

▶ HYPERSENSITIVITY PNEUMONITIS

Hypersensitivity pneumonitis is inflammation of the alveoli and bronchioles caused by hypersensitivity that occurs with inhalation of or exposure to toxins or irritants to the lungs. Acute hypersensitivity pneumonitis usually occurs with rapid onset upon exposure to a new chemotherapy (Bleomycin, Bortezomib, Docetaxel, Paclitaxel, Methotrexate, Oxaliplatin, or Procarbazine), antibiotics, or inhalation of toxic environmental factors. Hypersensitivity pneumonitis seen with chemotherapy agents is usually accompanied by fever, peripheral eosinophilia, and alveolitis seen via bronchoscopy. Other signs and symptoms include cough, dyspnea, chest tightness, myalgias, headache, chills, and fever.

Diagnostic tests for hypersensitivity pneumonitis include chest x-ray and CT, PFTs, blood tests to aid in detecting exposure to allergens, bronchoscopy, and VATS for open lung biopsy. Treatment includes corticosteroids, bronchodilators, and immunosuppressants; oxygen therapy, and elimination of the allergen since continued exposure can lead to permanent lung damage such as fibrosis. In addition, mold and bacteria in the environment should be minimized.

▶ IMMUNE CHECKPOINT INHIBITOR-INDUCED PNEUMONITIS

The use of immunotherapy agents for the treatment of various cancers is rapidly increasing. This category of drugs includes the immune checkpoint inhibitors, which are known to cause immune-related adverse effects such as inflammatory responses in multiple organs. Risk factors for immune checkpoint inhibitor-induced pneumonitis include the diagnosis of non-small cell lung cancer, history of chest radiation therapy, history of lung conditions (e.g., COPD, ILD), poor or decline in PFTs, and history of smoking.

Although pneumonitis is a rare adverse reaction of checkpoint inhibitor therapy, the patient should be closely monitored for early signs and symptoms that may be similar to ILD. Initial symptoms include nonproductive cough, dyspnea, decreased activity tolerance, rales, fever, and chest pain. Diffuse alveolar damage leads to tachypnea and hypoxemia.

Diagnostic tests include chest CT, which may show ground-glass opacities; lab studies, which may show elevated inflammatory markers (e.g., C-reactive protein, ESR); PFTs; and bronchoscopy with bronchoalveolar lavage (BAL).

TREATMENT

Immune-related pulmonary toxicity can be life-threatening and may require withholding treatment with checkpoint inhibitors until the pneumonitis is resolved. Pneumonitis can recur when rechallenged with immunotherapy and can be fatal if untreated. Patients are treated with a 6- to 8-week course of corticosteroids, which should be gradually tapered after resolution of pneumonitis. Tocilizumab has been noted to reduce systemic inflammatory response in treating immune-related adverse events that were refractory to corticosteroids. Bronchodilators may also be prescribed for the treatment of COPD. Supportive treatment includes oxygen therapy.

▶ RADIATION PNEUMONITIS

Generally, the lungs react to radiation treatment or stereotactic body radiotherapy by becoming inflamed, which is manifested by diffuse alveolar damage within the field of chest radiation. This is radiation pneumonitis and can eventually lead to fibrosis of the lungs in severe cases of tissue damage. Radiation pneumonitis and radiation fibrosis are both dose-limiting toxicities of radiation therapy. Risk factors include the dose of radiation >40 Gy, the total volume of lung tissue being irradiated, radiation to lower lobes of the lungs (could be related to greater oxygenation, perfusion, and ventilation in these areas), concurrent chemotherapy treatment, prior chemotherapy agents used, poor pulmonary function, and pulmonary hypertension.

The early or acute phase of radiation pneumonitis can occur up to 12 weeks after completing radiation and can last up to 6 months. Mild alveolar damage may be reversible with the recovery of structure and function. Patients are usually asymptomatic but may present with cough, dyspnea, low-grade fever, and chest discomfort. Unresolved acute phase of radiation pneumonitis can progress to the chronic phase with fibrosis and can last from the 6th to 12th month after completing treatment. Patients can be asymptomatic and may have progressive signs such as worsening dyspnea, nonproductive cough, and pulmonary hypertension resulting in cor pulmonale.

Radiation-induced pleural changes include inflammation within the pleura resulting in pleural effusions. These effusions may be detected up to 6 months after completing radiation treatment, tend to be small, and usually resolve spontaneously. Other pleural changes include pleural thickening. Pulmonary necrosis is caused by high doses of radiation therapy and is a complication that is rarely seen. This condition occurs late and is irreversible.

When appropriate, shrinking the bulky tumor with induction chemotherapy prior to initiating radiation therapy will decrease the lung treatment field and volume of lung tissue that will be exposed to radiation. However, administering pulmonary toxic chemotherapy or immunotherapy agents will not decrease the risk of developing lung toxicities. The side effects of chest radiation therapy depend on the dose of the radiation, the number of treatments, other comorbidities the patient may have, and their general state of health (Box 22.3). The side effects of chemotherapy can compound those of radiation therapy and vice versa.

Box 22.3 Side Effects of Radiation Therapy

- Nonproductive cough
- Dyspnea
- Chest discomfort
- Pleuritic pain
- Low grade fever
- Dysphagia
- Heartburn
- Chest hair and skin changes
- Fatigue
- Nausea
- Myelosuppression

▶ DIAGNOSTIC TESTS

Chest x-ray may show opacities, pleural effusion, or atelectasis. A chest CT scan is more sensitive than a chest x-ray and may show ground-glass opacities with consolidation known as the "halo" or "reversed halo" sign, depending on the configuration. May also show alveolar opacities, pulmonary necrosis, chronic pleural effusions. Other diagnostic tests include bronchoscopy with lavage and lung biopsy.

TREATMENT

Treatment for radiation pneumonitis is dependent upon the lung condition diagnosed. Techniques used in radiation therapy to minimize toxicities include using advanced delivery systems to provide precise therapeutic doses to the target area while attempting to spare surrounding healthy structures as much as possible. Currently, there is no effective treatment for radiation fibrosis. Corticosteroids should be prescribed for treatment of the acute phase, for anti-inflammatory effects, to help treat symptoms, and to prevent progression to the chronic phase. Doses should be tapered after the resolution of symptoms. Prophylactic antibiotics should be prescribed for patients with refractory pneumonitis (e.g., trimethoprim-sulfamethoxazole to prevent *Pneumocystis jiroveci* pneumonia). Decongestants, cough suppressants, bronchodilators, and NSAIDs can also be used. Oxygen therapy should be provided for supportive treatment

RADIOPROTECTANT AGENTS TO REDUCE THE RISK OF RADIATION PNEUMONITIS

Amifostine

Radioprotectant agents can be used to protect healthy normal tissues against damage from radiation. Currently, amifostine is the only radioprotectant available to help reduce radiation toxicity in cancer patients. Amifostine has been studied as a radioprotectant for radiation pneumonitis with positive results as well as being administered subcutaneously to reduce side effects, but further data are needed. See Box 22.4 for the proper administration of amifostine. Side effects of amifostine include nausea/vomiting, sleepiness, hypotension, dyspnea, skin reactions, allergic/hypersensitivity reactions, and hypocalcemia.

Box 22.4 Proper Administration of Amifostine

- ■ **Amifostine in the radiation patient with head and neck cancer:**
  - ● Dose is 200 mg/m² IV over 3 min prior to each radiation treatment.
  - ● Must be administered within 15 to 30 min PRIOR to each radiation treatment.
  - ● Blood pressure should be monitored before infusion, after, and as indicated.
- ■ **Amifostine in the chemotherapy patient:**
  - ● Dose is 910 mg/m² IV over 15 min prior to each chemotherapy treatment.
  - ● Must be administered within 30 min PRIOR to each chemotherapy treatment.
  - ● Prolonged infusion >15 min will result in a higher incidence of side effects.
  - ● Blood pressure should be monitored at baseline, every 5 min during the infusion, and after as indicated.
- ■ Amifostine CANNOT be administered to dehydrated patients. Patients should be adequately hydrated prior to receiving amifostine.
- ■ Patients should WITHHOLD antihypertensive medication 24 hours prior to receiving amifostine. Patients who must continue their antihypertensive medications CANNOT receive amifostine.
- ■ Support hypotension with normal saline IV bolus via a separate IV line.
- ■ It is recommended to administer antiemetics prior to the amifostine infusion.
- ■ Patients should remain SUPINE during the amifostine infusion.

Clarithromycin

Clarithromycin (CAM) is an antibiotic with immunomodulatory effects prescribed for inflammatory respiratory diseases (e.g., diffuse panbronchiolitis, cystic fibrosis). It has also been noted that CAM improved pulmonary function and frequency of exacerbations in patients with COPD, asthma, bronchiectasis, and chronic sinusitis. Side effects of CAM include hepatotoxicity, QT prolongation, *Clostridium difficile* associated diarrhea, and exacerbation of myasthenia gravis.

CAM has been studied as prophylactic therapy for the prevention of radiation pneumonitis following stereotactic body radiotherapy with positive results. CAM has also been noted to significantly reduce the severity of radiation pneumonitis. At this time, it is still unknown what the CAM dosage and duration should be. It is recommended that further prospective studies be performed (Takeda et al., 2018).

CONCLUSION

The oncology nurse plays a key role in managing patients with actual or potential for pulmonary toxicity through assessment, monitoring, management, and treatment. Educating the patient and caregiver on signs and symptoms, treatment, prophylactic measures, and when to report to the provider are all paramount for clinical recognition of these potentially life-threatening complications.

Cancer treatment plans that include pulmonary toxic drugs and radiation therapy should be determined on an individual basis, taking into consideration the patient's general state of health, performance status, and medical history. Treatment and supportive care should focus on relieving symptoms, slowing the progression of the complication, improving quality of life, and reducing mortality. The goal should be on achieving positive patient outcomes, supporting the patient to gain control of their breathing, and optimizing their level of functioning.

The bibliography and references for this chapter are available on ExamPrepConnect; see inside front cover for access instructions.

1. All of the following diagnostic tests would be ordered for the diagnosis of radiation pneumonitis, EXCEPT:

   A. Chest CT scan
   B. Pulmonary function tests
   C. Bronchoscopy with lavage
   D. Chest x-ray

2. Which agents are used prophylactically against radiation pneumonitis?

   A. Amifostine
   B. Dexrazoxane
   C. Clarithromycin
   D. Amifostine and clarithromycin

3. All of the following orders are appropriate for a patient who is about to receive the first dose of bleomycin, EXCEPT:

   A. Echocardiogram
   B. PFTs prior to initiating treatment
   C. A test dose of 2 units IV
   D. Complete blood count

4. What is the MOST appropriate treatment for a patient with pulmonary veno-occlusive disease?

   A. Warfarin
   B. Prostacyclins
   C. Digoxin
   D. Oxygen therapy

5. Which of the following is the MOST appropriate education for the nurse to provide a patient with pulmonary complications?

   A. Encourage discussions with a psychosocial counselor
   B. Schedule an appointment with the dietician
   C. Use extra pillows to raise the head and upper body while sleeping
   D. Schedule an appointment with the financial counselor

(See answers next page.)

1. B) Pulmonary function tests
Pulmonary function tests (PFTs) measure lung volume, capacity, rates of flow, and gas exchange. PFTs are used for assessment purposes and do not aid in the differential diagnosis of radiation pneumonitis; chest CT, bronchoscopy with lavage, and chest x-ray aid in the diagnosis.

2. D) Amifostine and clarithromycin
Amifostine and clarithromycin are used prophylactically against radiation pneumonitis. Dexrazoxane is a cytoprotectant for the heart, not the lungs.

3. A) Echocardiogram
PFTs, test dose, and CBC are all required prior to administering the first dose of bleomycin. An echocardiogram is not necessary prior to initiating treatment with bleomycin.

4. D) Oxygen therapy
Oxygen therapy is a supportive therapy appropriate for the treatment of PVOD. Warfarin, prostacyclins, and digoxin are all treatments for pulmonary hypertension and would be inappropriate for the patient with PVOD.

5. C) Use extra pillows to raise the head and upper body while sleeping
Using extra pillows will increase oxygen saturation by elevating the head and increasing ventilation. Although scheduling a session with psychosocial, dietary, and financial counselors is important, it does not have a direct effect on pulmonary complications.

Cardiovascular Side Effects

● INTRODUCTION

Cardiovascular side effects are the direct and indirect damage of cardiac cells due to exposure to the various categories of cancer treatment. Pre-existing cardiovascular disease can contribute to the possibility of these side effects and toxicities. Cardiovascular toxicities can occur months and even years after treatment has been completed. The most common types of cancer treatments that can cause injury or damage to the cardiovascular system include systemic chemotherapy, targeted therapy agents, radiation therapy to the mediastinal and pericardial area, and a combination of treatment modalities. This chapter examines the most common cardiovascular side effects that can occur due to cancer treatment.

● CARDIOMYOPATHY

Cardiomyopathy is damage to the cardiac muscle in which it can become abnormally enlarged, thickened, or stiffened. As a result, the heart is unable to pump blood efficiently, which can cause arrhythmias and congestive heart failure (CHF). Chemotherapy-induced cardiomyopathy can occur during treatment up to years after completing therapy and may be seen with a decrease in the left ventricular ejection fraction (LVEF). Thus, pretreatment baseline cardiac function with a multi-gated acquisition (MUGA) scan must be established and include regular monitoring during treatment and if the patient has signs and symptoms of cardiomyopathy. The most common signs and symptoms of cardiomyopathy are fatigue, weakness, dizziness and lightheadedness, hypertension, and tachycardia.

▶ TREATMENT

Treatment for cardiomyopathy includes:

1. Medications
   a. Diuretics rid the body of excess fluid and salt, thereby relieving edema and dyspnea (e.g., furosemide, spironolactone).
   b. Angiotensin-converting enzyme (ACE) inhibitors relax the blood vessels to lower the blood pressure and reduce the cardiac workload (e.g., enalapril, lisinopril, losartan).
   c. Beta-blockers slow down the heart rate thus, lowering the blood pressure (e.g., carvedilol, metoprolol).
   d. Calcium channel blockers cause arterial vasodilation thus, reducing pressure on the heart and optimizing its ability to pump (e.g., nifedipine, amlodipine).
   e. Antiarrhythmics control abnormal heart rhythms (e.g., amiodarone).
   f. Digoxin
   g. Anticoagulants reduce the risk for developing blood clots (e.g., aspirin, warfarin).

The bibliography and references for this chapter are available on ExamPrepConnect; see inside front cover for access instructions.

2. Invasive procedures:

    a. Left ventricular assist device (LVAD) is used for weakened hearts and helps pump blood from the ventricles to the rest of the body to provide circulation to vital organs.

    b. Implantable cardioverter-defibrillator (ICD) monitors heart rhythm and is like a pacemaker.

    c. A heart transplant is the final alternative when the cardiac condition progressively worsens, and medications and devices become less effective. However, oncology patients may not be candidates for this type of treatment due to a cancer diagnosis.

▶ CARDIOMYOPATHY WITH ANTHRACYCLINES

It is standard practice with chemotherapy administration to include a record of total cumulative doses of anthracyclines administered to a patient to ensure that the maximum lifetime dose of 400 mg/m^2 is not exceeded. Cardiomyopathy, in this case, is dose-dependent. A change in treatment with anthracyclines or discontinuation of therapy should be strongly considered when there is a reduction of >20% in the LVEF from baseline, there is a confirmed LVEF decrease <50% during treatment, and/or the patient exhibits signs and symptoms of cardiomyopathy or heart failure.

There is less risk for cardiotoxicity when anthracyclines are administered via continuous intravenous (IV) infusion versus the bolus method because of the lower peak plasma level of the drug in the blood. A central venous access device is required for continuous IV infusion of any anthracycline because of the vesicant properties of these cytotoxic agents. The risk for cardiotoxicity is decreased when pegylated liposomal formulations of anthracyclines are administered. The presence of the liposomes reduces drug exposure of the anthracyclines to the cardiac tissues. Because of the liposomal formulation, there is a higher incidence of infusion-related and hypersensitivity reactions. These agents are all administered via IV infusion, and vesicant precautions with monitoring of IV sites must be observed.

Dexrazoxane (Zinecard®) is a cardioprotectant agent that can be administered to minimize the incidence and severity of cardiomyopathy and reduce QT prolongation when treating with anthracyclines such as doxorubicin. It is administered intravenously over 15 minutes, just *prior* to the anthracycline. It should only be administered when a patient's cumulative dose of doxorubicin has reached 300 mg/m^2 and will continue with doxorubicin therapy. Dexrazoxane may interfere with the antitumor activity of the chemotherapy regimen; therefore, it is not initially included with the chemotherapy cycles.

● CONGESTIVE HEART FAILURE

Congestive heart failure (CHF) is a condition in which the heart is unable to pump blood effectively at a rate that is adequate to perfuse the body as well as meet the metabolic needs of the body, leading to pressure and volume. The additional workload and stress on the heart increases, which can ultimately cause enlargement of the heart, thrombi, and ischemia of the cardiac tissue. Risk factors for CHF include chemotherapy, targeted therapy, and chest irradiation; comorbidities such as diabetes, hypertension, coronary artery disease, and obesity; smoking; and substance abuse.

Patients with CHF may present with cough, fatigue, shortness of breath, pulmonary edema, pleural effusion, ascites, and lower-extremity edema. Diagnostic testing includes blood work with BNP, chest x-ray, EKG, echocardiogram, exercise stress test, cardiac CT and MRI, coronary angiogram, and myocardial biopsy.

▶ TREATMENT

Treatment for CHF includes:

1. Medications

   a. Angiotensin-converting enzyme (ACE) inhibitors are vasodilator drugs, thereby lowering the blood pressure, improving blood flow, and decreasing the cardiac workload on the heart (e.g., enalapril, lisinopril, and captopril).

   b. Angiotensin II receptor blockers (ARB) may be an alternative for patients who are unable to tolerate ACE inhibitors (e.g., losartan and valsartan).

   c. Beta-blockers decrease the heart rate and cardiac workload, reduce blood pressure, increase blood flow, and improve symptoms of heart failure. (e.g., carvedilol, metoprolol, and bisoprolol).

   d. Diuretics are used to control fluid overload and control hypertension (e.g., furosemide, hydrochlorothiazide, and spironolactone).

   e. Positive inotropes are used to improve the strength of cardiac contractions in patients with severe heart failure (e.g., dobutamine and norepinephrine).

   f. Digoxin is used to decrease the heart rate and to treat arrhythmias such as atrial fibrillation (AFib) and atrial flutter.

   g. Anticoagulants (e.g., aspirin).

   h. Nitrates are vasodilators and improve cardiac output by decreasing left ventricular filling pressure (e.g., nitroglycerin, isosorbide dinitrate).

2. Invasive procedures

   a. Coronary bypass surgery

   b. Heart valve repair or replacement

   c. Implantable cardioverter-defibrillator (ICD)

   d. Cardiac resynchronization therapy (CRT) is achieved via a biventricular pacemaker which sends electrical impulses to both ventricles to allow more efficient and coordinating pumping action.

   e. Ventricular assist device (VAD)

   f. Heart transplant

● ARRHYTHMIAS

Cancer treatment-induced arrhythmias can be caused by drugs that alter the cardiac conduction or by direct damage to the cardiac tissue via ischemia, inflammation, or radiation therapy. Arrhythmias can result from cardiomyopathy and lead to CHF and stroke due to thrombi formation. Arrhythmias can occur during treatment, or they can be a chronic effect after treatment has been completed.

It is common for cancer treatment plans to include combinations of chemotherapy, targeted therapy, and radiation. Cancer patients may also have been treated with multiple regimens due to the progression of the disease. All of this makes arrhythmia risk assessment, identification of the causative agent, and management extremely challenging. Other risk factors that can predispose the cancer patient to develop arrhythmias are cancer-related cardiac conditions such as primary cancer, metastasis to the heart, and cardiac amyloidosis; pre-existing cardiac conditions such as hypertension, CHF, and coronary artery disease; antiemetics; and electrolyte imbalances from vomiting, diarrhea, and anticancer agents such as cisplatin and cetuximab.

Arrhythmias do not always cause signs or symptoms and may be discovered by happenstance during a routine physical examination. Some people may be asymptomatic with a heart rate <50 bpm, and others may experience fatigue, syncope, lightheadedness. Common signs and symptoms include fluttering in the chest, bradycardia, skipped or irregular heartbeat, tachycardia, palpitations, and chest pain or pressure. Diagnostic tests used for arrhythmias include EKG and Holter monitoring.

▶ TREATMENT

Normal electrolyte levels are necessary for optimal cardiac function. Abnormal levels must be corrected to help decrease the incidence or prevent the exacerbation of arrhythmias. Other treatment includes:

1. Medications: Beta-blockers, calcium channel blockers, antiarrhythmic agents, and anticoagulants
2. Implanted devices: Pacemaker for bradycardia, ICD
3. Cardioversion: Can restore normal heart rhythm by either delivering synchronized shocks during a cardiac cycle or by using antiarrhythmic medications.
4. Catheter ablation: Is accomplished by inserting a flexible catheter into a major vein and then advanced toward the heart. Energy sources such as radiofrequency ablation (heat) or cryoablation (cold) are used to destroy the area of the heart that is the source of the faulty electrical pathway causing the arrhythmia. This procedure is used when pharmacologic methods are ineffective.

● QT PROLONGATION

Many cancer drugs, including conventional as well as targeted therapies, have the potential to cause life-threatening arrhythmias and QT prolongation. Additionally, cancer itself can place the patient at risk for electrolyte imbalances, thus compounding the possibility of causing QT prolongation. QT prolongation can put the patient at risk for life-threatening ventricular arrhythmias, torsade de pointes (TdP), and sudden death. In the event of severe QT prolongation, prompt treatment is necessary to prevent any arrhythmias and cardiac symptoms which can lead to syncope.

▶ KEY FACTS

- Normal QT interval is <400–440 milliseconds or 0.4–0.44 seconds.
- Women have a longer QT interval than men.
- The lower the heart rate, the longer the QT interval.
- The faster the heart rate, the shorter the QT interval.

A person with QT prolongation may very well be asymptomatic. Oftentimes, the condition is detected on an EKG. Signs and symptoms of QT prolongation are related to ventricular arrhythmias—presyncope (lightheadedness, feeling faint), syncope (actual fainting), dizziness, palpitations, dyspnea, and chest pain.

Arsenic trioxide is used to treat refractory or relapsed acute promyelocytic leukemia (APL). The cardiac conduction abnormalities that have been observed with arsenic trioxide include QTc prolongation, atrioventricular block, as well as torsade de pointes (TdP), which can quickly progress to ventricular fibrillation. Arsenic trioxide should not be administered to a patient with pre-existing ventricular arrhythmia or QTc prolongation.

▶ TREATMENT FOR QT PROLONGATION

Depending on the severity of QT prolongation, cancer treatment may continue with careful monitoring and repletion of electrolytes. The patient's list of other medications that are associated with QT prolongation will need to be reassessed periodically and be modified if possible. The causative agent may be held until a safe QTc interval is restored. Further interventions include:

- Correct any electrolyte abnormalities and monitor electrolytes at least weekly. Treat conditions that can cause electrolyte imbalances, such as diarrhea and vomiting.
- Monitor QT intervals in EKGs. EKGs may be performed weekly. Report QT prolongation to the provider.
- Avoid using other medications that can also cause QT prolongation or consider using an alternate drug.
- Consider dose reduction in the medication that is causing the QT prolongation.
- Beta-blockers to reduce arrhythmias.
- Pacemaker placement for bradycardia.
- Implantable cardiac-defibrillator (ICD) placement for severe arrhythmias or history with sudden cardiac death.

● HYPERTENSION

According to the 2020 International Society of Hypertension Global Hypertension Practice Guidelines published by the American Heart Association, hypertension in the adult is defined as blood pressure at or above 140/90 mmHg taken in an office or clinic setting during at least two visits at 1- to 4-week intervals. Normal blood pressure is less than or equal to 120/80 mmHg. Hypertension can be induced by cancer treatment with targeted therapy agents such as VEGF inhibitors (e.g., Bevacizumab) and TKI (e.g., Sorafenib, Sunitinib).

Vascular damage and increased cardiac workload due to hypertension can lead to myocardial infarction, heart failure, and stroke. Uncontrolled hypertension can cause an increase in intraglomerular pressure thus impairing glomerular filtration, which can lead to proteinuria. Proteinuria in the presence of hypertension can indicate declining renal function or the beginning of end-stage renal disease. Depending on the extent of proteinuria and/or decreased glomerular filtration rate, treatment with the causative medication may be placed on hold or discontinued. The vascular endothelial growth factor (VEGF) is one of the most important pathways responsible for normal endothelial cell function in angiogenesis. Inhibiting the VEGF pathway leads to the suppression of new blood vessel formation thus, starving the tumor of nutrients and oxygen from the blood supply as well as preventing metastasis. Due to this alteration in the vascular system, hypertension is a known side effect of certain targeted therapy agents such as the VEGF inhibitor, bevacizumab, and TKI agents such as sunitinib and sorafenib. The incidence of hypertension while undergoing treatment with these agents can be as high as 80%.

It is important to monitor the blood pressure regularly and treat hypertension effectively to prevent any cardiovascular and cerebrovascular complications as well as end-organ damage. The goal is to avoid delaying or discontinuation of the causative cancer therapy agent. Dose reduction or withholding treatment until hypertension is controlled is recommended.

The patient with hypertension may or may not be symptomatic or show any signs of hypertension (e.g., headaches, changes/loss in vision, epistaxis). A patient with symptoms of hypertension may have already been experiencing an elevated blood pressure for an extensive period of time. The blood pressure in a patient with a hypertensive crisis can be as high as 180/120 mmHg and can result in organ damage and life-threatening complications. Signs and symptoms include severe headache with confusion and blurry vision, severe chest pain, and dyspnea. This patient would require emergency treatment with intravenous antihypertensives, such as nitroglycerin, esmolol, and hydralazine.

▶ TREATMENT

The goal for the treatment of hypertension is to control and maintain the blood pressure within normal levels. Management of hypertension requires individualizing treatment for each patient as well as monitoring for adherence with antihypertensive medications.

1. Medications
   a. ACE inhibitors should be used with caution in patients with renal impairment (e.g., captopril, lisinopril).
   b. ARBs (e.g., losartan, valsartan)
   c. Beta-blockers (e.g., atenolol, metoprolol)
   d. Dihydropyridine calcium channel blockers (e.g., amlodipine, nifedipine)
   e. Thiazide diuretics (e.g., hydrochlorothiazide)
   f. Loop diuretics (e.g., furosemide)

Instruct the patient to check their blood pressure at least once a day. Patients should report any abnormal results and symptoms of hypertension to their provider. Lifestyle changes include maintaining a healthy weight, a well-balanced diet, and a reduction in sodium (<1500 mg a day).

● THROMBOEMBOLISM

Thromboembolism is the formation of a blood clot that was dislodged from another site resulting in obstruction of a blood vessel. Venous thromboembolism (VTE) includes deep vein thrombosis (DVT) and pulmonary embolism (PE). Cancer therapies such as vascular endothelial growth factor (VEGF) inhibitors and BCR-ABL tyrosine kinase inhibitors (TKI) can cause endothelial damage which contributes to thrombosis. Oncology patients who have central venous catheters placed for their intravenous treatments are also at risk for thrombus formation. Hormone replacement therapy (HRT) can also increase the risk for blood clots. The types of cancer with the highest risk of thrombosis include brain, lung, gastric, pancreatic, gynecologic, and multiple myeloma.

Signs and symptoms of DVT include swelling, pain and tenderness, and skin redness and warmth. Signs and symptoms of PE include dyspnea, tachypnea, palpitations, pleuritic chest pain, and cough. Diagnostic tests for thromboembolism include D-dimer studies, duplex ultrasound or Doppler echocardiogram of extremity, chest x-ray, ventilation perfusion (V/Q) scan, spiral CT scan, pulmonary angiogram, echocardiogram, and MRI.

▶ TREATMENT

Treatment for thromboembolism includes:

1. Medications
   a. Prophylactic anticoagulant therapy is recommended for the patient at risk for thromboembolism either to prevent or to reduce recurrence of thrombus formation. The presence of thromboembolism can delay the patient's treatment.
   b. Anticoagulant therapy may be oral, intravenous, or subcutaneous, depending on the indication and/or severity of the thrombotic event.
   c. The patient should be monitored for recurrent VTE and complications of bleeding. The patient's risk of bleeding may be compounded by cancer treatment that may have thrombocytopenia as a side effect.
2. Inferior vena cava (IVC) filter may be placed in combination with anticoagulant therapy in the case of acute venous thromboembolism.

The nurse should instruct the patient to report signs of bleeding to the provider, use compression stockings, exercise regularly, avoid sitting for long periods of time, lose weight (if obese), and quit smoking.

● MYOCARDIAL ISCHEMIA

Myocardial ischemia is caused by reduced blood flow from the narrowing of or blocked arteries, thus compromising oxygen delivery to the heart. Myocardial ischemia secondary to treatment with chemotherapy may be related to vasospasm of the coronary arteries. Radiation therapy to the chest (particularly left-sided) may induce damage to the coronary artery endothelium causing coronary artery disease. There may also be impaired regenerative capacity of endothelial cells resulting in vascular damage. These factors can contribute to thrombus formation. Decreased oxygen-carrying capacity due to anemia from either disease or chemotherapy treatment may be a risk factor for myocardial ischemia predisposing the patient to develop arrhythmias. Severe or prolonged ischemia can lead to myocardial infarction and even death of cardiac tissue. Other factors that can increase the cancer patient's risk of developing myocardial ischemia include the history of myocardial infarction, coronary artery disease, and cardiomyopathy; smoking; diabetes; and hypertension.

Some patients can be asymptomatic of any signs or symptoms of myocardial ischemia ("silent ischemia"). Common signs and symptoms include angina; pain in the shoulder, arms, back, neck, or jaw; palpitations; dyspnea; and nausea and vomiting. Severe chest pain requires immediate care. Complications can result in myocardial infarction, arrhythmias, and heart failure.

Diagnostic tests include EKG, echocardiogram, stress test to detect coronary artery disease, angiography, cardiac CT scan and chest x-ray, cardiac biomarkers (e.g., troponin, creatine kinase (CK), and CK-MB).

▶ TREATMENT

Treatment for myocardial ischemia includes:

1. Medications: Anticoagulants, ACE inhibitors, beta-blockers, calcium channel blockers, nitrates, statins, and antianginals (e.g., ranolazine, ivabradine)
2. Invasive procedures:
   a. Coronary angioplasty to unblock arteries
   b. Coronary artery bypass surgery
   c. Catheter-based revascularization procedure. This should be used with caution due to the risk for bleeding from dual antiplatelet therapy (treatment with two antiplatelet agents) and stent placement.
3. Healthy life choices can help reduce risk or treat myocardial ischemia. The patient at risk should be encouraged and supported with the following:
   a. Smoking cessation
   b. Managing other health conditions such as diabetes, hypertension, high cholesterol
   c. Eating a healthy diet
   d. Exercising regularly
   e. Achieving or maintaining a healthy weight
   f. Stress management
   g. Limiting alcoholic intake

PERICARDIAL EFFUSION

Normally, 15 to 50 mL of clear, straw-colored pericardial fluid occupies the pericardial space. This fluid acts as a lubricant as well as a barrier against infection and inflammation. Pericardial effusion is the accumulation of excessive amount of fluid in the pericardial space. This abnormal fluid may be serous, bloody, or purulent. Risk factors include metastatic disease, especially lung, breast, and esophageal cancers, renal cell carcinoma, malignant melanoma, leukemia, and Hodgkin's and non-Hodgkin's lymphoma; cardiac tumor; radiation therapy to the chest area; and chemotherapy agents such as high-dose cyclophosphamide, doxorubicin, busulfan, and cytarabine, as well as tretinoin for acute promyelocytic leukemia.

The patient with pericardial effusion may be fatigued, anxious, restless, and even confused. Symptoms may manifest gradually or rapidly and depend on how quickly fluid accumulates in the pericardial sac. The most common signs and symptoms include dyspnea on exertion, orthopnea, tachypnea, chest pain or pressure, and cough.

Diagnostic tests for pericardial effusion include chest x-ray, which may show an enlarged cardiac silhouette, EKG, echocardiogram, ultrasound of the heart, CT scan, and cardiac MRI.

▶ TREATMENT

Treatment for pericardial effusion depends on the underlying cause of the pericardial effusion as well as symptom management. If the etiology is due to a malignancy, the treatment would include chemotherapy and/or radiation therapy, and the pericardial fluid may reaccumulate, requiring placement of a drain. If the cause is due to inflammation, anti-inflammatory agents, corticosteroids, aspirin, or colchicine may be prescribed. Measures to support blood pressure and improve cardiac output include administering intravenous fluids and vasopressors. Treatment procedures are employed if systemic therapy is not sufficient such as:

a. Pericardiocentesis may be performed for diagnostic and therapeutic reasons. For instance, the presence of malignant cells in the cytology will confirm that the pericardial effusion is caused by the malignancy.

b. Pericardiostomy may be performed to create a pericardial window for fluid drainage or to instill a sclerosing or chemotherapy agent.

c. Percutaneous balloon pericardiotomy is where a catheter is placed in the pericardial space, and the balloon tip is inflated to allow drainage of fluid into the pleural space for reabsorption to occur.

d. Pericardiectomy is also known as pericardial stripping, where a portion or all the pericardium is removed to free the heart from being constricted.

e. Surgical pleuropericardiotomy involves surgical drainage of the pericardial fluid into the pleura.

f. Pericardio-peritoneal shunt creation drains the pericardial effusion into the peritoneal cavity.

● RADIATION-INDUCED CARDIOTOXICITY

Radiation therapy (RT) can cause radiation-induced cardiotoxicity (RIC) when used to treat cancers of the breast, lung, esophagus, and lymphomas in the mediastinal area. Cardiovascular changes can occur during RT and up to years after completing RT. Toxicity can occur at doses between 4,000 and 7,000 cGy depending on heart exposure being either full or partial. To help minimize organ toxicities, the radiation treatment team spends much time collaborating, planning, and calculating the total RT dose that would be received by each organ and surrounding structures within the treatment field. To reduce the incidence of RIC, the focus would be on minimizing the RT dose to the heart by using advanced RT delivery methods. This may involve using proton or carbon ion-charged particles. Using CT-guided images for field planning can help minimize radiation exposure to the heart.

Alterations in the conduction system of the heart caused by RT can manifest in EKG changes, including atrioventricular block and QT prolongation. RT can also cause malfunctions of pacemakers, ICDs, and CRT devices.

Pericarditis and pericardial effusion can develop within weeks after RT and is treatable, whereas damage to heart structures such as valves, pericardium, and myocardium can manifest as symptoms of dysfunction and CHF up to 20 years after RT.

Children and young adults are especially at high risk for developing RIC if they have received doses >30 Gy since their organs were still developing at the time of treatment.

▶ DIAGNOSTIC AND SCREENING TOOLS FOR RADIATION-INDUCED CARDIOTOXICITY

Diagnostic and screening tools include:

1. An echocardiogram may be performed every 2 years for asymptomatic patients and more often for those who are symptomatic or clinically indicated.
2. Coronary CT angiogram is used to evaluate any calcification in the cardiac structures.
3. Cardiac MRI enables detection of any coronary, valvular, and pericardial changes as well as any scarring or fibrosis.
4. Invasive catheterization can be performed to complement or confirm imaging findings.

TREATMENT FOR RADIATION-INDUCED CARDIOTOXICITY

Treatment for RIC largely depends on the symptoms and findings from physical examinations and diagnostic tests. Therefore, treatment approaches are individualized based on the diagnosis with the goal of reducing morbidity and mortality.

● CONCLUSION

In addition to educating patients on signs of cardiotoxicity and symptom management, patients should be encouraged to maintain a treatment diary to help track long-term effects after having completed cardiotoxic cancer therapy. Patients should be counseled and supported in adopting a healthier lifestyle. Routine cardiac assessments should continue even after cancer treatment has been completed since the patient can still be at risk for cardiovascular complications later in life. This is especially necessary for those who were treated for cancer as children or adolescents.

Managing this type of patient calls for a multidisciplinary approach to provide care that will result in a positive outcome and optimal quality of life. A cardio-oncology consult may be necessary for caring for the compromised patient.

Vigilant cardiovascular monitoring is paramount when caring for the patient receiving cardiotoxic cancer therapy. It is the responsibility of oncology nurses to be aware of any pre-existing cardiovascular disease their patients may have prior to initiating cardiotoxic therapy. Nurses should be knowledgeable about cancer treatments that can increase the risk of cardiotoxic side effects.

Nurses must follow the standard of care by making certain that pretreatment assessment of cardiac function has been completed. Patient safety and accurate assessment skills are paramount in caring for this population. Reducing mortality, relieving symptoms, improving quality of life, and the patient's ability to perform daily activities are of utmost priority.

The bibliography and references for this chapter are available on ExamPrepConnect; see inside front cover for access instructions.

1. All the following are risk factors for cardiac issues with cancer treatment, EXCEPT:

    A. Chemotherapy and biotherapy treatment for breast cancer
    B. Mediastinal radiation therapy for Hodgkin's lymphoma at 12 years of age
    C. Poor oral hygiene
    D. History of renal insufficiency

2. Which of the following nursing interventions must be completed prior to administering anthracycline chemotherapy?

    A. Dexrazoxane is ordered for the patient's first cycle of chemotherapy with doxorubicin
    B. A MUGA scan is ordered and results with an LVEF of 55%
    C. A cardio-oncology consultation
    D. A patient-centered family meeting regarding end-of-life issues

3. All the following should be monitored in patients receiving arsenic trioxide therapy for acute promyelocytic leukemia, EXCEPT:

    A. Troponin and CK-MB levels
    B. EKG
    C. Chemistry panel
    D. Patient's course of antibiotics

4. All of the following medications are appropriate for a patient with a history of myocardial ischemia, EXCEPT:

    A. Warfarin
    B. Nitroglycerin
    C. Furosemide
    D. Beta blocker

5. A multiple myeloma patient, who has been receiving a treatment regimen consisting of carfilzomib, lenalidomide, and dexamethasone, informs the nurse of swelling, pain, and warmth in the left calf area for the past 7 days. The nurse anticipates that the provider will order:

    A. Venous Doppler ultrasound
    B. MUGA scan
    C. EKG
    D. CBC

1. C) Poor oral hygiene

Cardiotoxic agents used to treat breast cancer include an anthracycline such as doxorubicin, cyclophosphamide, paclitaxel, pertuzumab, trastuzumab, and thoracic radiation therapy. Mediastinal radiation therapy can cause damage to heart structures and coronary vessels. The organs of a 12-year-old would still be developing, thus predisposing this patient to stunted cardiac development as well as cardiac problems later in life. A history of renal insufficiency may be a contributing factor in uncontrolled blood pressure. Poor oral hygiene is not a risk factor for cardiac issues with cancer treatment.

2. B) A MUGA scan is ordered and results with an LVEF of 55%

Dexrazoxane is not initially included with the first chemotherapy cycle and may be ordered when the cumulative dose of doxorubicin reaches 300mg/m². A cardio-oncologist may be consulted when the patient begins to experience signs and symptoms of cardiotoxicity from cancer treatment. Family meetings may be held at any time for a variety of reasons, such as at the time of diagnosis, discussing treatment options, or if the status or health of the patient changes.

3. A) Troponin and CK-MB levels

Patients receiving arsenic trioxide therapy for acute promyelocytic leukemia should be monitored with EKG and chemistry panel. In addition, their course of antibiotics should be monitored. Troponin and CK-MB are biomarkers for myocardial injury and are not necessary for monitoring QT prolongation.

4. C) Furosemide

An anticoagulant such as warfarin and a nitrate such as nitroglycerin, along with a beta-blocker, is used to treat or prevent myocardial ischemia. Furosemide, a diuretic, may be prescribed for the patient with congestive heart failure.

5. A) Venous Doppler ultrasound

A venous Doppler ultrasound is a diagnostic test used to check the circulation in the extremities and will show any blockages or clots in the veins. MUGA scan, EKG, and CBC would not be used for a patient with signs of blockages or clots.

Gastrointestinal Side Effects

INTRODUCTION

Gastrointestinal (GI) toxicities apply to the entire GI tract, from the mouth to the rectum. GI side effects can be mild to severe and can impact significantly impact the patient's nutritional status. The side effects and toxicity are a direct result of healthy epithelial cells being damaged by chemotherapy agents, radiation therapy, and the disease itself.

SIDE EFFECTS OF THE MOUTH

There are several changes and damage that can occur in the mouth, including taste changes, xerostomia (dry mouth), and mucositis.

▶ TASTE CHANGES

Taste changes refer to altered or loss of taste modalities in the taste receptors that are located throughout the tongue (Figure 24.1).

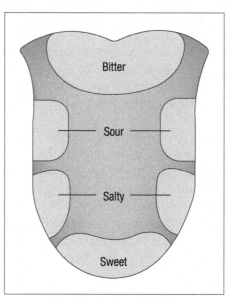

Figure 24.1 Taste receptors on the tongue.

Taste changes can be caused by chemotherapy agents (patients may complain of a metallic taste), prolonged exposure to radiation therapy, lesions in the oral mucosa, a wide range of medications, smoking, chronic hepatitis, and altered renal function. It is common in older adults.

The bibliography and references for this chapter are available on ExamPrepConnect; see inside front cover for access instructions.

Treatment includes lemon juice or chewing gum prior to eating a meal, good oral hygiene, avoiding eating with metal silverware, and the following medications:

- Zinc replacement: Promotes diffusion of taste stimuli to taste buds
- Pilocarpine: Increases saliva production
- Bethanechol: Increases taste perception

▶ XEROSTOMIA

Xerostomia is a dry mouth. It is most often related to radiation therapy damage specific to head and neck cancers. In addition, it can be caused by the removal of cancerous salivary glands, as well as supportive medications such as narcotics, anticholinergics, antihistamines, antidepressants, and many other drugs.

For treatment, patients should be instructed to increase their fluid intake, chew gum or suck on hard candy to increase salvation production (sugar-free gum recommended to prevent caries), and avoid mouth breathing when possible, caffeine, alcohol, tobacco, spicy foods, sugary drinks, and candy. They should moisturize their lips regularly, use saliva substitutes such as Biotene and Oasis Moisturizing Mouth Spray, brush their teeth with fluoride toothpaste. They should also use room humidifiers.

▶ MUCOSITIS

Mucositis is irritation, redness, ulcers, and pain in the mouth and/or tongue. It can also cause bleeding and thick saliva. Severe mucositis usually accompanies neutropenia, which makes the signs and symptoms more significant and concerning. Mucositis can be a dose-limiting side effect and grossly interfere with nutritional status. In addition, it places the patient at risk for secondary fungal infections such as candidiasis. The sores and irritation can extend to the esophagitis, causing the patient not to be able to swallow. Mucositis can be severe enough that it impairs the patient from eating any food or drink, as well as the development of excruciating pain.

Mucositis can be caused by chemotherapy agents such as doxorubicin, high-dose melphalan, and 5-fluorouracil, radiation therapy to the head and neck, bone marrow transplant, and long-term steroid use. Other risk factors include poor dental hygiene and poor-fitting dentures, dehydration, history of smoking and alcohol use, and comorbid conditions such as HIV, diabetes, and acute kidney disease.

Preventive measures should be taken to reduce the incidence and severity of mucositis. It is recommended that some patients chew on ice chips while the chemotherapy is infusing to protect the cells from being damaged from the chemotherapy medications (cryotherapy). Amifostine can be administered prior to radiation therapy to protect the oral mucosal, and caphosol can be administered prior to stem cell transplant and chemotherapy.

▶ **EXAM TIP**

Amifostine can cause severe and acute-onset hypotension. Monitor patients closely after administration.

Treatment for mucositis can include:

- Medicated mouth rinses, lozenges, and sprays: peridex, magic mouthwash, Benadryl elixir, Cepacol lozenges, chloraseptic sprays, baking soda mouth rinse
- Medications for pain: Narcotics, nonsteroidal anti-inflammatory drugs (NSAIDs), steroids
- Anti-fungal medications: Nystatin swish/expectorant, baking soda mouth rinse
- Antibiotics (if co-infection and accompanied by neutropenia)
- Total parental nutrition
- Palifermin: Should not be used with heparin

● SIDE EFFECTS OF THE STOMACH

▶ NAUSEA AND VOMITING

Nausea and vomiting (N/V) is the most common side effect of many chemotherapy agents. Nausea is the unsettling feeling in the stomach, also described as a queasy sensation. Vomiting is the sensation to throw up the contents within the stomach. Some patients may feel a sense of relief after vomiting. Often the patient does not vomit but experiences continued nausea. Uncontrolled N/V can lead to severe dehydration, electrolyte imbalances, anorexia, and cachexia.

The pathophysiology of N/V involves a complex process within the nervous system and numerous receptors in the brain and GI system, which invoke the N/V response. The physiological process begins when the central vomiting center (CVC), a receptor in the medulla, is triggered. There are five neurotransmitter receptor sites that are of primary importance in the vomiting reflex:

1. M1: Muscarinic
2. D2: Dopamine
3. H1: Histamine, which activates the vestibular system
4. 5-Hydroxytryptamine (HT)-3: Serotonin
5. Neurokinin 1 (NK1) receptor: Substance P

N/V is more common in females and individuals younger than 50 years of age. Other factors that contribute to N/V in the oncology population include types and dose of chemotherapy regimen, radiation, primary malignancy (e.g., brain tumors, brain metastasis), supportive medications (e.g., narcotics, antibiotics), history of motion sickness and emetics gravidarum, alcohol use in patients who are unaccustomed or sensitive to alcohol, bowel obstruction, vestibular dysfunction, and electrolyte imbalances.

TYPES OF NAUSEA AND VOMITING

There are six types of nausea and vomiting:

1. Acute N/V: Occurs within 24 hours of receiving chemotherapy and peaks approximately 5 to 6 hours after administration of chemotherapy agent.
2. Delayed N/V: Occurs 24 hours or more after receiving chemotherapy. It is commonly seen with higher doses of chemotherapy and regimens with multiple days of treatment.

3. Anticipatory N/V: Occurs before administration of the causative agent, usually after the third to fourth cycle. This is a conditioned response that is triggered by senses, including smell, sound, and sight. For example, a patient scheduled for cycle 4 of chemotherapy immediately becomes nauseous after entering the oncology clinic.

4. Chronic N/V: Continued N/V that is associated with advanced cancers, primary GI disorders, and supportive medications such as narcotics and antibiotics. The exact mechanism is not well understood.

5. Breakthrough N/V: Occurs in between the prescribed antiemetic prophylactic treatment. This type of N/V requires rescue with additional antiemetic agents.

6. Refractory N/V: Uncontrolled N/V despite the administration of antiemetic prophylaxis and/or rescues failed in earlier cycles.

> ▶ **EXAM TIP**

Know the different categories of N/V.

TREATMENT

Antiemetic drugs have evolved over the past two decades. Table 24.1 describes the different medications used to treat N/V.

Table 24.1 Anti-Nausea Medications for Oncology Patients

Drug Classification	Examples of Medications	Indications
5-HT3 serotonin receptor antagonists	Ganssetron, ondansetron, palonosetron	Acute and chronic N/V; prophylaxis
Neurokinin-1 receptor antagonists	Aprepitant	Delayed N/V
Dopamine antagonists: Phenothiazines Butyrophenones Benzamides	Prochlorperazine Haloperidol Metoclopramide*	Acute and breakthrough N/V Refractory N/V; end-of-life care Breakthrough N/V
Glucocorticoids	Dexamethasone**	Prophylaxis
Antihistamines	Hydroxyzine, diphenhydramine, meclizine	Prophylaxis; motion sickness
Anticholinergics	Scopolamine (M1)	Motion sickness; end-of-life care to decrease secretions
Benzodiazepines	Lorazepam, alprazolam	Anticipatory N/V

*Risk for extrapyramidal side effects.
**Anti-inflammatory properties; exact mechanism of action not well understood.

In addition to the traditional medications, there are alternative and complementary options that can be helpful to oncology patients, such as acupuncture. Nutritional options include ginger, tea, lemon-flavored hard candies, dry crackers, cola and ginger ale, and electrolyte replacement drinks such as Pedialyte and Gatorade.

SIDE EFFECTS OF THE LARGE INTESTINES AND RECTUM

▶ CONSTIPATION

Constipation is one of the most common side effects that can occur in oncology patients. It is defined as the inability to expel stool. The patient experiences hard stools accompanied by persistent straining. In some cases, it can lead to hemorrhoids from the pressure of straining.

Constipation can be caused by primary abdominal cancers (e.g., colon, ovarian, uterine), radiation therapy, medications such as opioids, chemotherapy, and vinca alkaloids, and poor dietary intake of fiber.

> ▶ **EXAM TIP**
>
> Know the different types of laxatives and their mechanisms of action.

Constipation can be treated by numerous types of laxatives, each of which have a unique mechanism of action (Table 24.2). In some cases, with severe uncontrolled constipation, multiple laxatives may be prescribed.

Table 24.2 Types of Laxatives Used to Treat Constipation

Type of Laxative/Mechanism of Action	Examples	Side Effects/Notes
Bulk forming (fiber supplements): Increases fiber; induces bowel movements	Calcium polycarbophil (Fibercon), methylcellulose (Citrucel), psyllium (Metamucil), wheat dextrin (Benefiber)	Bloating flatus, abdominal cramping Increase in fluids required to offset potential negative effects and exacerbation of constipation
Osmotic laxatives: Absorbs water into the large intestines; stimulates the bowel	Polyethylene glycol (Miralax), magnesium hydroxide (Milk of Magnesia), magnesium citrate, lactulose (Cephulac, Constulose, Duphalac, Kristalose)	Bloating, abdominal cramping, nausea Use with caution in patients with kidney dysfunction and the elderly
Stimulant laxatives: Stimulates the large intestines and bowel	Bisacodyl (Correctol, Ducodyl, Duloclax), sennocides (Senokot)	Abdominal cramping, diarrhea, belching, nausea
Stool softeners: Increases water into the stool to soften and decrease straining	Docusate (Colace, Surfak)	Long-term use can cause electrolyte imbalances

▶ DIARRHEA

Diarrhea is defined as more than three watery stools in a 24-hour period. Assessment of the stool is critical and includes consistency, color, odor, water, and presence of blood or mucus. Diarrhea is a common side effect of many chemotherapeutic agents, including 5-fluorouracil, irinotecan, cyclophosphamide, and capecitabine. Capecitabine, in particular, can cause life-threatening diarrhea. It can also be caused by different forms of radiation therapy, including brachytherapy for female reproductive cancers and male prostate cancer and external beam radiation targeted at the abdominal area, and targeted therapies such as tyrosine kinase inhibitors (TKIs), epidermal growth factors (EGFRs), and monclonal antibodies (MoAB). Oncology patients who are on multiple antibiotics can be at higher risk for diarrhea. Risk is also increased in individuals with a history of bowel Disorders (e.g., Crohn's disease and irritable bowel syndrome) and those with infections such as *Clostridioides difficile.*

Treatment for diarrhea includes:

1. Medications
   i. Imodium (OTC)
   ii. Opioid antidiarrheals (prescriptions required): Loperamide and opium of tincture (severe cases)
   iii. Octreotide (synthetic somatostatin analog) injection
2. Nutritional measures
   a. BRAT diet: Bananas, rice, apples, toast
   b. Oral hydration: Supports electrolyte replacement
   c. IV nutrition if the patient cannot maintain oral nutrition: Hyperalimentation or feeding tubes

● NUTRITIONAL DYSFUNCTION

Nutritional dysfunction can occur with cancer patients due to the diagnosis (especially head and neck and gastric malignancies) and treatment regimens. Nursing assessment is vital, including assessing the patient's comorbidities, reviewing health history and nutritional status, and monitoring medications to prevent morbidity and mortality.

Patients who receive combination chemotherapy and radiation therapy, particularly with head and neck cancers, should consult with a nutritionist to ensure proper intake of calories and protein-rich foods is achieved daily. Some patients may require oral, enteral, and/or parenteral nutritional supplements during or after treatment. Nutritional dysfunction includes cachexia and anorexia.

Cachexia is muscle wasting that occurs when protein and caloric intake are not adequately maintained. It can be caused by primary malignancies, chemotherapy agents, radiation therapy, and comorbidities such as diabetes, COPD, and hypertension.

Anorexia is the loss of appetite resulting from a decrease in oral intake and calories. Over time, anorexia can result in the development of cachexia, fatigue, weakness, and weight loss. Patients in advanced stages of cancer are at increased risk for anorexia symptoms, which ultimately correlates to higher morbidity and mortality.

Anorexia has a wide range of causes, including:

- Underlying tumor accompanied with dysphasia
- Underlying concurrent or post-chemotherapy, surgery, biotherapy, or radiation treatment-related symptoms: nausea or vomiting, early satiety, diarrhea, constipation, dysphagia, mucositis, ascites, taste/smell alterations, pain, and inability to perform activities of daily living

- Electrolyte abnormalities: Hypokalemia, hypercalcemia, hyponatremia, uremia
- Medications: Opioids, antibiotics, iron
- Psychosocial issues, financial difficulties, and decreased support system

▶ TREATMENT

Treatment for cachexia and anorexia can include:

- Appetite stimulants
  - Megestrol acetate (Megace)
  - Medroxyprogesterone
  - Corticosteroids: Dexamethasone (Decadron), methylprednisolone (Medrol), and prednisolone (Prednisone)
  - Dronabinol: (Marinol)
- Antiemetic and gut motility stimulator: Low-dose metoclopramide (Reglan)
- Nutrition
  - Total parental nutrition (TPN): Given through central line catheter over a period of time to replace the nutritional caloric deficit
  - Enteral feedings: Oral or g-tube feedings

Nursing interventions for cachexia and anorexia include the following:

1. Assess for dehydration: dry mouth, poor skin turgor, decreased or dark-colored urine.
2. Evaluate and replace electrolytes.
3. Consult with a speech and swallow therapist if dysphagia is suspected.
4. Evaluate for psychosocial, socioeconomic contributing factors.
5. Maintain a daily log of weight and caloric intake.
6. Request nutritional consult.
7. Encourage five or six small meals per day.
8. Recommend high-protein, high-calorie, and low-fat snacks.
9. Encourage nutritional supplements such as shakes, smoothies, or supplements.

The bibliography and references for this chapter are available on ExamPrepConnect; see inside front cover for access instructions.

1. A patient diagnosed with colon cancer is receiving the first dose of 5-fluorouracil chemotherapy. The MOST appropriate nursing intervention is to:

   A. Offer lemon candies
   B. Plan to start cryotherapy
   C. Administer caphasol
   D. Administer increased IV fluids

2. A patient diagnosed with ovarian cancer complains that she has been constipated for the past 3 days and has nausea and abdominal pain (6/10). The nurse's BEST initial question is:

   A. "What is your normal pattern bowel movements?"
   B. "Are you passing any flatus?"
   C. "What did you eat in the past 24 hours?"
   D. "Are you taking any medications?"

3. All of the following are 5-HT3 serotonin receptor antagonists, EXCEPT:

   A. Dolasetron
   B. Granisetron
   C. Olanzapine
   D. Palonosetron

4. Which of the following chemotherapy agents causes the highest risk for diarrhea?

   A. Doxorubicin
   B. Gemcitabine
   C. Capecitabine
   D. Thalidomide

5. Palifermin should not be administered with which of the following medications?

   A. Lovenox
   B. Heparin
   C. Morphine
   D. Tylenol

1. B) Plan to start cryotherapy

This patient is susceptible to taste changes due to chemotherapy. Cryotherapy (chewing ice during chemotherapy) causes vasoconstriction and decreases the exposure of the oral cavity membranes to mycotoxin agents. Lemon candy will alter the taste temporarily. Caphasol serves as a barrier, not as a vasoconstrictor, and is used in stem cell transplant patients. Increased fluids will not protect the oral mucosal.

2. B) "Are you passing any flatus?"

In ovarian cancer patients, obstruction should always be ruled out. If the patient is not passing flatus, it may be a sign of obstruction. Medications may be contributing to the constipation, but that can be explored after obstruction is ruled out. It is also important to know the patient's daily habits and food consumption in the past 24 hours, but they are not the priority questions when there is constipation and pain.

3. C) Olanzapine

Olanzapine is an antipsychotic used to treat schizophrenia. Dolasetron, granisetron, and palonosetron are 5-HT3 serotonin receptor antagonists used to treat nausea and vomiting.

4. C) Capecitabine

Capecitabine has a high potential to cause life-threatening diarrhea. Gemcitabine causes myelosuppression, doxorubicin causes cardiotoxicity, and thalidomide causes peripheral neuropathy.

5. B) Heparin

Heparin is contraindicated with palifermin as it increases the effects of palifermin. Lovenox, morphine, and Tylenol are not contraindicated with palifermin.

Genitourinary Side Effects and Hepatotoxicity

INTRODUCTION

Genitourinary (GU) complications are common in oncology patients. GU side effects can be caused by the disease itself, chemotherapy agents, radiation, or a combination of all three. In some cases, renal and bladder complications from cancer and cancer therapies can be life altering for the patient and may be difficult to treat. This chapter addresses the most common GU side effects—urinary incontinence and hemorrhagic cystitis. In addition, it will address nephrotoxicity and hepatotoxicity. The kidneys and liver act as the filter to eliminate wastes from the body. Chemotherapy and biotherapy are excreted from the kidneys and the liver, leading to nephrotoxicity and hepatotoxicity, which will also be addressed.

URINARY INCONTINENCE

Urinary incontinence is the inability to maintain urine in the bladder. It affects both genders, and symptoms can range from mild to severe, as well as be temporary or pose long-term complications. There are several forms of incontinence:

- Stress incontinence: Leaking of urine during specific activities such as laughing, exercising, sneezing, and coughing
- Overflow incontinence: Dribbling of urine when the bladder is full.
- Urge incontinence: The acute-onset need to void.
- Continuous incontinence: The inability to control the bladder.

Malignancies are a primary risk factor for urinary incontinence, including primary bladder, urethra gynecologic, prostate, colorectal, brain and spinal cord, lung, and esophageal cancers. Surgical treatments for various cancers can cause temporary or permanent nerve damage and alter the function of the bladder, including prostatectomy, partial removal of the bladder, and gynecologic and colorectal surgeries. In addition, radiation can cause inflammation and nerve damage that can alter the function of the bladder. Both external and internal radiation can cause urinary incontinence, specifically brachytherapy for the prostate, rectal, and gynecologic cancers.

▶ TREATMENT

There is a multitude of treatment options, including behavioral, medical, and surgical interventions:

- Behavioral strategies: Decrease fluid intake, bladder training (e.g., toilet schedules, double voiding to completely empty the bladder), increased physical activity, and Kegel exercises.

The bibliography and references for this chapter are available on ExamPrepConnect; see inside front cover for access instructions.

- Medications:
  - Alpha-blockers: Tamsulosin (Flomax), alfuzosin (Uroxatral)
  - Anticholinergics: Oxybutynin (Ditropan), tolterodine (Detrol)
  - Beta-3 adrenergic agonist: Mirabegron (Myrbetriq)
  - Topical estrogen (female patients): Rejuvenates the tissues in the vaginal and urethral area
- Medical devices to stabilize the bladder and hold in the urine (female patients): Urethral inserts, pessaries
- Surgery (female patients): Sling procedure, bladder neck suspension

HEMORRHAGIC CYSTITIS

Hemorrhagic cystitis (HC) is the acute inflammation of the lining of the bladder. In severe cases, it can cause bleeding with blood clots, which requires immediate medical attention. The primary causes for HC are chemotherapy and radiation. Chemotherapy medications are metabolized in the kidneys, and the byproducts, acrolein, are spontaneously developed and act as caustic chemicals that aggravate the lining of the bladder. Patients receiving combined chemotherapy with cyclophosphamide and/or ifosfamide plus radiation are at the highest risk for developing HC, for example, patients with lymphoma, testicular, and breast cancers. BCG, which is used to treat bladder cancer, can also cause HC, as can busulfan and thiotepa, although the incidence is much lower.

Radiation has the ability to destroy blood cells within the bladder, which can lead to scarring, ulcerations, and severe irritation weeks to months post-radiation treatments. Patients receiving internal or external radiation for prostate, cervical, and bladder cancers are at the highest risk for HC. HC can also be caused by infection and bone marrow transplantation due to the elevated dosages of chemotherapy agents.

The most common signs and symptoms are urinary frequency, pain, burning, urinary retention. Hematuria HC is graded based on the amount of blood in the urine:

1. Grade 1: No visible blood in urine (microscopic blood may be present)
2. Grade 2: Visible blood in urine
3. Grade 3: Visible blood in urine with small clots
4. Grade 4: Significant amount of blood in the urine with large clots that require immediate removal

▶ TREATMENT

Treatment includes increased fluid Intake to flush the bladder, especially when receiving cyclophosphamide and ifosfamide. Mesna (IV/oral), a uro protector, can be administered after elevated doses of cyclophosphamide and combined for bone marrow transplant doses, as well as given concomitantly with ifosfamide, to decrease the effects of acrolein byproduct as the drug is metabolized. Mesna binds to the acrolein to decrease the damage to the bladder. Antibiotics can be administered if a comorbid infection is present. The most common antibiotics to treat urinary tract infections are trimethoprim/sulfamethoxazole, cephalexin, ceftriaxone, fosfomycin, and nitrofurantoin. Bladder irrigations are recommended for grade 3 and 4 HC, and patients with moderate to severe pain can be administered narcotics.

NEPHROTOXICITY

Nephrotoxicity is a concern for many chemotherapy agents and may be a dose-limiting side effect. Chemotherapy can cause a direct effect on the glomerular filtration rate, electrolyte changes, and, in severe cases, acute kidney failure. It can cause temporary or permanent kidney damage. Risk factors for nephrotoxicity include comorbid renal issues (renal stones, diabetes, overuse of nephrotic agents) and renal, prostate, and cervical cancers. The chemotherapy and biotherapy agents that pose the greatest risk for nephrotoxicity include:

- Cisplatin
- Carboplatin: Ordered based upon AUC (area under the curve); the two formulas are the Cockcroft–Gault formula and the Jelliffe formula
- Ifosfamide
- Methotrexate (high-dose)
- Mitomycin
- Nitrosoureas: BCNU, CCNU
- Interferons
- Interleukin-2

A chem screen to monitor kidney functions should be assessed closely, and BUN and creatinine levels and electrolytes should be drawn on a regular basis when high-risk chemotherapy agents are being administered, regardless of the disease process.

Initial signs and symptoms occur when changes in the BUN and creatine are noted. Severe signs and symptoms that indicate acute kidney failure include peripheral edema, decreased urinary output, fatigue/weakness, SOB, nausea/vomiting, abnormal heart rate, angina, electrolyte imbalances (hyperkalemia, hypernatremia, hypermagnesemia, hypocalcemia). Signs of end-stage renal disease include confusion, seizures, and coma.

▶ TREATMENT

Prevention is key, which requires close monitoring of kidney function and adjustment of chemotherapy doses based upon the BUN and creatinine levels. Electrolyte balance should be maintained, and fluids should be increased fluids to replace lost fluids. It is important to maintain accurate intake and output and provide calcium supplements and replacement. Amifostine, a chemo protectant, may be prescribed to prevent kidney dysfunction due to cisplatin. Dialysis is reserved for acute kidney failure.

HEPATOTOXICITY

Hepatotoxicity is damage to the liver. Risk factors include primary hepatic cancer, prior hepatic dysfunctions, and use of chemotherapy and biotherapy agents such as crizotinib, cyclophosphamide, cytarabine, dactinomycin, etoposide, gemcitabine, ifosfamide, irinotecan, methotrexate, 6-mercaptopurine, sorafenib, and procarbazine.

Liver functions should be diligently assessed to prevent dysfunction. Liver function is monitored by the bilirubin blood levels. Elevated bilirubin levels indicate that the liver is not filtering and working properly. Additionally, alkaline phosphate (AP), alanine aminotransferase (ALT), aspartate aminotransferase (ALT), and lactate dehydrogenase (LDH) are lab values that are used to assess the functionality of the liver.

As with all side effects, hepatotoxicity can range from mild to severe. Common signs and symptoms include itching, jaundice of the sclera and skin, abdominal distention, pain in the right upper quadrant, N/V, unintentional weight loss, unexplained fever, rash, dark-colored urine, and uncontrolled bleeding.

▶ TREATMENT

There is no specific treatment for hepatotoxicity; however, symptomatology should be treated accordingly. For example, if the patient is experiencing severe 3+ pitting edema, they should be administered diuretics. Supportive medications include diuretics to decrease the fluid distention and pain medication, which must be titrated accordingly to avoid further insult to the already damaged liver. If possible, the causative agent should be discontinued or the dose adjusted based upon the liver and kidney function.

The bibliography and references for this chapter are available on ExamPrepConnect; see inside front cover for access instructions.

1. Which two medications act as chemo protectants?

   A. Caphosol and lasix
   B. Caphosol and mesna
   C. Mesna and amifostine
   D. Amifostine and caphosol

2. A patient is receiving gemzar and carboplatin for lung cancer. The nurse will closely monitor which of the following lab values?

   A. CBC and glucose levels
   B. CBC, ALT, AST, and LDH
   C. CBC, BUN, and creatinine
   D. CBC, PT, PTT, and BUN

3. All of the following are side effects of hepatotoxicity, EXCEPT:

   A. Increased abdominal girth
   B. Sclera jaundice
   C. Hypernatremia
   D. Rashes

4. Which agents pose the highest risk for hemorrhagic cystitis?

   A. Gemzar and mitomycin
   B. Cyclophosphamide and ifosfamide
   C. Cyclophasmide and mitomycin
   D. Ifosfamide and gemzar

5. Which of the following agents is hepatotoxic?

   A. Lasix
   B. Inderal
   C. Irinotecan
   D. Morphine

(See answers next page.)

1. C) Mesna and amifostine
Mesna and amifostine are chemoprotective agents. Caphosol is a prevention measure to protect against mouth sores for bone marrow transplant patients.

2. C) CBC, BUN, and creatinine
CBC, BUN, and creatinine monitoring is required to administer carboplatin, a drug that is nephrotoxic and must be dosed based upon AUC. ALT, AST, LDH, PT, and PTT are monitored for liver side effects.

3. C) Hypernatremia
Increased abdominal girth, sclera jaundice, and rashes are signs and symptoms of hepatotoxicity. Hypernatremia is a sign of nephrotoxicity.

4. B) Cyclophosphamide and ifosfamide
Cyclophosphamide and ifosfamide are the primary causative agents for HC.

5. C) Irinotecan. Irinotecan is hepatotoxic
Inderal and morphine do not cause liver toxicity. Lasix can cause kidney issues.

Neurological Side Effects

INTRODUCTION

Neurological toxicities are effects caused by cancer therapies, chemotherapy, immunotherapy, and radiation therapy. The neurotoxic effects can cause vascular complications, seizures, mood disorders, cognitive dysfunctions, and peripheral neuropathies.

The nervous system is composed of the brain, spinal cord, and the peripheral nervous system. There is also the blood–brain barrier and blood–nerve barrier, which protect the central nervous system (CNS) from the neurotoxic effects related to chemotherapy and immunotherapy. Neurotoxic side effects are the direct and indirect damage of nerve cells due to exposure to chemotherapy and radiation therapy. These effects are usually temporary but can also cause permanent symptoms occurring in varying grades. Comorbid conditions combined with chemotherapy can enhance potential adjustments to treatment doses or selection of chemotherapy agents. In some individuals, neurotoxic effects are present due to comorbidities such as diabetes, specifically peripheral neuropathy.

The nervous system is comprised of the peripheral nervous system, which is the link between the cranial and spinal nerves branching out from the brain and spinal cord to all parts of the body. Myelinated neurons have layers of Schwann cells, which are large glial cells; these cells are essential in the development, maintenance, function, and regeneration of peripheral nerves. The myelin acts as an electrical insulator; when it is damaged, the electrical signals are interrupted, affecting the nerve cell function (Cavaletti et al., 2015). The peripheral nervous system is divided into autonomic and sensory functions.

The sensory nerves are responsible for touch, pain, and temperature; the motor nerves are responsible for coordination and movement; and the autonomic nerves control blood pressure and involuntary muscle movement (Grisdale & Armstrong, 2016). Damage to the peripheral nervous system results in loss of motor or sensory function, paralysis, pain, ileus, urinary retention, constipation, and impotence.

CEREBELLUM TOXICITY

Toxicity to this system primarily affects the cerebellum, the part of the brain that acts as a center for treating sensory information relating to body position, coordination of muscle movements, and maintenance of body posture. Chemotherapy agents are the primary cause of cerebellum toxicity; however, total brain irradiation can also be a causative agent. Table 26.1 describes the most common chemotherapy agents responsible for cerebellum toxicity.

The bibliography and references for this chapter are available on ExamPrepConnect; see inside front cover for access instructions.

Table 26.1 Chemotherapy Agents That Cause Cerebellum Toxicity

Chemotherapy Agent	Cancers
Cytarabine (ARA-C)	Leukemia
Cyclophosphamide (Cytoxan)	Many malignancies, including breast, lung, lymphoma, ovarian
5-Fluorouracil	Many malignancies, including breast, colorectal, and head and neck
Ifosfamide (Ifex)	Many malignancies, including breast, lung, lymphoma, and sarcomas
Methotrexate	Leukemia, lymphoma, and breast cancer
Taxol (Paclitaxel)	Breast, lung, and ovarian cancer
Thalidomide (Thamilde)	Multiple myeloma
Velcade (Bortezomib)	Multiple myeloma and lymphoma
Vinblastine (Oncovin)	Breast, lymphoma, and lung cancer patients

Signs and symptoms of cerebellum toxicities include posterior reversible encephalopathy syndrome (PRES), which is an acute rapid neurological situation that presents with headaches, seizures, altered mental status, visual changes, hypertension (not always). Other possible symptoms include seizures, ataxia (unsteady gait), impaired coordination of legs and arms, slurred speech, and headache.

▶ TREATMENT

There is no standardized treatment for acute cerebellar syndrome; however, symptom management is essential. The first treatment response is either to discontinue the chemotherapy or to reduce the dose. The remainder of treatments is symptom management, which includes medications to treat individual symptoms. For example, with PRES presenting with hypertension, antihypertensive medications will be prescribed. A wide range of antiseizure medications can be prescribed, including carbamazepine (Carbatrol and Tegretol), gabapentin (Neurontin), phenytoin (Dilantin), and lamotrigine (Lamictal). Steroids such as dexamethasone and methylprednisolone can be prescribed to decrease the inflammatory response.

⬤ PERIPHERAL NEUROPATHY

Peripheral neuropathy (PN) is a common toxicity caused by many chemotherapy agents. PN occurs due to the less competent blood nervous system barrier and mostly affects the dorsal root ganglia, which has easy access to nerve fibers and neurons (Cavaletti et al., 2015). Chemotherapy-induced peripheral neuropathy (CIPN) is the response of the peripheral nervous system insult imposed by the exposure to neurotoxic chemotherapy agents (Table 26.2). In addition, diabetes and peripheral vascular disease are also risk factors for patients receiving these agents.

Table 26.2 Chemotherapy Agents That Cause Chemotherapy-Induced Peripheral Neuropathy

Chemotherapy Agent	Cancers
Platinum-based agents: Oxaliplatin (Eloxatin)* carboplatin (Paraplatin), cisplatin (Platinol)	Colorectal and pancreatic cancer (oxaliplatin) Lung, ovarian, bladder, breast, and testicular cancer (carboplatin and cisplatin)

(continued)

Table 26.2 Chemotherapy Agents That Cause Chemotherapy-Induced Peripheral Neuropathy (*continued*)

Chemotherapy Agent	Cancers
Taxanes: Cabazitaxel (Jevtana), docetaxel (Taxotere), paclitaxel (Taxol)	Breast, lung, ovarian, and pancreatic cancer Prostate cancer (cabazitaxel)
Vinca alkaloids: Vincristine (Oncovin), vinblastine (Velban), vinorelbine (Navelibine)	Many malignancies, including lung, bladder, and testicular cancer; lymphomas
Immunomodulatory drugs (IMiDs): Thalomide (Thalmid), lenolidomide (Revlimid), pomalidomide (Pomalyst)	Multiple myeloma
Proteasome inhibitors (PI): Bortezomib (Velcade)	Multiple myeloma

*Oxaliplatin neurotoxicities are induced and aggravated by cold; they can cause transient cold-induced pharyngolaryngeal dysesthesia, which is a feeling of difficulty in breathing and swallowing.

CIPN presents with either or both sensory, motor, and autonomic symptoms. Sensory symptoms include paresthesia, which is the feeling of burning, tingling, numbness, or skin-crawling sensation on the skin, and dysesthesia, which is the feeling of prickling, burning, or a feeling of ice-cold hands or feet. They can result in diminished awareness of the posture, altered gait and balance, altered body movements, and diminished vibratory and cutaneous sensation. Motor symptoms include muscle atrophy, weakness, and difficulty with activities of daily living (ADL), such as dressing, writing, and driving. Autonomic symptoms include urinary retention, constipation, alterations in blood pressure, and sexual dysfunction.

▶ TREATMENT

The primary treatment for CINP is to adjust the dose of or discontinue the causative chemotherapy agent. Symptom management is accomplished with lifestyle changes, a variety of medications, and complementary measures.

- Lifestyle changes: Encourage the patient to remain active and engage in physical therapy; avoid smoking, alcohol, and the cold, wear protective clothing, especially during the winter months.
- Pain medications
  - NSAIDs and narcotics (e.g., tramadol and oxycodone): They work on different pathways and receptors to block the pain caused by the nerve damage and may be used in combination.
  - Antiseizure medications: Gabapentin (Neurontin) and pregabalin (Lyrica) can also be used to reduce nerve pain by working on different nerve pathways.
  - Tricyclic antidepressant: Doxepin and nortriptyline can be beneficial.
  - Serotonin–norepinephrine reuptake inhibitors (SNRIs): Duloxetine (Cymbalta) and venlafaxine (Effexor XR) help to restore balance of serotonin and norepinephrine in the brain.
  - Topical pain medications: Capsaicin and lidocaine patches.
- Complementary measures: Transcutaneous electrical nerve stimulation (TENS) applied on the area of concern for 30 minutes daily or as determined by the physical therapist/provider; acupuncture.

● CHEMO BRAIN

Chemo brain is defined as a fogginess or decreased mental acuity that is associated with chemotherapy, radiation, and surgical procedures specific to the brain, as a result of inflammation. Risk factors include primary brain tumor and comorbid conditions such as diabetes, hypertension, extreme fatigue, and history of anxiety, depression, or alcohol and drug abuse. It is common in older adults and postmenopausal women.

Signs and symptoms of chemo brain include difficulty concentrating, loss of interest in reading, and difficulty with ADLs. Unfortunately, many of the cognitive issues can remain post treatment (Henderson et al., 2019). Patients who are emotionally stable are better able to cope with the challenges that can occur during their medical and psychosocial care.

▶ TREATMENT

There are no medications currently available to treat the cognitive changes associated with chemo brain; however, there are behaviors that can be implemented to increase brain activity, including staying active, keeping a routine, avoiding distractions and alcohol, engaging in mental games (e.g., puzzle, word games, matching games), using a daily planner, and decreasing stress with mediation, yoga, and breathing exercises.

● OTOTOXICITY

Ototoxicity is direct damage to the vestibulocochlear nerve caused by platinum-based chemotherapy agents (Carboplatin and Platinol). It is a progressive condition that begins with the loss of high-frequency sounds. Chemo-induced ototoxicity is often associated with permanent sensorineural hearing loss.

In addition to the use of Carboplatin and Platinol, risk factors include the history of hearing issues and tinnitus, older age, use of supportive medications such as antibiotics and loop diuretics, and use of antimalarials. Signs and symptoms can occur during and post treatment and include decreased hearing, tinnitus, continually asking individuals to repeat themselves, dizziness, balance issues, difficulty sleeping, altered mental status and changes in memory, social isolation, and difficulties with activities of daily living.

▶ TREATMENT

The most effective treatment is early identification of the hearing loss and hearing evaluation, including a baseline audiogram. In addition, the causative agent should be dose-adjusted or discontinued. Some patients may benefit from auditory rehabilitation, physical therapy, and, in severe cases, hearing aids. Patients should be instructed to monitor for numbness or tingling in the fingers or toes before each treatment, as well as for changes in hearing. Patients should be encouraged to exercise regularly; lose weight if overweight or obese; and quit smoking.

● PAIN

Pain, which is an individual and subjective experience, is common in oncology patients. It can be caused by the disease process, treatment (radiation and surgery), procedures (including diagnostic testing), arthritis, and fibromyalgia. Nociceptive pain (physiologic pain) is characterized by the normal response to painful stimuli from direct damage to the tissues. Neuropathic pain, pathophysiologic pain that is defined as the abnormal processing of stimuli via the nervous system, is caused by direct damage to the central and peripheral nervous system. Pain can be protective to the body by acting as a warning sign; however, it also has the ability to be maladaptive or dysfunctional, resulting in chronic pain.

Types of pain include:

■ Nociceptive pain: Related to an injury or muscle strain. It does not cause nerve damage, just irritation of the nerve.
■ Inflammatory pain: Related an inflammatory process, such as a sprained ankle or rheumatoid arthritis
■ Neuropathic pain: Related to irritation or damage to nerves (e.g., peripheral neuropathy); can be caused by spinal issues, diabetes, and chemotherapy.
■ Functional pain: Interferes with everyday activities; typically does not have a clear etiology.
■ Acute pain: Sudden onset and typically related to a soft tissue injury or a surgical procedure; typically lasts fewer than 12 weeks.
■ Chronic pain: Typically associated with an unhealed injury, complications of a trauma, injury, or surgery; typically lasts longer than 12 weeks.

Signs and symptoms of pain include the inability to concentrate, decreased/loss of appetite, muscle spasms, numbness and tingling, depression, and sleep disturbances. A patient can express pain verbally using the universal pain rating scale (0–10) or non-verbally, with signs such as facial grimacing or frowning; writhing or constant shifting positions to obtain comfort; moaning, groaning, and or crying; irritability; guarding area of pain; and limited movement.

▶ TREATMENT

Treatment of pain involves both non-pharmacologic and pharmacologic interventions. Nonpharmacologic interventions include transcutaneous electrical nerve stimulation (TENS), acupuncture, massage, reflexology, and distraction (e.g., music, deep breathing, meditation). See Table 26.3 for pharmacological pain management.

Table 26.3 Pharmacologic Pain Interventions

Pharmacological Intervention	Medications	Notes
Narcotics	Oxycodone (Percocet), hydromorphone (Dilaudid), morphine sulfate immediate release (MSIR), long-acting morphine sulfate (MS Contin), long-acting oxycodone (Oxycontin)	Usually the first line for acute, short-term pain related to primary cancer and treatments

(continued)

Table 26.3 Pharmacologic Pain Interventions (*continued*)

Pharmacological Intervention	Medications	Notes
Nerve blocks	Combination of a local anesthetic and steroid injected around the nerves surrounding the spinal column	Used to stop pain signals from reaching the brain
Nonsteroidal anti-inflammatory drugs (NSAIDs)	Celecoxib (Celebrex), meloxicam (Mobic), indomethacin (Indocin), Ketorolac (Toradol), Ibuprofen (Advil, Motrin), naproxen (Aleve)	Should be used with caution as they can disrupt the platelets
Norepinephrine reuptake inhibitors (SNRIs)	Duloxetine (Cymbalta), venlafaxine (Effexor)	Most commonly used class of antidepressants to treat neuropathic pain
Tricyclic antidepressants (TCAs)	Amitriptyline (Elavil), nortriptyline (Pamelor)	Older class of drugs used to treat neuropathic pain; not used as first-line therapy due to cardiac side effects Anticholinergic effects; use caution in the elderly

Patients should be encouraged to keep a diary of side effects, record any changes in activities of daily living, engage in open communication with their provider, and take prescribed medications appropriately.

CONCLUSION

Oncology nurses need to be knowledgeable about the risk of neurological toxicities. Safety in caring for the oncology patient population is imperative, reducing the risk of harm and enabling continued enjoyment and sustained quality of life.

The bibliography and references for this chapter are available on ExamPrepConnect; see inside front cover for access instructions.

1. All of the following agents can cause neurotoxicity, EXCEPT:

   A. Vinblastine (Velban)
   B. Paclitaxel (Taxol)
   C. Gemcitabine (Gemzar)
   D. Doxorubicin (Adriamycin)

2. Which of the following statements BEST describes the difference between acute and chronic pain?

   A. Acute pain requires the administration of narcotics, and chronic pain occurs immediately after a surgical procedure
   B. Acute pain requires the administration of narcotics, and chronic pain occurs for 3 months or more
   C. Acute pain requires NSAIDs, and chronic pain occurs immediately after a procedure
   D. Acute and chronic pain occurs immediately after a surgical procedure or trauma

3. Oxaliplatin can cause which of the following toxic events?

   A. Acute laryngeal spasms, cold intolerance, and peripheral neuropathy
   B. Acute laryngeal spasms, cold intolerance, and pulmonary fibrosis
   C. Cold intolerance, nausea/vomiting, and pulmonary fibrosis
   D. Cold intolerance, cardiac changes, and pulmonary fibrosis

4. Which of the following chemotherapy agents can cause ototoxicity?

   A. Paclitaxel (Taxol)
   B. Vinblastine (Velban)
   C. Cisplatin (Platinol)
   D. Vincristine (Oncovin)

5. Which of the following nursing measures should be implemented when caring for a patient receiving a platinum-based chemotherapy agent?

   A. Monitor CBC, AST, ALT, and potassium
   B. Monitor CBC, BUN and creatine, and strict I & Os
   C. Monitor BUN, AST, ALT, and I & Os
   D. Monitor potassium, magnesium, and BUN

6. A 50-year-old breast cancer patient with a history of depression and anxiety disorder completed her fourth cycle of chemotherapy. The patient is complaining of forgetfulness and difficulty working with numbers at her job. The nurse suspects that the patient is experiencing:

   A. Ototoxicity
   B. Peripheral neuropathy
   C. Chemo brain
   D. Hypoxia

1. D) Doxorubicin (Adriamycin)
Vinblastine, paclitaxel, and gemcitabine can cause neurotoxicity. Doxorubicin causes cardiac toxicities.

2. B) Acute pain requires administration of narcotics, and chronic pain occurs for 3 months or more
Acute pain can occur immediately after a surgical procedure or trauma and typically lasts fewer than 3 months.

3. A) Acute laryngeal spasms, cold intolerance, and peripheral neuropathy
Oxaliplatin can cause laryngeal spasms, cold intolerance, and peripheral neuropathy. Pulmonary fibrosis can be caused by bleomycin, and doxorubicin can cause cardiac changes.

4. C) Cisplatin (Platinol)
Paclitaxel, vinblastine, and vincristine are not known to cause ototoxicity.

5. B) Monitor CBC, BUN and creatine, and strict I & Os
When caring for a patient receiving a platinum-based chemotherapy agent, the nurse should monitor CBC, BUN and creatine, and strict I & Os. It is not necessary to monitor AST and ALT, which measure liver function, potassium, and magnesium.

6. C) Chemo brain
Chemo brain is a cognitive side effect from chemotherapy that can be exacerbated when a patient has a history of depression or anxiety. Signs and symptoms include mental fogginess, memory issues, and difficulty with job-related tasks. Peripheral neuropathy is damage to the peripheral nerves, and hypoxia is decreased oxygenation to the brain.

Oncologic Emergencies

INTRODUCTION

Oncologic emergencies are urgent or emergent conditions arising from the cancer disease process or the treatment of cancer. Sometimes these conditions are the reasons that patients first seek care, ultimately resulting in a cancer diagnosis. Other times, oncologic emergencies can be seen during the treatment process and indicate a progression of the disease.

Oncologic emergencies are classified into metabolic or structural emergencies, which often dictates the assessment and choice of care. Metabolic emergencies are defined as alterations in electrolytes, laboratory values that can cause life-threatening issues. Structural emergencies are identified as changes within the organs of the body, such as the spinal column, heart, and other vital organs.

Nurses who work with oncology patients need to understand the pathophysiology of oncologic emergencies and which patients are at risk. Nurses further need to be able how to recognize the most common signs and symptoms and anticipate appropriate monitoring, interventions, and treatment for this dynamic patient population. This chapter addresses the most common metabolic and structural oncologic emergencies.

METABOLIC-RELATED EMERGENCIES

▶ HYPERCALCEMIA

Hypercalcemia is the most common type of metabolic oncology emergency. It occurs when more calcium is available in the vascular plasma than the kidneys can excrete, or the bones can reabsorb. The source of the calcium can be endogenous from bone loss due to the disease process or mediated by hormone or pseudo hormone secretions from cancer itself, such as increased levels of parathyroid hormone (PTH) or PTH-related protein (PTHrP) levels. In cancer patients, the condition can be complicated by dehydration, leading to the greater relative concentration of serum calcium or impaired mobility leading to greater bone loss and calcium release. Both dehydration and mobility issues are common comorbidities in oncology patients. Hypercalcemia is usually associated with advanced disease.

Hypercalcemia is most often seen in patients with leukemia, lymphoma, or multiple myeloma. It is also commonly seen in breast cancer or squamous cell lung cancer, especially with bone metastases. Symptoms vary depending on the degree of hypercalcemia as well as the individual patient and comorbidities. Common symptoms include decreased appetite, nausea, abdominal pain, constipation, headache, fatigue, muscle weakness and pain, depression, seizures (severe), coma (severe), cardiac arrhythmias (severe), and myocardial infarction. The severity of symptoms generally correlates with the degree of hypercalcemia and is often dependent on how quickly the calcium level rises:

The bibliography and references for this chapter are available on ExamPrepConnect; see inside front cover for access instructions.

- Mild hypercalcemia: Calcium level greater than normal but <12 mg/dL. The patient is often asymptomatic or accompanied by only mild symptoms. Patients can usually be treated with a restriction in oral calcium and vitamin D intake.
- Moderate hypercalcemia: Calcium levels between 12 and 14 mg/dL. Patients with mild to moderate hypercalcemia usually respond well to symptom management hydration and medications used to increase the renal excretion of calcium.
- Severe hypercalcemia: Calcium levels >14 mg/dL. Considered critical and emergent, especially if rapid onset. It may cause cardiac dysrhythmias such as bradycardia, shortening of the QT and ST interval, and can lead to myocardial infarctions, seizures, or even death.

TREATMENT FOR HYPERCALCEMIA

Treatment for hypercalcemia includes:

- Hydration: Aggressive hydration if severe levels of calcium are noted
- Antiemetics: For symptom management
- Diuretics: Non-thiazide loop diuretics help improve renal calcium excretion
- Bisphosphonates (zoledronic acid [Reclast], pamidronate [Aredia]): Initiates bone reabsorption and inhibits tumor-related osteoclasts.
- Calcitonin: Acts by decreasing calcium reabsorption in the kidneys.
- Denosumab: Used in patients when bisphosphonates and calcitonin are ineffective or are contraindicated due to renal insufficiencies.

NURSING MANAGEMENT

Nursing management includes assessment and ongoing monitoring of the patient's mental, neurologic, and cardiovascular status. The patient's electrolytes, including phosphorus, magnesium, potassium, as well as calcium levels, should be examined, and any abnormalities should be communicated to the appropriate healthcare provider and replacement of electrolytes if required.

▶ TUMOR LYSIS SYNDROME

Tumor lysis syndrome (TLS) is another metabolic abnormality that occurs as a result of the large-scale rapid degradation of tumor cells. It is often a direct result of treatments such as biotherapy, chemotherapy, or radiation. Although less frequent, it can also be the result of surgical intervention such as a debulking procedure. During tumor lysis syndrome, the cell membrane is destroyed or ruptures, leading to the release of intracellular material, including nucleic acids, into the circulating plasma volume. This causes the release of formerly intracellular contents into the blood, resulting in elevated levels of serum potassium and phosphate. The breakdown of the nucleic acid increases uric acid levels in the blood. The uric acid forms crystals in the renal tubules of the kidney. This process is further exacerbated by hyperphosphatemia from the large intracellular phosphate release. The phosphates bind with serum calcium, forming crystals that also deposit in the renal tubules causing potential additional acute renal injury and decreasing serum calcium levels. The major complication of tumor lysis syndrome is acute kidney injury.

It can occur in patients with acute leukemias, Hodgkin's disease, high-grade non-Hodgkin's lymphoma (NHL), myelofibrosis, and blastomas located in the liver and /or brain. It is less commonly seen in blast crises with chronic leukemias or after treatment of large chemosensitive solid tumors. TLS can occur spontaneously in highly proliferative malignancies due to increased cell turnover from the tumor itself.

According to the classification system of Cairo and Bishop (2005), laboratory findings consistent with TLS are defined as the presence of two or more of the following electrolyte abnormalities: elevated uric acid levels, hyperkalemia, hyperphosphatemia, or hypocalcemia. Signs and symptoms include fatigue/weakness, peripheral neuropathy, irritability, nausea/vomiting, decreased cloudy urine production, muscle cramping, and pain.

> ▶ **EXAM TIP**
>
> Know and recognize the signs and symptoms of tumor lysis syndrome.

TREATMENT

If TLS is not appropriately treated, it can lead to delirium, acute cardiac arrhythmias, and seizures. Treatment includes:

- Hydration: Increase fluids to flush the kidneys and excrete the toxins released from the tumor lysis.
- Allopurinol: It is normally initiated as a preventive measure in high-risk patients 2 to 3 days prior to the commencement of therapy. Allopurinol blocks the formation of uric acid and crystals; however, it is not the drug of choice in the treatment of acute TLS because it is slower acting.
- Diuretics: Used to increase urine production and the renal secretion of potassium. Most commonly diuretics used are furosemide (Lasix) and mannitol (Resectisol).
- Rasburicase: Oxidizes uric acid into allantoin, which is more easily excretable. In addition, it usually lowers uric acid levels within 24 hours; therefore, it is the drug of choice in the treatment of acute TLS.
- Dialysis: May be prescribed if the above treatments are ineffective and the kidneys are not functioning.

NURSING MANAGEMENT

The best treatment for tumor lysis syndrome is prevention and a focus on at-risk patients prior to the appearance of complications. Pre-hydration and allopurinol prior to the administration of chemotherapy, close monitoring of patient's electrolytes and frequent communication as well as early recognition and intervention by nurses all are effective strategies in the prevention of tumor lysis syndrome and its complication. Nursing interventions include assessing the patient's clinical and via laboratory criteria for the diagnosis of tumor lysis syndrome. Nurses not only need to be aware of abnormal lab values but also need to be sensitive to individual trends, such as when a patient's lab values deviate from an established baseline.

▶ SYNDROME OF INAPPROPRIATE ANTIDIURETIC HORMONE SECRETION

Syndrome of inappropriate antidiuretic hormone secretion (SIADH) occurs due to the overproduction of antidiuretic hormone (ADH), the hormone that regulates urine concentration via water reabsorption in the kidneys. The excess production of ADH causes the body to retain too much water leading to fluid volume overload, dilutional hyponatremia, decreased urine output, increased urine specific gravity, and fluid-based weight gain.

Various medications and conditions are linked to SIADH and the overproduction of ADH, including antibiotics, antidepressants, brain malignancies, infections, and head traumas. In oncology patients, the malignancy itself may be the source of the non-pituitary ADH, with bronchogenic carcinomas being the most common. Signs and symptoms include:

- Early stage: Sodium levels <135mEq/L but >120mEq/L.
  - Thirst, anorexia, lethargy, drowsiness, or fatigue, headaches, and muscle cramps.
- Moderate stage: Sodium levels between 120 and 110 mEq/L.
  - Confusion, restlessness, irritability, muscle weakness, spasms, and/or cramps.
- Severe stage: Sodium levels <110 mEq/L are considered critical and life-threatening. Patients with severe hyponatremia can experience seizures, coma, or even death.
  - N/V, tremors, depressed mood/confusion, personality alterations, seizures, and coma.

TREATMENT

Treatment includes IV hydration and medications:

- Mild hyponatremia: Oral fluid restriction, isotonic IV hydration, diuretics
- Moderate hyponatremia: Demeclocycline, lithium, urea, salt tabs
- Severe hyponatremia: Hypertonic saline solution with close monitoring of labs and infusion rates.

NURSING MANAGEMENT

The patient's sodium level must be corrected slowly in order to avoid central pontine myelinolysis and long-term neurologic damage. Long-term treatment of SIADH focuses on identifying and correcting the underlying cause. Nursing interventions for patients with SIADH include beginning IV infusions, fluid restrictions with strict input and output measurements, possible high sodium diet, or oral sodium supplementation. Safety is a priority with frequent neurologic assessments, seizure prevention protocols as well as emotional and supportive care for the patient and family members.

▶ SEPSIS/SEPTIC SHOCK

Cancer and cancer treatments place oncology patients at increased risk for infection. Disruption to the mucosal and skin integrity compounded with immunosuppression from the treatment options, as well as the use of long-term indwelling central venous catheters, all serve to dramatically pose a risk of infection. Infections during treatment may delay or compromise the primary goal for a cure. Systemic inflammatory response syndrome is the result of insult or injury. Sepsis is SIRS with confirmed infection process.

Sepsis can occur from an infectious or a noninfectious event. Gram-negative bacteria are the most common causes of sepsis, including *Escherichia coli, Enterobacter, Klebsiella,* and *Pseudomonas.* It can also be caused by gram-positive bacteria (*Staphylococcus, Streptococcus, Corynebacterium, and Clostridium difficile*), and virus and fungi.

Septic shock is a clinical progression of sepsis when the body's systemic immune response with or without support is insufficient to control the invading agent. Septic shock is associated with gram-negative bacteria due to the bacterial release of endotoxins resulting in increased vascular permeability, which leads to hemodynamic instability, altered metabolism, hypotension, and abnormal coagulation.

Cytotoxic drugs that have the highest risk of inducing neutropenia include anthracyclines, taxanes, topoisomerase inhibitors, platinum-based agents, gemcitabine, vinorelbine, and cyclophosphamide/ifosfamide. Neutropenic patients are at the greatest risk for sepsis and septic shock. Neutropenia is defined as an absolute neutrophil count (ANC) of <1500/μL, while severe neutropenia is defined as an ANC of <500/μL. Neutropenia alone is not considered an oncologic emergency. However, neutropenic fever is one of the most common complications of cancer treatment. Febrile neutropenia is defined as a single oral temperature of ≥38.5°C (101.3°F) or a temperature of greater than 38°C (100.4°F) sustained for over a 1-hour period in a neutropenic patient (Alsharawneh et al., 2020). The rate of neutrophil decline, the timing in relation to chemotherapy, the type of chemotherapy, other immunosuppression therapy, especially concurrently administered of corticosteroids as part of the treatment protocol, impaired liver function at initiation of therapy all serve to complicate a neutropenic cancer patient's prognosis, condition, and progression to septic shock.

Symptoms of shock include warm, often flushing skin and increased respirations with decreased oxygenation and a widening pulse pressure progressing to destabilizing hypotension. It is manifested by two or more of the following:

- Temperature >100.5°F
- Heart rate >90 beats/min
- Respiratory rate >20 breaths/min or $PaCO_2$ <32 mmHg
- WBC >12,000 cells/mm³ or < 4,000 cells/mm³ (indicating neutropenia)

TREATMENT

Treatment for sepsis/septic shock includes:

- Antibiotics: Timely administration of antibiotics is key with a goal of initiating empirical therapy within one hour of patient assessment. Broad-spectrum mono-therapy or dual coverage depending on patient presentation. Common agents include piperacillin (Tazabactam), imipenem (Cilastatin), meropenem, ceftazidime, and cefepime.
- Granulocyte colony stimulating factors (CSF): Prophylaxis with agents such as Neupogen (filgrastim) or Neulasta (pegfilgrastim) when neutropenia is expected to occur following a course of chemotherapy.
- Fluid resuscitation:
  - Crystalloids (normal saline or ringers lactated): 500 to 1000 mL bolus until BP >90 mmHg systolic up to 6 to 10 L.
  - Colloids (Albumin): Mobilize extracellular fluid into the intravascular space.
- Vasopressors: Dopamine; norepinephrine can be added if dopamine is not effective.

NURSING MANAGEMENT

Antibiotics and colony-stimulating factors should be administered in a timely manner. The nurse should teach the patient the signs/symptoms of infection and encourage good hygiene.

▶ HYPERSENSITIVITY

A hypersensitivity reaction is caused when exposure to an antigen, such as a chemotherapeutic agent, results in the formation of an antibody. A second exposure to the same or similar antigen triggers an immediate and vigorous IgE antibody-mediated response by the immune system resulting in the release of histamines from basophils and mast cells. Because antibodies were produced in ample supply after the initial exposure, the reaction usually occurs very swiftly upon second exposure. Certain chemotherapeutic agents are at a high risk of reaction because they produce what is known as an anaphylactoid response. Anaphylactoid reactions are different from anaphylactic reactions because a prior exposure is not necessary. The chemotherapy agent itself, not the IgE antibodies, causes the immune response. Anaphylactoid and anaphylactic reactions have the same signs and symptoms and are treated in the same manner. Epinephrine is used as a first-line agent in severe reactions. Other common medications used to treat hypersensitivity reactions include antihistamines, corticosteroids, and bronchodilators. Some evidence suggests that combining H1 and H2 blockers may be more effective than H1 blockers alone. Hypersensitivity allergic reactions have been reported with countless chemotherapy drugs and can vary from mild localized reactions to severe reactions that can be life-threatening.

Hypersensitivity risk is increased in patients with a history of allergies. Chemotherapy agents such as L-asparaginase, paclitaxel, rituximab docetaxel, teniposide, procarbazine, cytarabine, and carboplatin can cause hypersensitivity, as can biotherapy agents such as monoclonal antibodies (MABs), rituximab, and daratumumab.

> ### ▶ EXAM TIP
>
> Hypersensitivity reactions most commonly manifest after first treatments, except with carboplatin, in which reactions can occur after the seventh treatment.

Based upon head-to-toe assessment, signs and symptoms include:

- Dermatologic: Flushing, pruritus, urticaria, angioedema
- Neurologic: Agitation, confusion, dizziness
- Respiratory: Stridor, cough, wheezing, tachypnea, hoarseness, tightness in the chest, decreased air movement, diminished breath sounds, tightness, tickling, scratchy throat
- Cardiovascular: Chest discomfort, tachycardia, hypotension, dysrhythmias

TREATMENT

Prevention is the most important nursing intervention in chemotherapy-related hypersensitivity reactions, and nurses play an integral role in this aspect of care. Patient education regarding signs and symptoms is vital. Pre-medications include steroids, antihistamines, and antiemetics (H2 blockers such as Pepcid). Treatment for acute reactions includes steroids, antihistamines, and antiemetics, epinephrine (severe reactions, anaphylaxis), and bronchodilators such as albuterol (moderate to severe reactions).

NURSING MANAGEMENT

The following steps should be taken if a hypersensitivity reaction is suspected:

1. Stop the infusion immediately and convert to rapidly infusing normal saline.
2. Assess the patient and their airway.

3. Initiate O$_2$ and rapid response (if severe anaphylaxis reaction noted).

4. Obtain vital signs.

5. Stay with the patient and continue to monitor the patient's status.

6. Contact the healthcare provider.

7. Administer rescue medications as directed.

▶ DISSEMINATED INTRAVASCULAR COAGULATION

Disseminated intravascular coagulation (DIC) is a disruption of normal coagulation that is secondary to malignancy. DIC is frequently associated with malignancies such as leukemias, especially the myelogenous leukemias, or mucin-secreting adenocarcinomas. These cancers alter the extrinsic coagulation pathway and the over expressions of tissue factor (TF). The hallmark of DIC is simultaneous clot formation and diffuse hemorrhaging resulting in widespread microvascular thrombosis, hypoxic tissue injury, consumption of platelets, and coagulation factors. The most common cause of DIC is sepsis associated with gram-negative organisms via the intrinsic coagulation pathway from damage to the vascular endothelium often caused by the source of the infection. Endotoxins released from the bacteria can contribute to the activation of the clotting cascade. Nurses must be acutely aware of the possibility of DIC in patients presenting with neutropenic fever, where the condition must be managed in conjunction with addressing both the underlying infection and with consideration for the patient's decreased neutrophil count. Table 27.1 provides the clinical definition of DIC.

Table 27.1 Clinical Definition of DIC

Lab Values	Description
Prothrombin time (PT)	>13.5 s
Partial thromboplastin (PTT)	>35 s
Platelet count	<140,000*** with an increased in fibrin split product

▶ EXAM TIP

There is no definitive test for DIC.

Patients with leukemias, especially acute promyelocytic leukemia, are at risk as are patients with mucin-secreting adenocarcinomas (pancreas and prostate). It is less commonly seen in ovarian, kidney, stomach, and gallbladder cancers. Signs and symptoms of DIC (based upon a head-to-toe assessment) include:

- Dermatologic: Petechiae, purpura or ecchymosis
- Neurologic: Headache, nausea/vomiting, confusion, or mental status changes
- Eyes: Vision changes, conjunctival or scleral hemorrhage
- ENT: Bleeding from nose, gums, and/or mouth
- Respiratory: Tachypnea, hemoptysis, frothy bright red blood, diminished breath sounds, chest discomfort, desire to cough

- Cardiovascular: Vital sign changes (tachycardia and hypotension), changes in peripheral profusion, or signs of acute blood loss
- GI/GU: Hematemesis, epigastric pain, coffee-ground emesis, melena or tarry stools, rectal or vaginal bleeding

TREATMENT

The cause—infection or cancer—should be treated. Blood products such as platelets, cryoprecipitate, and fresh frozen plasma may be administered. Anticoagulants such as heparin may be used in slow-progressing DIC. In severe acute DIC, fibrinolytic agents such as aminocaproic acid (Amicar) can be used when bleeding is not stopped with supportive blood products.

NURSING MANAGEMENT

Nursing management of DIC patients is complicated and multifactorial. The desired outcome is to minimize bleeding, decrease clotting and promote circulation. The nurse should monitor for signs of bleeding and clotting, administer supportive medications and blood products, and closely monitor the patient's vital signs, oxygenation, and appropriate lab values.

● STRUCTURAL-RELATED EMERGENCIES

▶ CARDIAC TAMPONADE

Cardiac tamponade results from a compression of the heart that occurs when blood or fluid accumulates inside the pericardial sac. A pericardial effusion can occur without causing tamponade. Tamponade can also be caused by pressure from inflammation of the pericardial sac, such as pericarditis from either an infection or as a result of radiation treatment to the chest wall. This can occur when the heart is exposed to increased amounts of radiation, only when the heart is inside the radiation field. A pericardial infusion can result in increasing pressure which decreases left ventricular function, stroke volume, and eventually collapses cardiac output.

It can occur in patients with cancers of the thorax, including lung, breast, melanoma, lymphomas, or leukemias. Primary tumors of the pericardium are rare but commonly cause cardiac tamponade, where the treatment is a surgical intervention to decrease pressure in the pericardial sac. It can also occur in patients with a history of radiation to the chest and in those receiving cardiotoxic agents such as doxorubicin, daunorubicin, or cyclophosphamide.

Symptoms of a pericardial effusion depend on the rate of fluid accumulation, with many patients never developing symptoms. Up to 50% of oncology patients experience some form of cardiac effusions during the course of their disease. Slower effusions that progress over time may be able to accommodate larger volumes of fluid with fewer symptoms. The classic symptoms of cardiac tamponade include:

- Dyspnea, chest pain, and palpitations
- Muffled heart sounds
- Nonproductive cough or even hiccups
- Hypotension and jugular vein distension are common with rapid accumulations

■ Tachycardia

■ Engorged neck veins

■ Peripheral edema

TREATMENTS

Treatment for cardiac tamponade includes:

■ Surgery: Shunts and windows are especially common when the source of fluid has not been eliminated.
  ● Pericardiocentesis: Removal of the fluid
  ● Pericardial shunt: Placement of internal indwelling catheter to redistribute the fluid and avoid it from accumulating in the pericardial sac
  ● Pericardial window: Removal of the piece of the pericardium in order for the fluid to drain
■ Medications: Medical interventions may be the only treatment utilized if effusions do not warrant more aggressive treatment or the patient's status limits interventions.
  ● Corticosteroids: Used to decrease inflammation
  ● Diuretics: To pheresis fluids
  ● Chemotherapy agents: To decrease the tumor burden
■ Radiation therapy: External beam radiation to decrease the size of a tumor

Medical interventions may be the only treatment utilized if effusions do not warrant more aggressive treatment or the patient's status limits interventions.

NURSING MANAGEMENT

If cardiac tamponade is suspected, the nurse should ensure the following:

1. Monitor for signs and symptoms of cardiac effusion.
2. Assess cardiac and lung sounds.
3. Monitor vital signs.
4. Initiate immediate treatment.
5. Place the patient in Fowler's position, which increases cardiac output.
6. Administer O_2 therapy.
7. Educate patient regarding life-threatening situation if left untreated.

▶ SPINAL CORD COMPRESSION

Spinal cord compression is the mechanical compression of the dural sac of the spinal cord, and the most common area to be involved is the thoracic region. The majority of cases are associated with metastatic bone lesions to the vertebrae. The cancers with the highest incidence of spinal cord compression are breast, lung, prostate, renal, primary spinal cord cancers, and brain cancers (glioma, astrocytoma, or ependymoma). In addition, patients with metastatic spinal lesions are also at risk for pathologic fractures, which can result in pieces of broken vertebrae impinging on the dural sac. A spinal cord compression is classified as a life-threatening oncologic emergency and, if left untreated, can lead to permanent upper or lower extremity paralysis.

Signs and symptoms include spinal pain, especially upon palpation of the involved vertebrae, pain that interrupts sleep, numbness, tenderness, weakness in hands, legs, or feet (bilaterally but not always symmetrical), and bowel or bladder difficulties.

TREATMENT

Treatment focuses on the reduction of the compression and maintaining upper and lower extremity function. Improvements are unlikely, but maintenance of function is paramount. Interventions such as radiation or a surgical procedure for cord compression are usually aimed at eliminating symptom progression and often determined by the degree of radiosensitivity, tumor location, and type.

- Corticosteroids: Dexamethasone is usually the first line as a bolus and then 24-hour dosing to reduce the inflammatory response and symptom management
- Pain medications: Narcotics or NSAIDs
- Radiation therapy: External beam radiation to the area of the compression or fracture
- Surgery: Decompression of the vertebrate that is affected by the cancer

NURSING MANAGEMENT

The nurse should ensure the following:

1. Assess neurologic function of upper and lower extremities.
2. Administer pain medications when appropriate.
3. Administer steroids bowel and bladder function regularly.
4. Educate patients regarding the importance of immediate care if signs/symptoms of cord compression occur.

● SUPERIOR VENA CAVA SYNDROME

Superior vena cava syndrome (SVC) is caused by an obstruction of blood flow that decreases the return of blood from the brain and upper body. The superior vena cava sits retro to the supraclavicular lymph nodes inside the chest cavity. Extrinsic or external to the vessel obstructions are common. There are various causes for SVC, for example, an acutely enlarged lymph node can lead to constriction. Additionally, mechanical pressure from a solid tumor can lead to either compression or obstruction. Intrinsic or internal vascular obstruction is most often the result of a thrombus or possibly an intraluminal injury. In rare cases, invasive tumors that penetrate the vessel wall are both intrinsic and extrinsic obstructions. The increased vascular congestion from the vessel constriction leads to reduced cardiac output and increased vessel permeability, resulting in both edema and hypoxia. Lung cancer and lymphomas are the most common malignant causes of superior vena cava syndrome. It can also be caused by breast cancers, metastatic tumors, and central venous catheters.

Signs and symptoms of SVC include facial edema, swelling of the neck, distended neck and chest vessels, headache, and dysphagia. The condition can often be visualized on a chest x-ray but is usually confirmed with computed tomography (CT) of the chest to determine the type, location, and level of vessel compression.

TREATMENT

Treatment is aimed at reducing the compression. Targeted chemotherapy can be used to decrease the tumor burden, steroids can be used to reduce the inflammatory response, and diuretics are used in some cases to decrease the fluid. Antithrombic agents should be prescribed to prevent clot formation. External beam radiation to the tumor that is causing the constriction can also be utilized.

NURSING MANAGEMENT

SVS is most commonly seen later in the course of the disease and can be life-threatening if not treated promptly. The nurse should assess the cardiac and respiratory status on a regular basis, educate the patient of signs/symptoms of SVC syndrome, administer medications as prescribed, and keep the patient's head of the bed elevated.

▶ INCREASED INTRACRANIAL PRESSURE

Increased intracranial pressure (ICP) is a potential neurologic oncologic emergency most frequently seen with primary and metastatic brain tumors. The brain is protected by the skull and has a fixed volume which is comprised of the brain, blood, and cerebrospinal fluid. Any change with these relative portions can result in increased intracranial pressure.

Causes related to increased cerebral volume are most frequently due to the expansion and growth of tumors. However, increases in cerebrospinal fluid volume or vascular volume are also common. Malignances have the ability to create independent blood supply, which increased both cerebral volume and vascular volume, thus resulting in ICP. In addition, the tumor burden changes the blood–brain barrier, contributing to the ICP. Increased intracranial pressure can also be the result of cerebral edema triggered by radiation therapy, surgical removal of a brain tumor, chemotherapy/biotherapy agents, increased ammonia levels, and stroke.

Changes in cerebrospinal fluids, including increased production or mechanical impedance of the dynamic fluid flow due to the position of a brain or spinal tumor, are also other possible causes of increased volume in the skull chamber. Brain herniation is a particularly devasting neurovascular complication of increased intracranial pressure from which there are limited options for meaningful recovery.

Patients most at risk include those with primary brain tumors, metastatic brain lesions, meningeal cancers, Ommaya reservoir complications, the impedance of cerebrospinal fluid, infections, and intracranial bleeds. Regardless of etiology, patients may present with headache, especially one that worsens with position change, cough, or other transient changes. The presentation of Cushing's reflex (hypertension, bradycardia, and irregular breathing) is particularly ominous and indicative of ischemia or imminent herniation (Lin & Avila, 2017). Other symptoms include nausea, vomiting (especially spontaneous vomiting), vision changes, focal neurologic deficits, sensory changes, and plegias.

TREATMENT

Treatment for ICP includes:

- Medications: Steroids to decrease the inflammatory process, anticonvulsants to prevent seizures, diuretics (mannitol, furosemide [Lasix]), and pain medications if required
- Radiation therapy: Stereotactic surgery or external beam

- Surgery: Placement of shunt
- Chemotherapy and biotherapy agents: To treat primary tumor and decrease the size of the lesion (if possible)

NURSING MANAGEMENT

Nursing interventions for a patient with increased intracranial pressure include frequent neuro assessment, including assessment of eyes, vision, and oculomotor function; head-of-bed elevation to 45 degrees, administration of medications as prescribed, and emotional support and active listening.

▶ MALIGNANT PLEURAL EFFUSION

A malignant pleural effusion (MPE) is an abnormal accumulation of fluid containing cancer cells in the pleural space. The fluid in the pleural space decreases the lungs' ability to expand as well as diaphragmatic compliance. It is seen in patients with lung cancer, breast cancer, and non-Hodgkin's lymphoma. Signs and symptoms include chest discomfort and pain, nonproductive cough, shortness of breath that is usually exacerbated when the patient is supine, and paroxysmal nocturnal dyspnea.

TREATMENTS

Surgical options include surgical thoracentesis, which can be used diagnostically or therapeutically; thoracoscopy with biopsy to identify the cause of the effusion or to obtain tissue for a marker; and pleurodesis, which is a fusion of the pleural space by a sclerosing agent. Sclerosing agents include bleomycin, thiotepa, doxycycline, minocycline, 5-fluorouracil, and talc. A chest tube, or indwelling pleural catheter (IPC), can be placed to allow for ongoing drainage of fluid from the pleural space.

NURSING MANAGEMENT

The nurse should assess respiratory status frequently, maintain chest tube, and educate the patient regarding the management of the chest tube, especially if sent home with the catheter.

▶ EXTRAVASATIONS

An extravasation occurs when there is an accidental release of a vesicant usually a chemotherapeutic drug into the tissue surrounding a blood vessel. An extravasation is different and more serious than a peripheral infiltration which usually involves the leaking of medication, irritant, or fluid out of a blood vessel.

Patients receiving a known vesicant are at the highest risk of an extravasation including dacarbazine, doxorubicin, daunorubicin, idarubicin, vinblastine, vincristine, dactinomycin, or mitomycin. Early symptoms of a vesicant extravasation include localized pain at the site of the infusion, itching, burning, redness, or swelling. Later symptoms include signs of deep and progressive tissue damage such as skin discoloration, mottling, blistering, necrosis, and skin sluffing.

TREATMENT

The infusion should be stopped at the first sign of an extravasation. The nurse should attempt to aspirate as much of the vesicant as possible and apply heat or cold (agent dependent). Long-term treatment may include plastic surgery and skin grafting.

NURSING MANAGEMENT

Infiltrations may cause pain at the insertion site, along the vein and possible inflammation in the surrounding tissue, but a vesicant is caustic and can cause extensive tissue damage beneath the dermis (Doellman et al., 2019). Although extravasation is more likely to occur with peripheral IV infusions, these complications can develop with central venous catheters or implanted infusion devices. The effects are more difficult to assess and sometimes devastating because of the volume involved and because these devices are below the subcutaneous tissue as well as more likely to be delivering vesicant medications. Nurses need to be sure to closely monitor any infusion for signs of infiltration or extravasation, especially when infusing a vesicant, by assessing for continuous blood return during a vesicant infusion. Damage is progressive, which often leads to a false sense of security when initial assessments yield mild tissue damage. The full extent of the tissue damage may not be apparent for days or weeks after the injury. Therefore, nurses need to be vigilant in assessing any possible venous access site or device when extravasation is suspected or believed to be possible.

● CONCLUSION

Oncologic emergencies can have devastating outcomes for patients and their families. The assessment skills of the nurse in recognizing oncologic emergency and the clinical judgment of the nurse in knowing when to intervene are an essential part of comprehensive clinical cancer care. When nurses are aware of the pathology, the presenting signs and symptoms, the appropriate assessments, and nursing interventions, they are better equipped to promote the best possible outcomes for cancer patients that experience complications.

The role of the nurse in oncologic emergencies also very much focuses on prevention. Knowing which patients are at risk and engaging the patient in proper education and preparation also helps to treat oncologic emergencies by preventing them from occurring. The goal of cancer treatment is to cure the disease. In the absence of this option, prolonged survival with optimal quality of life become the goal. Nurses in all areas of care can assist patients with early recognition of emergent situations and timely intervention to promote a patient's survival, as well as maintain a patient's functionality and quality of life.

The bibliography and references for this chapter are available on ExamPrepConnect; see inside front cover for access instructions.

1. The nurse is assessing a patient with metastatic non-small cell lung cancer. During the assessment, the patient reports new back pain with intermittent numbness and tingling in their hands. The nurse's BEST action is to:

   A. Explain to the patient that this is a normal side effect of chemotherapy
   B. Educate the patient about the signs and symptoms of peripheral neuropathy related to chemotherapy
   C. Communicate the finding to the appropriate provider
   D. Contact the provider to initiate pain management consult as this is a new issue for this patient

2. The nurse is monitoring a patient during their first infusion of rituximab. The patient's baseline vitals were HR 78, BP 125/80, 37°C, RR 16, 99%. The patient reports a tight sensation in the chest, shortness of breath, and a scratchy feeling in the throat. Their vitals are currently HR 95, BP 100/60, 38°, RR 22, 94%. The nurse's priority intervention is to:

   A. Decrease the rate of infusion by 50%
   B. Contact the provider for an order of acetaminophen
   C. Continue with the infusion and monitor the patient
   D. Stop the infusion, initiate fluids and supplemental oxygen

3. A patient with metastatic breast cancer to the brain comes to the clinic for cycle 3 of lapatinib and trastuzumab. The patient complains of a headache that worsens while coughing and has not been relieved by acetaminophen for the last 2 days. The nurse contacts the provider and anticipates an order for which of the following interventions?

   A. Oral dexamethasone
   B. MRI of the head
   C. Oral oxycodone
   D. EKG

4. A nurse is reviewing the laboratory values of a patient with *Pseudomonas* infection, including platelets 55,000/mm³, prothrombin time 21 seconds, partial thromboplastin time 43 seconds, and fibrinogen 100 mg/dL. What oncologic emergency is causing the changes in lab values?

   A. Hypercalcemia
   B. SIADH
   C. DIC
   D. Tumor lysis syndrome

5. Which of the following symptoms would lead the nurse to suspect cardiac tamponade in a lymphoma patient with a history of chest radiation?

   A. Vasodilation and flushing
   B. Hypertension and widening pulse pressure.
   C. Shortness of breath and bradycardia
   D. Agitation and tachycardia

1. C) Communicate the finding to the appropriate provider
Patients with lung cancer are at risk of spinal cord compression. This patient is exhibiting signs and symptoms of this oncologic emergency, including back pain and numbness and tingling in extremities. The nurse should communicate the finding to the appropriate provider as spinal cord compression is an oncologic emergency.

2. D) Stop the infusion, initiate fluids and supplemental oxygen
The patient is exhibiting signs and symptoms of a hypersensitivity reaction. The nurse should immediately stop the infusion, initiate fluids, and apply O_2 therapy. After those interventions, the nurse should contact the provider. Decreasing the infusion rate requires a provider order, and continuing is not an option at this point in time. If left untreated, the patient could have anaphylaxis.

3. B) MRI of the head
A headache that worsens when coughing and is unrelieved by pain medication could be a sign of ICP. The nurse should anticipate an MRI order to determine if the patient has ICP. If ICP is confirmed, steroids (e.g., dexamethasone) will likely be prescribed. Oxycodone and EKG are not indicated for this patient.

4. C) DIC
The patient's laboratory values are indicative of DIC: prothrombin time >13.5 seconds, partial thromboplastin >35 seconds, and platelet count <140,000.

5. D) Agitation and tachycardia
Cardiac tamponade constricts blood flow (vasoconstriction), which causes hypotension, not hypertension. Patient may have shortness of breath but not bradycardia.

Part V
Survivorship and End-of-Life Care

Cancer Survivorship

INTRODUCTION

"Cancer survivorship" encompasses physical, psychosocial, and economic issues, including follow-up care, treatment effects, secondary malignancies, and quality of life following the treatment phase of cancer. Patients, their families, friends, and caregivers are considered in regard to survivorship. With advances in screening, early detection, and treatment options, patients are living longer following a cancer diagnosis. The 5-year relative survival rate for all cancers combined is 70% among White adults and 63% among Black adults (American Cancer Society, 2019). In this chapter, we review the unique concerns and considerations faced by cancer survivors.

CARE FOR CANCER SURVIVORS

Care for cancer survivors can be particularly complex as survivors may need to follow up with multiple specialists depending upon the course of their treatment, may require extensive psychosocial support, and may experience long term-side effects because of their treatment (Ganz, 2009). Concerns and complications experienced by cancer survivors are often dependent on the cancer the patient had and the treatment they received; however, common concerns experienced by survivors include (Ness et al., 2013):

- Residual physiologic effects: Fatigue, sleep disturbance, peripheral neuropathy, hair and skin changes, bowel and bladder changes, impaired body image
- Impaired concentration and memory
- Fertility
- Sexuality
- Financial toxicity
- Fear of recurrence
- Emotional/spiritual concerns

In 2006 the Institute of Medicine (IOM) report, *From Cancer Patient to Cancer Survivor: Lost in Transition,* presented 10 recommendations for cancer survivors which focused on the importance of follow-up care and addressing the long-term issues associated with survivorship; those recommendations include (Striker et al., 2011):

1. Review of recovery from treatment-associated toxicities
2. Recommendations for cancer screening, tests, and examinations
3. Information on psychosocial effects of cancer and survivorship (marital/social relationships, sexual function, work, insurance, ongoing need for psychological support)
4. Information on possible long-term treatment side effects
5. Information on signs and symptoms of secondary cancers

The bibliography and references for this chapter are available on ExamPrepConnect; see inside front cover for access instructions.

6. Information on insurance and employment implications, referral to legal aid and financial assistance programs
7. Specific recommendations to maintain a healthy lifestyle including diet, exercise, and cancer prevention techniques
8. Information on genetic counseling if appropriate
9. Information on known chemoprevention strategies for secondary malignancies if appropriate
10. Referrals for follow-up with healthcare providers such as primary care providers and support groups

⬤ RECURRENCE

Fear of cancer recurrence (FCR) is one of the most common concerns among people with cancer. Almost 99% of cancer patients report fear of recurrence that interferes with their quality of life following the treatment phase of cancer (Chen et al., 2018). Fear of cancer recurrence can be experienced by both patients with curable disease who fear their disease returning and patients with advanced cancer who fear progression. (Butow et al., 2018).

Characteristics of fear of recurrence include being preoccupied with worry and intrusive thoughts about the potential for recurrence, poor coping mechanisms, unable to perform essential daily activities due to excessive worry and anxiety, and trouble planning future events (Lebel et al., 2016).

Risk factors for experiencing fear of cancer recurrence include patients with a new diagnosis, age, severe side effects of treatments, and underlying psychological disorder (Butow et al., 2018).

Table 28.1 describes the most common malignancies and risks of recurrence.

Table 28.1 Recurrence Rates for Common Cancers

Common Cancer	Rate of Risk of Recurrence
Bladder	50% (after cystectomy)
Breast	30%
Colorectal	17%
Glioblastoma	Approximately 100%
Hodgkin's lymphoma	10%–13%
Lymphoma, DLBCL	30%–40%
Melanoma	15%–41%; 87% if metastatic
Ovarian	85%
Pancreatic	36%–46%

Source: From Belvins Primeau (2019).

▶ REDUCING FEAR OF CANCER RECURRENCE

Finding positive ways to manage the fear of cancer recurrence is essential for cancer survivors. Evidence has demonstrated the positive effects psychosocial interventions, such as mindfulness-based stress reduction (MBSR), cognitive behavioral therapy (CBT), meditation exercises, can have on reducing anxiety, uncertainty, and depression as well as improving the overall quality of life (Chen et al., 2018). It is important for oncology nurses to acknowledge the emotional implications of a cancer diagnosis and respond appropriately to emotional cues such as nonverbal signs of anxiety or emotional distress. Oncology nurses should be comfortable speaking openly and asking questions about patients' fear of cancer recurrence and directing patients to appropriate resources such as educational pamphlets or support groups (Butow et al., 2018).

Oncology nurses can help their patients cope more effectively by establishing rapport with both the patient and their loved ones. Developing a trusting relationship helps the patient and family feel comfortable with the information provided, know that the nurse will advocate on their behalf and promote the patient's best interest. In addition, the oncology nurse needs to create a relationship with both the patient and the person(s) the patient chooses to support them throughout their cancer journey. Encouraging a "team"-based approach where the patient's support system is included can help to optimize patient outcomes and promote better coping, healthy behaviors, and improved quality of life (Northouse, 2012).

Support groups can be vital to cancer survivors. Finding and knowing information about acceptable online support groups can offer cancer patients the ability to connect with others who are experiencing similar emotions in the comfort and safety of their own home. Online support groups are popular in rural areas to connect with others regardless of their physical location. In addition, the computer can provide more comfort and potential engagement rather than being in a face-to-face support group. Cancer survivors may need direction on how to find appropriate resources; therefore, it is important for oncology nurses to be familiar with the available resources and reputable websites.

FINANCIAL TOXICITY

Oncology nurses need to be aware of the signs and symptoms of financial toxicity. Finances can be disrupted with a major illness such as cancer. Souza et al. (2016) identified at-risk patients for financial toxicity included:

- Patients with disabilities
- Patients who are unemployed
- Non-White patients experience higher degrees of financial toxicity compared to White patients
- Patients who require three or more hospital stays

In addition, cancer patients and their families can have a tremendous financial burden due to surgical procedures, treatments, and daily medications. The most common financial concerns include lengthy hospital stays, multiple physician visits, numerous co-payments, medications and medical supplies, and diagnostic tests. Concerns can extend to hotel accommodations if living far away from the hospital and parking fees, as well as childcare issues and loss of wages or jobs.

The oncology nurse plays an important role in helping to address the impact of the financial burden associated with cancer care. The oncology nurse must assess financial toxicity as it correlates to other symptoms such as fatigue, pain, sleep disturbance, anxiety, and depression. Patients experiencing financial toxicity often report a diminished quality of life and increased symptom burden.

ONCOLOGY NURSE NAVIGATORS

Oncology nurse navigators are a valuable resource in helping to coordinate care, overcome barriers, facilitate timely access to treatment, and assist in helping the patient to find the most affordable options. Nurse navigators need to be astutely aware of the potential resources available for their patients. To successfully assist the cancer survivor, the nurse navigator needs to be able to perform the following:

1. Make referrals to patient assistance programs (PAPs). These are programs funded by charities, advocacy groups, and pharmaceutical companies designed to offset copays or expenses associated with a diagnosis, treatment, and/or drugs (Mcmullen, 2019).
2. Assisting patients in contacting their insurance companies. It is essential to help guide patients in inquiring about biosimilar or generic medications when appropriate (McCain, 2012).
3. Refer the patient to specialty pharmacies for specific medications. Specialty pharmacies are becoming increasingly common in oncology and are most often used for medications that are expensive to purchase. The term "specialty" refers to a special population, in this case, oncology, and is associated with complex management or strict administration guidelines. Specialty pharmacies receive drugs directly from the wholesale distributor, thereby reducing the cost of the medications (Schwartz et al., 2010).

▶ INSURANCE ISSUES

Cancer survivors unfortunately often struggle to access healthcare regardless of their insurance status. Inadequate insurance coverage can contribute to the financial burden patients and their loved ones may face. The major barriers to understanding health insurance policies include:

- **Inadequate healthcare coverage:** Approximately 35% (61 million Americans) are either uninsured or underinsured. Patients who are underinsured are more likely to forgo healthcare unless they deem it essential (Schoen et al., 2005). This is particularly important for cancer survivors who are advised to adhere to strict follow-up and screening schedules.
- **Insurance rules and regulations:** Many insurance policies have dictated who and where the care be delivered. Some policies also have specific guidelines of what diagnostic tests and procedures can be provided. Often an approval process is required to obtain authorization for the recommended and ordered tests and procedures. Nurse navigators and healthcare providers are instrumental in explaining these rules and regulations to the patient as well as continuing to advocate for the patients.
- **Limited health literacy:** Consumers who later become patients often find themselves lacking adequate coverage to meet their healthcare needs because they do not have a thorough understanding of the healthcare plan. Often individuals selected or chose to select a less expensive and less comprehensive plan to save money, not knowing their healthcare needs would increase or become a major problem. An estimated 40% of Americans carry high-deductible healthcare plans with deductibles of at least $1,300 per individual (Edward, 2020).
- **Difficulties with the English language:** Patients that speak English as a second language and/or are unable to speak or understand English tend to have more difficulties with comprehending the healthcare policies.

By closely collaborating with the patient, their family members, and the multidisciplinary team, the oncology nurse can assist the cancer survivor in finding the most cost-effective options to meet their needs, thereby improving outcomes.

FAMILY AND SOCIAL SUPPORT

Family and friends play an important role in helping to promote positive outcomes for patients in both the active and post-treatment phases of cancer survivorship; however, a diagnosis of cancer can have a dramatic effect on not only the person diagnosed but their family and friends.

Even though family members may experience their own emotional distress due to the care diagnosis, they often become primary caregivers for their loved ones, which creates an added strain. Family and social relationships can change because of the restrictions that cancer treatments can cause, for example, inability to engage in social activities, gather at holidays, to see extended family and young children. Lastly, the perceptions and beliefs of the patient and family members may differ. As the patient becomes more restricted because of cancer/treatment, cancer patients and their loved ones have different opinions/values on sensitive topics related to the disease, and caregivers become overburdened by their responsibilities (Northouse, 2012).

Mazanec et al. (2014) documented that patient's family members were more likely to report higher levels of distress than patients at the completion of cancer treatment. Caregivers may also experience physical symptoms of distress such as fatigue, difficulty sleeping, weight gain, and depression (Skalla et al., 2013). Despite the distress the family and friends of the patient may face, cancer survivors have identified support from their family and friends as the top two supportive care needs (Zebrack et al., 2007). It is important for the oncology nurse to have an awareness of the potential unmet needs patients' family members and caregivers may experience. The oncology nurse should assess for signs of physical and emotional distress in patients' family members and friends, and be aware of support services that may help to alleviate some of the caregivers' burden. Some examples of support services that may be helpful to caregivers include transportation for doctor visits, financial assistance, help with daily housekeeping, emotional support, and visiting nursing services.

COMMUNITY RESOURCES

Community resources have also proven to be an effective means of improving the overall quality of life and alleviating anxiety. While community-based interventions can be a valuable resource, it is important for the oncology nurse to recognize that preferences on environment and method of support can vary among participants. Interventions targeting effective communication and coping strategies can be effective in decreasing feelings of anxiety and depression and improving caregiver's self-confidence and self-care practices. Examples of interventions that may be helpful to both the survivor and their loved ones include expressive writing, individual counseling or mentoring sessions, exercise programs, and religious/spiritual rituals (Roux et al., 2015).

The oncology nurse plays an essential role in helping to promote healthy relationships as patients transition from the acute to the post-treatment phase of a cancer diagnosis. It is important for the oncology nurse to assess both the patient and their loved ones for signs and symptoms of distress and evaluate their needs and dynamics to appropriately tailor recommendations to meet the needs of their patients and their loved ones.

REHABILITATION

Patients may experience functional limitations secondary to cancer treatment, such as impaired mobility, peripheral neuropathy, and activity intolerance. Rehabilitation can help to minimize functional impairments, improve physical functioning, and promote independence. Physical exercise has proven to be an effective long-term rehabilitation intervention that is associated with improved outcomes such as reduced pain and fatigue and improved quality of life (Mcneely et al., 2016).

It is important for the oncology nurse to strategically plan conversations regarding exercise rehabilitation for a time when the patient is most receptive. In the early stages of a cancer diagnosis, patients often experience heightened levels of fear and anxiety. A patient may be more responsive and open to discussing exercise rehabilitation during the survivorship phase of a cancer diagnosis; however, it is important for the oncology nurse to recognize that patients may have already developed preventable treatment-related complications by the post-treatment phase. If appropriate, the oncology nurse should aim to work discussions regarding rehabilitation measures into each office visit or hospitalization (Schumacher & McNiel, 2018).

Oncology nurses are often one of the first in the healthcare team to identify a patient's functional limitations. Nurses can choose to use a clinical screening tool to screen for functional limitations. Nurses should also consider the potential of poorly controlled symptoms or treatment-related side effects such as shortness of breath, fatigue, pain, lymphedema, and peripheral neuropathy as potential cause of a patient's functional limitations (Mcneely et al., 2016). Exercise modalities, duration, and intensity should be tailored to suit survivors' individual needs. Some examples of exercises that are appropriate for almost all cancer survivors include (Haas et al., 2016):

- Resistance training (using light weights or resistance bands)
- Flexibility and stretching exercises to promote movement and minimize the chance of injury
- Core-strength training
- Light aerobic exercises (recommended 150 minutes/week)

Additional rehabilitation interventions have been classified as "likely to be effective" in managing cancer-related fatigue include psychoeducational intervention, relaxation breathing with/without imagery, cognitive behavioral therapy for improved sleep, yoga, structured multidimensional rehabilitation, meditations mindfulness-based stress reduction, and cognitive behavioral stress management (Mitchell et al., 2014).

FOLLOW-UP CARE

With the number of cancer survivors growing, it is more important than ever that the unique needs of survivorship are thoroughly addressed. The role of the oncology nurse in helping to facilitate appropriate care for the cancer survivor as well as address their psychosocial needs cannot be underestimated. The oncology nurse is in a unique position to help improve patient outcomes by assisting in the creation and implementation of survivorship care plans, being patient advocates, and helping to bridge the gaps in healthcare that cancer survivors experience.

The bibliography and references for this chapter are available on ExamPrepConnect; see inside front cover for access instructions.

1. Which of the following patients is most likely to experience fear of cancer recurrence (FCR)?

   A. An 84-year-old retired female with a past medical history of HTN, diabetes, and depression who was treated for breast cancer in her 50s

   B. A 54-year-old male who works in construction with a diagnosis of small cell lung cancer who declined treatment

   C. A 22-year-old female college student with a past medical history of generalized anxiety disorder who was recently diagnosed and began treatment for diffuse large B-cell lymphoma

   D. A 62-year-old male with a past medical history of Lynch syndrome who was recently diagnosed with colorectal cancer

2. A male patient presents to the clinic for his seventh cycle of FOLFOX. As the nurse is beginning the treatment, the patient says, "I have only one more treatment left. I am afraid my cancer is going to come back once I stop chemo, and no one will know because I will not be seeing the doctor as frequently. Maybe I should schedule a standing weekly appointment with my doctor just to make sure everything is okay." The nurse's most appropriate response is:

   A. "There is no indication that you need to see your doctor that frequently."

   B. "You are almost done with treatment. Try thinking positively!"

   C. "If that would make you feel better, I would be happy to schedule the appointments."

   D. "It is normal to worry about your disease coming back; however, if these thoughts are making it difficult for you to function or concentrate, our hospital has a support group for cancer survivors that you may be interested in."

3. A patient has canceled their last two appointments for chemotherapy, so the nurse performs a follow-up phone call to check on the patient. During the conversation, the patient says, "I've had to cancel my appointments because I can't afford my insurance deductible." The nurse's most appropriate response is:

   A. "Perhaps one of your family members can lend you the money."

   B. "I will transfer you to the nurse navigator; they may be able to help you find resources to receive care."

   C. "Many cancer patients experience financial hardship. I am sorry you are having difficulties."

   D. "I understand. When you have the funds, please call the office back to make appointment for your treatment."

1. C) A 22-year-old female college student with a past medical history of generalized anxiety disorder who was recently diagnosed and began treatment for diffuse large B-cell lymphoma

Risk factors for FCR include existing psychologic disorders, new diagnosis, and decreased age. The other patients do not those criteria.

2. D) "It is normal to worry about your disease coming back; however, if these thoughts are making it difficult for you to function or concentrate, our hospital has a support group for cancer survivors that you may be interested in."

It is important for the nurse to acknowledge and validate the patient's concerns. Telling the patient that they do not have to see the doctor that frequently or to think positively does not acknowledge and validate the patient's concerns, nor does it demonstrate therapeutic communication techniques. The nurse should address the issue rather than simply scheduling the appointments.

3. B) "I will transfer you to the nurse navigator; they may be able to help you find resources to receive care."

Oncology nurse navigators can assist patients in identifying resources that can help provide access to healthcare. While it is appropriate to express empathy for the patient, the nurse should focus on helping the patient receive the care they need.

4. The nurse recognizes that the best time for the patient to start exercise rehabilitation is:

A. Upon the completion of cancer treatment
B. Midway through treatment to promote continued wellness
C. Only when the patient scores below a certain level on a functional screening assessment
D. Upon diagnosis

5. During a financial counseling visit at the oncologist's office, a patient recently diagnosed with colon cancer is told that they will be responsible for a $3,000 deductible before insurance will cover any costs, and that only 60% of costs will be covered. Additionally, the patient has a limited prescription plan that does not include coverage for specialty medications that may be required for treatment. The nurse recognizes that the patient is:

A. Uninsured
B. Eligible for copay assistance programs
C. Underinsured
D. Eligible for Medicaid

(See answers next page.)

4. D) Upon diagnosis

The goal of rehabilitation is to minimize functional limitations secondary to treatment and promote independence. Implementing an individualized exercise rehabilitation plan as early as possible (i.e., upon diagnosis) can help to maintain patient's pre-treatment activity level and reduce unpleasant treatment-related side effects such as cancer-related fatigue, anxiety, and pain.

5. C) Underinsured

If a patient has an insurance plan that requires them to meet high deductibles, offers limited coverage for prescriptions, or does not fully meet the healthcare needs of the patient, the patient is underinsured. Additional factors would need to be reviewed to determine if the patient is eligible for copay assistance programs or Medicaid.

End-of-Life Care

INTRODUCTION

End of life involves hospice care, which is a holistic approach to healthcare services that provides physiological, psychological, social support and care to the patients and their families who are facing death and cannot be cured at the current medical level (Fu et al., 2020). The main purpose of hospice care is to provide scientific and reasonable nursing services when the patient is dying and to reduce the patient's physical pain and the negative emotions of the patient and the family (Fu et al., 2020). Hospice care differs from palliative care in that its scope is limited to the care of patients who have a life expectancy of 6 months or less if the disease runs its normal course without curative intervention. The services are provided by a team of healthcare professionals who maximize comfort by reducing pain and addressing physical, psychological, social, and spiritual needs ("End of Life," n.d.). For patients with advanced cancer, in addition to their physical pain, they may also suffer from great psychological pain. Therefore, the application of hospice care to patients with advanced cancer has a positive impact on improving the quality of life and psychological status of patients (Fu et al., 2020).

Hospice care and palliative care both aim to provide better quality of life and relief from symptoms and side effects for people with a serious illness. Table 29.1 explains the differences between hospice and palliative care.

Table 29.1 Difference Between Hospice and Palliative Care

Hospice Care	Palliative Care
A type of care for the terminally ill and dying patients	A type of care aimed at promoting comfort for seriously ill patients, whether their condition is terminal or not
Bereavement services provided for up to 1 year after the death of the patient	Bereavement services are not always provided
Care is primarily delivered in the home	Care may be delivered in acute care, long-term care, or other settings
Patient chooses to forgo curative treatments	Palliative care is provided in conjunction with either curative or end-of-life treatments
Covered by the Medicare hospice benefit	May or may not be covered by Medicare or other health insurance plans
Life expectancy of patient is 6 months or less	Life expectancy is not a factor

The bibliography and references for this chapter are available on ExamPrepConnect; see inside front cover for access instructions.

● HOSPICE CARE

There are four different levels of hospice care within the Medicare Hospice Benefit:

1. **Traditional routine home care:** Care is delivered with intermittent visits from members of the interdisciplinary hospice team either at an individual's home, skilled nursing facility, or group home.

2. **Continuous home care:** Includes predominately nursing care, for at least 8 hours and up to 24 hours in a 24-hour period, beginning and ending at midnight. Either homemaker or hospice aide services or both may be covered on a 24-hour continuous basis during periods of crisis to maintain the terminally ill patient at home. The purpose of continuous home care is to achieve palliation and management of acute medical symptoms.

3. **Respite care:** The terminally ill individual is temporarily (5 days maximum) admitted into a professional care facility, such as a hospice inpatient unit or nursing home ("Respite Care," n.d.). This allows the caregiver to obtain some much-needed rest and time away from the rigorous demands of daily caregiving.

4. **General inpatient care (GIP):** Short-term care (5 to 7 days maximum) for pain control or acute/chronic symptom management cannot be provided in any other setting. Imminence of death is not an approved reason unless there is an unmanaged or skilled need. Eligible conditions include intractable nausea/vomiting that requires IV treatment; advanced, open wounds; unmanageable respiratory distress, and acute delirium with behavior issues causing the individual possible harm. GIP may be provided in any one of these three settings: hospital, inpatient hospice unit, or a skilled nursing facility ("Medicare Hospice," n.d.).

▶ THE MEDICARE HOSPICE BENEFIT

The Medicare Hospice Benefit provides a variety of services for terminally ill individuals, including nursing, medical social services, physician services, short-term inpatient care, medical appliances and supplies, home health aide and homemaker services, and counseling services for the patient and their family members up to 13 months after patient's death ("Hospice Benefits," n.d.). General hospice eligibility guidelines have been established by the Centers for Medicare & Medicaid Services. Many of the disease-specific criteria refer to scales such as the FAST scale for Alzheimer's and the Palliative Performance Scale, along with others. The information from the scales, the local coverage determinations, the disease-specific criteria, and the expected disease trajectory all help to make a case for hospice admission. A hospice provider must obtain a physician certification that an individual is terminally ill, and hospice services must be reasonable and necessary for the palliation or management of the terminal illness and related conditions ("Hospice Benefits," n.d.). A hospice plan of care must be established before services are provided and is paid for through Medicare Part A, Medicaid, the Department of Veteran Affairs, and private insurances ("End of Life," January 30, 2019). See Table 29.2 for the truth about common misconceptions about hospice.

Table 29.2 Common Misconceptions About Hospice

Myth	Fact
Hospice means giving up hope	Hospice does not mean giving up hope. Hospice maximizes quality of life, so the patient may live life as fully as possible for as long as possible. Patients and families receive the greatest benefit when hospice care is started early
Once a patient chooses hospice, they cannot change their mind	A patient can choose to stop hospice at any time and re-enter again later, provided they meet the criteria
Hospice patients are given so much medicine that they are out of touch, sleep too much, and become addicted to pain medication. In addition, pain medications such as morphine may make the patient die sooner	The goal of hospice is to make the patient comfortable, free of pain, and as alert as possible. Hospice follows orders on medications from the patient's physician. Morphine does not cause death
Hospice patients must be homebound	Hospice patients are encouraged to participate in their normal activities for as long as possible
Hospice patients are not fed, which makes them dehydrated and starves them to death	Not eating and drinking is a part of the dying process. Dehydration is not painful and may help to relieve symptoms such as pain and anxiety. Patient may eat if they are hungry and can safely swallow food
Since hospice care is only available for 6 months, patients should delay a long as possible	Hospice eligibility requires a prognosis of <6 months, but patients who survive that period can be re-certified for hospice as necessary
A patient needs Medicare or Medicaid to afford hospice care	Most insurance plans, HMOs, and managed care plans cover hospice care
Hospice pays room and board for skilled nursing facilities (SNF)	Hospice does not pay room and board. Only certain Medicaid plans or private insurance will pay SNF for room and board

> ▶ **EXAM TIP**
>
> Review complete hospice criteria on the Medicare website: https://www.medicare.gov/coverage/hospice-care.

▶ PHYSICAL DYING PROCESS

The dying process can be exceedingly difficult for both the patient and family members. It is important to recognize and understand the dying process, as well as be able to educate family members as it can potentially decrease the anxiety of the dying experience. Signs of the dying process include:

- Decreased appetite
- Increased fatigue and sleeping time
- Decreased respiratory rate; Kussmaul breathing patterns
- Decreased urination and bowel movements

- Hypothermia
- Confusion, hallucinations, and agitation
- Increased pain
- Isolation
- Burst of energy (typically 24 hours before death)

Regardless of where the patient is during this process, either at home or in a care facility, the primary goal is to provide a safe, comfortable, pain-free, peaceful death. Oncology nurses are key players in reaching this goal for the patient and, most importantly, the family members.

The bibliography and references for this chapter are available on ExamPrepConnect; see inside front cover for access instructions.

1. The Medicare Hospice Benefit covers:

   A. Admission in a clinical trial

   B. Durable medical equipment

   C. Transportation for radiation treatments

   D. Respite care lasting more than 7 days

2. A patient was sent home on hospice due to advanced and untreatable pancreatic cancer, with O_2 at 2 L, orders for morphine, and lorazepam for pain and anxiety. During the initial home visit, the nurse recognizes that which of the following situations poses the highest safety risk for patient and family?

   A. There is only one bathroom

   B. The are five entrance steps to the home

   C. The patient's wife is smoking in the living room

   D. There are four cats and two dogs living in the house

3. Which of the following service providers is not covered under the Medicare Hospice Benefit?

   A. Home health aide

   B. Homemaker

   C. Social worker

   D. Speech therapist

4. A patient's family tells the nurse that they are concerned that their loved one is starving because they have not had any food or water in the past 48 hours. The nurse's most appropriate response is:

   A. "Don't worry, starving the body is a normal part of the dying process."

   B. "Don't worry, this a normal body mechanism in the dying process."

   C. "I know this is hard to watch, but dehydration is a normal body mechanism in the dying process. We need to ensure that they are comfortable."

   D. "I know this hard to watch. We can call the physician to obtain an order for IV fluids."

5. All of the following are common physical symptoms in the dying process, except:

   A. Increased respirations

   B. Decreased appetite

   C. Increased fatigue

   D. Hypothermia

1. B) Durable medical equipment
The Medicare Hospice Benefit covers durable medical equipment. It does not cover admission in a clinical trial, transportation for radiation treatments, or respite care lasting more than seven days.

2. C) The patient's wife is smoking in the living room
Smoking is a fire danger because the patient has O_2 via 2 L. Sharing a bathroom is not an issue, nor is five steps to the house because the patient is already in the home. Animals can be comforting to a patient during the dying process.

3. D) Speech therapist
Speech therapy is a service that is not performed during end-of-life care; thus, it is not covered under the Medicare Hospice Benefit. Home health aides, homemakers, and social workers are covered under the benefit.

4. C) "I know this is hard to watch, but dehydration is a normal body mechanism in the dying process. We need to ensure that they are comfortable."
Validate the family member and explaining that dehydration is the body's normal mechanism in dying process. Options A and B are neither therapeutic, nor do they provide accurate medical information. IV fluids should not be used in hospice care as they prolong the dying process.

5. A) Increased respirations
Common symptoms of the dying process include decreased appetite, increased fatigue, increased pain, and hypothermia. Respirations are decreased, usually with Kussmaul's breathing patterns.

Part VI
Psychosocial Dimensions of Care

Psychosocial Issues Related to Oncology Patients

INTRODUCTION

There are many psychological issues that arise for oncology patients. Emotional stress of having a diagnosis of cancer and the numerous, complicated, and often difficult treatment options can lead to lead to fear and other negative emotions such as anxiety, depression, anger, and grief.

Each patient responds differently, depending on the foundation of their emotional stability. Some patients have preexisting psychiatric disorders and mental health issues. When underlying disorders are present, a cancer diagnosis can often exacerbate the emotional distress. Therefore, it is imperative to assess not only the physical well-being but also the emotional and psychosocial health of the patient to deliver high-quality holistic care.

FEAR

Fear is an emotion that can present during many facets of the cancer trajectory, including in regard to life-long complications, which can cause a substantial burden upon cancer survivors (Bowman et al., 2020). Fear is not isolated to a diagnosis; there is also fear of recurrence and death. In addition, fear can manifest into depression, anxiety, sleep disturbance, and poor quality of life. Table 30.1 describes the fear patients experience in relation to cancer diagnosis and treatments.

Table 30.1 Fears That Oncology Patients May Experience

Fears	Patient Concerns and Issues	Nursing Actions and Interventions
Diagnosis of cancer Difficult treatment options Dying Fear of unknown	Anxiety; depression; sleep disturbances; physical and emotional pain	Provide active listening and emotional support Deliver patient education Refer to other healthcare professionals, social workers, therapists, and psychiatrists Administer antidepressant, anti-anxiety, and antipsychotic agents as prescribed Encourage rest and exercise Discuss death and dying when appropriate Refer to hospice, if appropriate
Recurrence	Stress; anxiety; depression; sleep disturbances; nutritional status issues	Monitor nutritional intake Consult dietician Encourage rest and exercises Administer prescribed medications

(continued)

The bibliography and references for this chapter are available on ExamPrepConnect; see inside front cover for access instructions.

Table 30.1 Fears That Oncology Patients May Experience (*continued*)

Fear of pain	Severity and length; availability of pain medication	Administer pain medications, as prescribed, and supportive therapies to alleviate pain Refer to pain clinic Encourage alternative therapies (e.g., acupuncture, music, distraction techniques)
Disability Body image changes: hair loss, loss of body part, loss of ADL	Disfigurement; intimacy and sexuality; emotional distress; anxiety; anger; poor coping skills; depression	Provide active listening and emotional support Encourage patient to verbalize concerns Deliver patient education on how to handle body image changes (e.g., hair loss, mastectomy site, colostomy, loss of limb) Administer prescribed medications Refer to social workers, therapists, and psychiatrists
Loss of control	Depression; anger; anxiety	Administer prescribed medications Provide active listening and emotional support Refer to social work, Medicare, Medicaid, and other financial resources Refer for individual or group therapy Ensure that patient maintains current cancer treatment plan

ADL, activities of daily living.

ANXIETY AND DEPRESSION

Everyone at some point in their life experiences anxiety—changing to a new career, starting a new job, having a baby, moving, the list is endless. Signs and symptoms of anxiety include restlessness, fatigue, irritability, sleep problems (e.g., falling or staying asleep), worry, difficulty concentrating, and muscle tension (NIMH, 2018). Individuals who suffer from acute or chronic illness and those diagnosed with cancer often suffer from anxiety stemming from the many fears they may encounter (see Table 30.1). In addition, some of those individuals may already have generalized anxiety disorder (GAD), which is excessive worry and anxiety that is debilitating for more than 6 months (NIH 2018). GAD can cause the inability to have social interactions, attend work or school. Adding a cancer diagnosis to the situation can create havoc in an individual's life.

Depression is a mood disorder characterized by feelings of deep sadness, hopelessness, and despair. Cottone (2020) describes four types of depression:

1. **Situational depression:** Short-term, stress-related disorder triggered by a traumatic event(s); common with cancer diagnoses.

2. **Biological depression:** Caused by biological factors (neurotransmitters), genetic factors (family history), and/or abnormal hormones.

3. **Psychological depression:** Negative self-talk and unrealistic expectations of life.

4. **Existential depression:** Feelings of depression after a positive event, goal directed, and often associated with deep emotional issues.

Signs and symptoms of depression include persistent sad, anxious or empty mood; thoughts of death, suicidal ideation, suicide attempts; feeling of hopelessness, irritability, guilt, worthlessness or helplessness; loss of interest in hobbies or pleasure activities; fatigue; moving or talking more slowly; difficulty concentrating; restlessness; difficulty sleeping or under/oversleeping; appetite or weight changes; and headaches, digestive problems, cramps or other physical problems with no discernable cause (NIMH, 2018).

▶ TREATMENT

Treatment for anxiety includes group and individual therapy, relaxation exercises, physical exercise, and, in some cases, medications. Antidepressant medications are vital for patients suffering from depression. SSRIs, SNRIs, tricyclic antidepressants, and MAO inhibitors are treatment options. The SSRI and SNRI have decreased side-effect profiles; however, may take 4 to 6 weeks to become effective. See Table 30.2 for drug classes used to treat anxiety and depression.

Table 30.2 Drug Classes Used to Treat Anxiety and Depression

Drug Class	Common Medications	Indications	Notes
Atypical antidepressants	Bupropion (Wellbutrin XL/SR), mirtazapine (Remeron), vortioxetine (Trintellix), vilazodone (Vilbryd)	Depression	Bupropion also used for smoking cessation; increased potential for sexual side effects
Benzodiazepines	Alprazolam (Xanax), lorazepam (Ativan), clonazepam (Klonopin), diazepam (Valium)	Anxiety, short-acting episodes	Black box warnings: causes addiction, severe withdrawal, sedation and decreased respiratory rates Use diazepam with caution in the elderly
Beta-blockers	Atenolol (Tenormin), propranolol	Anxiety	Primarily used to treat hypertension
Monoamine oxidase inhibitors (MAOIs)	Tranylcypromine (Parnate), phenelzine (Nardil), isocarboxazid (Marplan)	Depression	First class of antidepressants; however, not used as first-line treatment due to drug and food interactions (e.g., SSRIs, pain medications, decongestants, herbal agents, aged cheeses, wine, pickles) Do not administer in combination with SSRIS
Selective-serotonin reuptake inhibitors (SSRIs)	Citalopram (Celexa), escitalopram (Lexapro), fluoxetine (Prozac), fluvoxamine (Luvox), paroxetine, (Paxil), sertraline (Zoloft)	Depression, anxiety	May take 4–6 weeks to become effective
Serotonin–norepinephrine reuptake inhibitors (SNRIs)	Duloxetine (Cymbalta), venlafaxine (Effexor XR)	Depression, anxiety, pain	May take 4–6 weeks to become effective
Tricyclic antidepressants (TCAs)	Amitriptyline (Elavil), imipramine (Tofanil), nortriptyline (Pamelor)	Depression, anxiety	Not used as first-line therapy due to increased side-effect profile

▶ NURSING INTERVENTIONS

Intense nursing care has been shown to reduce anxiety and depression and improve quality of life (Zhang et al., 2020). Nurse-led self-care activities and psychotherapeutic interventions have been shown to reduce anxiety in cancer patients (Hauffman et al., 2017) (Zweers et al.,

2016). Oncology nurses need to be astutely aware of any issues of potential acute self-harm. Depression scales should be used to assess and measure risk at every visit. Referral to the psychiatric department is mandatory if a patient expresses a plan for self-harm.

● GRIEF

Grief is the feeling of acute emotional pain related to a loss. It can occur due to death, divorce, ending of friendship/relationship, or the loss of a body part or appearance. In addition, individuals (particularly those with cancer) can suffer anticipatory grief, which is grief in anticipation of a possible or perceived loss (Rogalla, 2020). Common causes of grief for oncology patients include:

- Loss of bodily functions, such as speech, health, vision, and the ability to walk (Nguyen et al., 2019)
- Loss of body parts can change not just how patients normally function in their day-to-day life, but also how the body itself functions. For example, losing the ability to eliminate waste can necessitate the use of colostomy or urostomy bags, which results in reduced self-esteem (Bell, 2019). In addition, mastectomy patients struggle with the loss of the breast.
- Loss of self-care ability can have a severe impact on independence, requiring patients to rely on others for day-to-day living (Tzeng et al., 2019).
- Loss of self affects a patient's perceived identity (e.g., sexuality, masculinity/femininity, self-esteem, and perceived usefulness; Matheson et al., 2020).

Elisabeth Kübler-Ross is the leader of grief theory and developed the seminal Kübler-Ross Five-Stage Grief Model in 1969. The five stages of grief are:

1. Denial: Avoidance, confusion, shock, and fear.
2. Anger: Frustration, anxiety, and irritability.
3. Bargaining: Struggling to make sense of loss; retelling the story of the loss; a need to reach out to others.
4. Depression: Feeling overwhelmed, helpless, and anger, which leads to hostility.
5. Acceptance: Finally accepting the loss; the ability to explore new options and move into the future.

Many individuals experiencing grief move through the stages at different points in time. It is not uncommon for patients to vacillate between the stages until acceptance is met.

▶ EXAM TIP

Understand and recognize examples of the five stages of grief.

● CONCLUSION

Addressing both the physical and psychosocial needs of oncology patients takes time, patience, compassion, cultural awareness, knowledge, and self-awareness. To deliver safe high-quality care to not only the physical body but also the mind, the oncology nurse must utilize excellent communication and interpersonal skills, provide thorough patient education, and practice detailed documentation.

The bibliography and references for this chapter are available on ExamPrepConnect; see inside front cover for access instructions.

1. The nurse is speaking to the widow of a recently deceased cancer patient. The widow notes that she has decided to accept a new job in a different state. The nurse recognizes that the widow is experiencing which stage of grief?

   A. Anger
   B. Denial
   C. Acceptance
   D. Depression

2. Which class of medication is used to treat anxiety and hypertension?

   A. Selective-serotonin reuptake inhibitors
   B. Serotonin–norepinephrine reuptake inhibitors
   C. Benzodiazepines
   D. Beta-blockers

3. Which of the following patients is at the highest risk for feeling loss of control?

   A. A 24-year-old female diagnosed with lymphoma who is starting her career
   B. A 60-year-old male retired editor diagnosed with prostate cancer who was planning to move to Florida
   C. A 45-year-old male diagnosed with pancreatic cancer who has a history of biological depression
   D. A 70-year-old female diagnosed with breast cancer who has a history of diabetes

4. The correct order of the Kübler-Ross Five-Stage Grief Model is:

   A. Denial, anger, bargaining, depression, and anxiety
   B. Anger, bargaining, denial, depression, and anxiety
   C. Anxiety, anger, bargaining, denial, and depression
   D. Depression, anxiety, bargaining, anger, and denial

5. The nurse is reviewing an oncology patient's list of medications and is concerned about a potential drug–drug interaction. Which drug combination does the nurse question?

   A. Clonazepam (Klonopin) and sertraline (Zoloft)
   B. Tranylcypromine (Parnate) and sertraline (Zoloft)
   C. Mirtazapine (Remeron) and clonazepam (Klonopin)
   D. Amitriptyline (Elavil) and propranolol (Inderal)

1. C) Acceptance

Acceptance is the ability to accept the loss and develop a plan for the future. The patient's widow is demonstrating acceptance by taking a new job that requires a move to a different state. Individuals in the denial, anger, and depression stages do not yet accept the loss and are unable to make changes for the future.

2. D) Beta-blockers

Beta-blockers are primarily used for hypertension, but they can also be used to treat anxiety, particularly in patients with hypertension. Selective-serotonin reuptake inhibitors and serotonin-norepinephrine reuptake inhibitors target neurotransmitters in the brain and thus do not have any effect on the blood pressure. Benzodiazepines are used to treat short-term anxiety.

3. C) A 45-year-old male diagnosed with pancreatic cancer who has a history of biological depression

All of the patients are at risk for feeling loss of control; however, the 45-year male with a known history of depression is at the highest risk due to existing psychosocial issues. This patient may experience more difficulty coping with the fear and challenges of a new cancer diagnosis.

4. A) Denial, anger, bargaining, depression, and anxiety

The correct order for the five stages of grief (as developed by Elizabeth Kübler-Ross) is denial, anger, bargaining, depression, and anxiety.

5. B) Tranylcypromine (Parnate) and sertraline (Zoloft)

Tranylcypromine (Parnate) is a monoamine oxidase inhibitor (MAOI). MAOIs were the first class of antidepressants developed; however, they were not used as first-line treatment due to drug and food interactions—for example, SSRIs such as sertraline, pain medications, decongestants, herbal agents; aged cheeses, wine, pickles; pain medications, decongestants, herbal agents. All the other choices can be prescribed in combination.

Cancer and Sexual Health

INTRODUCTION

Sexuality has a significant impact on overall health and quality of life. According to the World Health Organization (2019), sexual health is linked to social, emotional, mental well-being and needs to be discussed in a respectful and positive manner. When a patient is diagnosed with cancer, sexuality is typically not at the forefront of concern. As cancer treatments improve and patients live longer, sexuality becomes a survivorship issue.

Cancer is often treated as a chronic illness, and once the immediate concerns of appropriate treatments, potential side effects, and survival status are addressed, patients will encounter "the new normal." Part of this new normal will inevitably include sexual health. It is important that healthcare providers address questions and concerns at the time of diagnosis or early during the treatment process. As treatment progresses, regular updates with patients about their sexual concerns validate their experience and can provide support to improve their quality of life. Patients need to feel empowered and autonomous regarding healthcare, and this includes sexual health.

The literature supports that oncology patients often have unmet sexual needs. However, the unmet needs can be addressed via education. The educational process has been determined as crucial strategy to ensure that patients are practicing safe sex without risking their health and treatment (Stabile, 2017). The sexuality issues for patients depend on the age, diagnosis, and recommended treatment options; however, most common topics of concern for patients include:

- Fertility preservation
- Contraceptive methods
- Risk of infection
- Body image/self-esteem
- Sexual dysfunction: Decreased libido and erectile dysfunction

BARRIERS FOR SEXUAL HEALTH DISCUSSIONS

It is imperative that oncology nurses develop confidence in discussing sexual health with patients in order for them to have knowledge of how cancer treatment will affect their sexuality; if patients do not have the proper information it will be difficult for them to practice autonomy, self-management, and safe sex practices.

Unfortunately, there is a discrepancy in which sexual health is often not discussed with oncology patients. There is a multitude of barriers between patient and provider that impede the discussions; most of these involve embarrassment, lack of knowledge, and lack of resources. Healthcare professionals must acknowledge that sexuality is a normal facet of

The bibliography and references for this chapter are available on ExamPrepConnect; see inside front cover for access instructions.

the human experience, and patients deserve the necessary information to provide a holistic approach to oncology care. Educating oncology patients about their sexual health and providing resources to ensure safe sexual activity during treatment improves quality of life.

TREATMENT-RELATED EFFECTS ON SEXUAL HEALTH

▶ SEXUAL FUNCTIONING

Local and systemic cancer treatments, including radiation, chemotherapy, surgery, and bone marrow/stem cell transplant, can have significant negative effects on sexual function and reproduction. Patients may experience decreased sexual desire, impaired sexual function, and loss of fertility. Table 31.1 explains the most common surgical procedures that are associated with sexual functioning.

Table 31.1 Surgical Procedures That Impair Sexual Functioning

Surgical Procedure	Physical/Mental Impact	Resulting Sexual Issue(s)
Cystectomy (male/female): Removal of the bladder/urethra due to bladder cancer	Altered sexual sensation; altered blood flow due to nerve-sparing techniques	Inability to obtain an orgasm due to decreased sensation
Head and neck surgeries (male/female): Range of procedures performed for nasal, skin, throat, thyroid, tongue, mouth, sinus, and laryngeal cancers	Altered appearance, which can have negative implications for self-image; reconstructive surgery can be helpful in achieving a more "normal" appearance	Inability to engage in oral sex; impaired speech and communication, which is important for intimacy
Hysterectomy/oophorectomy (female): Removal of the uterus, cervix, ovaries, and fallopian tubes due to reproductive cancers	Infertility	Sexual functioning is not compromised as the clitoris is not disturbed or removed
Mastectomy/lumpectomy (female): Removal of part or whole breast(s) due to breast cancer	Negative body image due to loss of breast, altered breast shape, and scarring; grief over loss of feminine self-image	Sexuality may be impacted due to negative body image and lack of nipple sensitivity
Bilateral orchiectomy (male): Removal of one or both testicles due to testicular cancer	Sexual disturbance and infertility	Decreased libido and inability to maintain an erection
Ostomies (male/female): Colostomies, urostomies, ileostomies performed for various cancers	Disruption of nerves and blood flow, which can lead to sexual dysfunction	Impaired sensation, vaginal dryness, and erectile dysfunction; altered body image
Prostatectomy (male): Removal of the prostate due to prostate cancer	Removal method plays a vital role in sexual functioning; no ejaculate released during orgasm	Post-procedure, loss of erectile function can lead to lowered libido; patients with good erectile function before surgery tend to recover function over time

> ## ▶ KEY FACTS

- Cancer surgery can result in nerve damage/changes in sensation and sexual functioning.
- Removal or damage to reproductive organs can cause infertility.
- Changes may be temporary or permanent.
- Sexual rehabilitation may help to resume/improve sexual functioning.

▶ FERTILITY

Chemotherapy, radiation, and bone marrow/stem cell transplant are primary causes of sterility in patients. These treatment options have the potential to affect healthy growing cells within the body, and reproductive organs are not exempted from being damaged. Patients who are diagnosed with cancer at a young age (adolescent/young adult: AYA) often have concerns about fertility, especially those who are not in relationships, who do not have a family or have immediate plans for a family. Clinical guidelines from the American Society for Clinical Oncology outlined that fertility preservation methods should be discussed with every newly diagnosed AYA patient prior to initiating treatment (Oktay et al., 2018). Therefore, it is important to discuss fertility preservation, answer questions, and develop a plan as soon as possible prior to the start of the treatment.

There are some cases where fertility issues can be avoided. For example, in ovarian and testicular cancers, if only one ovary/testicle is affected, the other may be spared to preserve fertility and continue proper functioning of the organ. However, it is still advisable to encourage the patients to proceed with sperm banking and/or egg harvesting resources, in the event that the remaining organ function fails.

HAZARDOUS AGENTS

Hazardous agents such as chemotherapy, certain biotherapies, immunotherapies, and targeted therapies, which have the potential to cause carcinogenicity, teratogenicity, reproductive defects, genotoxicity, and organ toxicity, are especially dangersous to oncology patients that are concerned about fertility and unborn fetus. There are several chemotherapy categories that pose a greater risk to fertility and the unborn fetus than others (Table 31.2). For example, thalidomide is an anti-cancer drug used to treat multiple myeloma, but initially the drug was utilized to combat morning sickness during pregnancy in the 1950s. It was soon discovered that this drug has teratogenic effects on a developing fetus.

Clinical Pearls

- AYA patients may have fertility concerns that should be discussed prior to starting treatment.
- Sperm and oocyte cryopreservation are options to preserve fertility; must be harvested before treatment.
- It may not always be an option to delay treatment.

Table 31.2 Fertility Risk With Hazardous Agents

Hazardous Agents that have Higher Risk for Fertility Issues	Hazardous Agents that have Lower Risk for Fertility Issues
▪ Busulfan (Busulfex) ▪ Carboplatin (Paraplatin) ▪ Carmustine (BiCNU) ▪ Chlorambucil (Leukeran) ▪ Cisplatin (Platinol) ▪ Cyclophosphamide (Cytoxan) ▪ Cytosine arabinoside (Cytarabine) ▪ Doxorubicin (Adriamycin) ▪ Ifosfamide (Ifex) ▪ Lomustine (Gleostine) ▪ Melphalan (Alkeran) ▪ Mitomycin-C (Mutamycin) ▪ Nitrogen mustard (Mechlorethamine) ▪ Procarbazine (Matulane) ▪ Temozolomide (Temodar) ▪ Avastin (Bevacizumab) ▪ Thalidomide (Thalomid) ▪ Lenalidomide (Revlimid)	▪ 5-Fluorouracil (5-FU) (Adrucil) ▪ 6-Mercaptopurine (6-MP) (Purinethol) ▪ Bleomycin (Blenoxane) ▪ Cytarabine (Ara C) ▪ Dactinomycin (Cosmegen) ▪ Daunorubicin (Cerubidine) ▪ Epirubicin (Ellence) ▪ Etoposide (VP-16) ▪ Fludarabine (Fludara) ▪ Gemcitabine (Gemzar) ▪ Idarubicin (Idamycin)

Thalidomide has the potential to cause severe birth defects such as musculoskeletal, hearing, and vision abnormalities (Hill, 2020). When thalidomide or a drug with similar properties is ordered, an extensive pre-screening must be performed prior to the dispensing and administration of these agents. The patient must sign a lengthy consent form as well as have a negative pregnancy test if female and of childbearing years. The consent also clearly documents that the patient and partner will agree to use appropriate contraception while receiving treatment. Even though fertility may be compromised during the treatment it is still possible to become pregnant, and contraceptive precautions must be encouraged as well as the opportunity to educate the patient and significant others of the dangers of pregnancy during treatment.

RADIATION THERAPY

Radiation therapy for cancer treatment can impact fertility based on the location of irradiation. The gamma rays that kill cancer cells preventing them from multiplying may also cause damage to healthy tissue. Pelvic and lower spine radiation can destroy sperm/eggs, and abdominal radiation can alter cervical and uterine tissue making it difficult to carry a pregnancy. Additionally, patients who receive brain radiation may have damage to the pituitary gland, which secretes certain hormones that affect fertility. Patients who undergo stem cell transplants may receive total body irradiation which can cause azoospermia and ovarian failure ("Alliance for Fertility Preservation | Fertility Preservation for Cancer Patients," 2019). Prior to radiation therapy, it is important to discuss options and methods for fertility preservation.

METHODS FOR FERTILITY PRESERVATION

Methods for fertility preservation include sperm banking and egg harvesting. Sperm banking must be done prior to initiation of chemotherapy treatments. Ideally, three semen specimens are acquired through masturbation, with the patient abstaining from ejaculation for 24 to 72 hours between collections. Cost for collection, analysis, and freezing of sperm varies, but the average cost is approximately $1,000. Annual storage fees may apply in the range of $150 to $300. Some facilities offer long-term discounts, especially for male cancer patients ("Alliance for Fertility Preservation | Fertility Preservation for Cancer Patients," 2019).

The process for harvesting eggs is similar to a preparation cycle for in vitro fertilization, as patients must self-inject hormones to stimulate the ovaries. Timing may vary, but generally injections are required for approximately 10 days prior to egg retrieval. Egg retrieval is a surgical procedure performed under anesthesia. The cost for freezing eggs can range from $8,000 to $15,000 or more with annual storage fees of approximately $500. This can depend on the location and storage facility. Estrogen levels may be elevated due to the hormone injections, which pose a risk for patients with a history of blood clots or hormone-sensitive tumors. Patients with hormone sensitive tumors may be treated with aromatase inhibitors to lower their estrogen levels ("Alliance for Fertility Preservation | Fertility Preservation for Cancer Patients," 2019).

▶ BARRIERS TO FERTILITY PRESERVATION

Although the recommendation is to encourage fertility preservation, unfortunately not all patients have the understanding and ability to pursue these options. Barriers to fertility preservation include lack of knowledge of fertility options, costs of cryopreserving sperm and oocytes, rapid onset of cancer diagnosis, need to immediately start treatment, and length of time for female cryopreservation. Nurses are instrumental in the education process for patients and families who are interested in fertility preservation. It is critical to advocate for the needs of these patients as well as provide emotional support throughout the process.

● PREGNANCY AND CANCER

Radiation, chemotherapy, biotherapy, immunotherapy, and targeted therapies can have severe chromosomal changes to a growing fetus. Chemotherapeutic agents are toxic and may cause genetic damage to an embryo resulting in miscarriage or birth defects (U.S. News & World Report, 2019). The rationale for avoiding pregnancies is due to the potential birth defects that could arise in the developing fetus. It is also important to remember that exposure to cytotoxic agents during the first trimester causes the greatest risk of chromosomal, genetic, and physical abnormalities to fetus. Therefore, patients receiving radiation and/or chemotherapy need to avoid becoming pregnant during treatment and several months after completing therapy.

▶ IMPORTANCE OF CONTRACEPTION EDUCATION

Contraception use in oncology patients has a twofold effect, the ability to prevent a pregnancy as well as the avoidance of sexually transmitted infections. Patients receiving cancer treatment must take precautions to avoid becoming pregnant and to prevent sexually transmitted infections (STIs). The forms of contraception that prevent STIs are called barrier methods such as condoms or dental dams. Condoms and dental dams are known to protect against chlamydia, gonorrhea, herpes, HIV, HPV, and syphilis. In addition, patients should use other forms of birth control to prevent pregnancy, such as oral contraception, an intrauterine device, or contraceptive implant. However, it is imperative to stress that these forms of contraception do not prevent sexually transmitted infections.

● SEXUAL DYSFUNCTION

Patients receiving cancer treatment may experience some degree of sexual dysfunction during and after treatment. Educating patients about changes they may undergo is an effective way to prepare them for any issues that may arise. There are physical and psychological implications of cancer treatment on sexual health. Since sexuality is a highly personal and sensitive subject, individuals may be hesitant to address and/or discuss concerns. Many healthcare professionals are inhibited by the misconception that patients are not interested in sexual health or believe the patient will be offended if discussed. In addition, health professionals avoid the subject of sexual health thinking that another clinician will address the topic.

There are multiple reasons for sexual dysfunction in the oncology patient. The sex and age of the patient, diagnosis, and treatment are factors in the type and severity of the dysfunction. Some common reason that patients do not engage in sexual health include:

■ Decreased libido
■ Experiencing nausea
■ Feeling fatigue
■ Negative body image
■ Feeling anxious and depressed

See Table 31.3 for physical causes of sexual dysfunction and related treatments.

Table 31.3 Physical Causes of Sexual Dysfunction

Sex	Physical Effects	Treatment
Female	Vaginal dryness, atrophy, itching, inflammation, lowered libido, nerve damage, and pain during intercourse; some of these side effects of treatment can make it difficult for women to reach orgasm	Vaginal moisturizers and lubricants Dilator therapy and pelvic floor exercises
Male	Erectile dysfunction, dry orgasm, retrograde ejaculation	Oral prescription medications, self-injectable treatment, intra-urethral suppositories, vacuum erection device, or inflatable penile implant

▶ PSYCHOLOGICAL EFFECTS

In addition to physical symptoms of altered sexual functioning related to cancer treatment, patients can experience psychological distress. Treatment may elicit feelings of anxiety and depression, which are further complicated when involving sexual relations. Patients who are anxious about their body image, grieving fertility changes, or worried about experiencing pain may have tension that makes it difficult to reach orgasm during sexual activity (U.S. News & World Report Health, 2019). Cancer treatment and depression can both lower libido, and patients often experience fatigue simultaneously. Patients who are fatigued, depressed, lacking sexual desire, and experiencing physical side effects of treatment may not feel up to expressing physical intimacy with a partner. This can lead to conflict and feelings of guilt within a relationship dynamic, which further isolates the patient from their partner. All these psychological factors weigh heavily on a patient's ability to function sexually. Discussion with the oncologist, counseling, and medication to treat anxiety and depression may be helpful.

Patients who have altered body image related to treatment often experience difficulty with intimacy in their "new" body. Accepting the change can be a difficult part of a cancer patient's journey, and there may be some degree of grieving regarding the loss of their old body image. Some physical changes such as an ostomy, mastectomy, weight loss/gain, alopecia, surgical scars, swelling, incontinence, central lines, and so on, can negatively impact a patient's self-image, putting them in a vulnerable psychological position when it comes to sexuality (Bates et al., 2016). Sex can be a way for patients to feel empowered and take back their physical body after being vulnerable in a medical setting. Safely engaging in sexual relations can enable a patient to gain confidence and feel in charge of their body despite their disease. Sex can also be an effective way to connect with a partner and facilitate feelings of intimacy.

● SAFETY DURING SEXUAL ACTIVITY

Patients who are undergoing cancer treatment are encouraged to prioritize safety during sexual activity. It is critical that oncology patients are aware of the risks of sexual contact during treatment such as partner exposure to chemotherapy, infection, bleeding, and so forth. Chemotherapy may lower blood counts, and patients with thrombocytopenia must exercise caution during sex. Depending on how low platelets are, patients are advised to use water- or silicone-based lubricants and practice gentle sexual contact, or possibly abstain from sex completely until counts recover (oncolink.org, 2018). If abstaining from sexual activity due to low platelets, this includes vaginal, anal, and oral penetration, as well as the insertion of sex toys. Patients with mucositis should abstain from oral sex, especially when platelets are low, to avoid pain and/or bleeding.

Additionally, low white blood cell counts due to immunosuppression from chemotherapy may require taking a hiatus from sexual intercourse due to increased risk of infection. It is recommended that when engaging in sexual activity during treatment, condoms or other barrier methods are utilized to reduce the risk of infection, regardless of whether another form of birth control is being used. Trace amounts of chemotherapy can be present in semen or vaginal fluids after treatment, and barrier methods (i.e., condom or dental dam) prevent partner exposure to chemotherapy (Peterson, n.d.).

Clinical Pearls

- Advise patients to use caution during sexual activity of any kind when blood counts are low.
- Educate patients about barrier methods that can help prevent infection and partner exposure to chemotherapy.

● INTIMACY

Having a healthy relationship with sex and intimacy can improve patients' overall health and quality of life (Flynn et al., 2016). Sexuality links aspects of mental health, physical health, and interpersonal relationships. Intimacy in a relationship is crucial for an oncology patient; cancer can make a person feel vulnerable and isolated, and it is helpful to have a trusting partner who is compassionate and supportive. Intimacy can be fostered through sexual activity, nonsexual affection, and creating an environment within the relationship for open, honest conversations.

Patients should have honest conversations with their partners about relationship expectations and what is manageable during this challenging time. Without these conversations, there may be feelings of guilt or resentment in the relationship. If a patient and their partner have decided to abstain from sexual activity, nonsexual intimacy is an excellent way to remain close to a loved one. If a patient and their partner choose to move forward with sexual activity during treatment, they should approach relations with patience and understanding of their new normal. Patients who feel anxious about physical intimacy may find it helpful to use masturbation as a tool to find what feels good and become comfortable with their body before sexually engaging with someone else. Communicating about this with their partner may alleviate some anxiety surrounding sexuality during treatment.

Providers consulting with oncology patients on the topic of intimacy should consider an individualized approach based on relationship dynamics, culture and values, preferences, emotional and physical support, and coordination of treatment (AACN, 2012). In situations where a patient has terminal cancer and is nearing the end of life, it is not uncommon for patients and their partners to experience anticipatory grief. It is important to express intimacy in a relationship even toward the end of life so as not to isolate the dying patient. In the right environment, end-of-life circumstances can promote growth in relationships as well as healthy closure (Hottensen, 2010).

▶ **KEY FACTS**

- Intimacy comes in many forms and contributes to overall health.
- Side effects of cancer treatment can impede sexual activity.
- Honest conversations between partners about expectations and expression of intimacy are helpful in fostering sexual health.
- Intimacy is needed toward the end of life to prevent isolation of the dying person and encourage closure.

SEXUAL HEALTH DISCUSSIONS

In order to properly educate oncology patients about sexual health, it is imperative to eliminate barriers impeding the discussion. These barriers include lack of time, privacy, knowledge, resources, and support. It has been proven in a 2019 study that face-to-face sexual health discussion does not significantly lengthen appointment times (Reese, 2019), so it is important for the healthcare professional to address the topic. There are assessments such as ALARM, BETTER, and PLEASURE that evaluate a patient's sexual functioning. In addition to these assessments, the PLISSIT model is an excellent approach to initiate sexual health discussions with oncology patients. This model includes four steps that may solve a variety of sexual health concerns even at the first level of intervention (Faghani, & Ghaffari, 2016).

1. **Permission:** Using sensitivity and patience, ask the patient's permission to discuss sexual health during their cancer treatment. Gauge their level of comfort and preferred method of learning.

2. **Limited Information:** Based on the patient's learning preferences, provide education about sexual health using written or online resources as well as a focused conversation.

3. **Specific Suggestions:** Depending on individual areas of concern, provide solutions for patients to experiment at home.

4. **Intensive Therapy:** After discussing issues and educating the patient, they may require intensive therapy. This can either be a plan developed with the oncologist, or patients can be referred to a counselor, physical therapist, or other provider.

A 2017 study showed that 48% of patients never discussed sexual health concerns with a provider despite 87% of the population citing the importance of sexual health to overall quality of life (Stabile, 2017). Attitudes toward discussing sexuality vary between patients and providers, but it is the duty of the healthcare worker to create a safe space where the conversation may occur. Clinicians must be mindful that the patient's culture, past experiences, and health status have influence on how they receive sexual health information. Some patients prefer face-to-face discussion, while others may learn more effectively using internet resources or reading an informational pamphlet. Patient driven suggestions for sexual health discussions include (Frederick, 2019):

- Creating an environment of privacy
- Provider initiating the conversation
- Destigmatizing topic; sexual health is a normal part of the human experience
- Continuing to address sexual health throughout treatment as needed, concerns may change as treatment progresses
- Modifying education to suit individual patients' needs and preferences
- Communicating with patient in a direct manner (Frederick, 2019)

Approaching this sensitive discussion nonjudgmentally and tailoring education to fit individual patient needs can help improve sexual functioning and quality of life.

CONCLUSION

Sexuality during cancer treatment is an important discussion to have with oncology patients. Barriers that prevent this conversation include embarrassment and lack of knowledge, time, or resources, but it is crucial to make time and reflect on one's own discomfort surrounding this topic. Patience, sensitivity, and understanding are techniques to approach the sexual health conversation. Patients are entitled to know about the local and systemic side effects that cancer treatment may have on their sexual function and reproduction. Educating patients about radiation, chemotherapy, and surgical therapies will prepare them for what they may expect and provide them with the resources necessary to deal with expected side effects.

The bibliography and references for this chapter are available on ExamPrepConnect; see inside front cover for access instructions.

1. Which of the following concerns is a patient MOST LIKELY to express after a prostatectomy?

   A. "I am having issues with erectile dysfunction"
   B. "I am experiencing nausea and vomiting"
   C. "I have no issues with urination"
   D. "I have a decreased libido"

2. The nurse is providing patient education to a newly diagnosed patient with an ostomy. The nurse will include which of the following points regarding sexual health?

   A. Appropriate times to change the ostomy appliance
   B. Concerns related to altered body image
   C. Dietary changes
   D. Pain medication

3. A 66-year-old male patient presents to the clinic post a radical prostatectomy. He has history of blood clots and is presently taking enoxaparin sodium (Lovenox) twice daily. The patient is concerned about his erectile dysfunction and is asking about treatments to increase sexual relations. Which of the following is NOT an appropriate treatment option?

   A. Vacuum erection device
   B. Ginkgo supplements
   C. Oral prescription medication
   D. Intra-urethral suppositories

4. In the PLISSIT model to initiate conversations regarding sexual health, the SS stands for:

   A. Standard sex
   B. Specific suggestions
   C. Standard suggestions
   D. Specific sex

5. Which of the following is the most important patient education concept discussing sperm banking with a patient?

   A. Cost
   B. Timing
   C. Procedure
   D. Resources

1. A) "I am having issues with erectile dysfunction"

After prostatectomy, it is common to have erectile dysfunction. Nausea and vomiting is not a complication of prostatectomy procedure. Patient often experience incontinence with this procedure. Patient may have decreased libido; however, the more common issue is the inability to have an erection.

2. B) Concerns related to altered body image

Discussion of altered body image is imperative in pursuing sexual health. The discussion of times to change of appliance and dietary changes are general information specific to the new ostomy and not directly related to sexual health. Pain medication is an individual discussion and depends on how many days post op of ostomy.

3. B) Ginkgo supplements

Ginkgo increases bleeding risk and is not a proven treatment for erectile dysfunction. Viable treatment options include oral prescription medications, vacuum erection devices, and intra-urethral suppositories.

4. B) Specific suggestions

PLISSIT stands for permission, limited information, specific suggestions, and intensive therapy. Specific suggestions include suggestions for the patient to experiment at home depending on the area of concern.

5. B) Timing

Timing is the most important factor for the patient and family to understand because a delay in treatment can cause a mortality issue. Cost, procedure, and resources are secondary education to the timing factor.

Part VII
Professional Performance

Standards of Professional Performance

INTRODUCTION

Oncology nurses are held to a high standard of caring for patients and their families. The oncology forefront is constantly changing with new treatments available at a rapid pace, and oncology nurses must maintain competency to practice professionally. Professional practice encompasses legal aspects, ethics, education, evidence-based practice, quality issues, communication, leadership, collaboration, evaluation, and resource utilization. Two sets of standards guide oncology nursing, one that provides standards of care and the other that guides performance.

Six oncology standards of care and ten standards of professional performance were devised by the Oncology Nursing Society (ONS), and the American Nurses Association (ANA) developed a Code of Ethics for Nurses with Interpretive Statements that guides nurses with values and duties to provide the highest ethical care to society (ANA, 2015). The ONS standards of care include the nursing actions expected to be performed competently by oncology nurses to provide quality cancer care and to promote professional development (Wickham, 2016). The standards also allow oncology nurses to continuously appraise quality and guide quality improvement, develop research questions, and generate new research projects. The six standards of care are:

1. **Assessment:** It collects holistic data regarding all aspects of patients' health.
2. **Diagnosis:** It verifies assessment information to identify and create a nursing diagnosis,
3. **Outcome identification:** It identifies expected outcomes for both the patient and the family based upon the nursing diagnosis.
4. **Planning:** It coordinates a holistic plan of care that is focused on the individual, which includes vital interventions to meet the outcomes identified.
5. **Implementation:** It aids the patient in meeting outcomes by implementing the necessary interventions.
6. **Evaluation:** It utilizes a systematic plan, the opportunity to evaluate patients' responses to interventions and identify the progress.

Standards of professional performance outline expectations in care for oncology nurses at any level of practice, from beginning to expert level, and in any oncology role or setting. This chapter outlines the standards of professional performance that provide the framework for oncology nursing and guide oncology nurses through the behaviors and knowledge necessary to provide ethical, equitable care, and to lead other oncology nurses as the healthcare arena continuously changes.

LEGAL CONCEPTS

Rules and regulations that govern nurses' practice are vital to patient protection as well as the nurse. Nurses' knowledge of the legal terms aids in reducing and/or eliminating the

---

The bibliography and references for this chapter are available on ExamPrepConnect; see inside front cover for access instructions.

chance of error and potential malpractice issues. Table 32.1 describes the key legal terms which are significant to all nursing specialties.

Table 32.1 Key Legal Terms and Definitions

Term	Definitions
Affordable Care Act	Legislation that provided access to healthcare and benefits at reasonable or no cost
Common Law	Law guided by the court system; decisions made in courts and then used again in other medical malpractice cases
Comparative Negligence	Malpractice term for how a jury compares degree of negligence of various defendants and determines an appropriate number of damages and or financial compensation
Contributory Negligence	Malpractice term for how a patient's conduct may have contributed to the cause of injury; in this case, the patient is not able to recover damages
Good Samaritan Laws	Law that protects people who provide care to a patient at the scene of an emergency
Nurse Practice Act	Provides the scope of practice for each nursing role and provides safe guidelines for nurses to follow while protecting the patients' rights
Patients' Bill of Rights	The right to know and understand what healthcare the provider and organization is performing, and the right to refuse care
State Board of Nursing	Develops rules and regulations on how to deliver care safely, accurately, and appropriately to patients; responsible for licensure and revoking license in the event of misconduct, drug, and alcohol abuse and/or any situation that causes a nurse to practice unsafely
Statute Law	Law that is written and has been passed by the Congress, Legislature, Governor, or President
Statute of limitation	The amount of time in which a legal action with a healthcare provider and/or organization must be initiated

▶ MALPRACTICE

Oncology nurses need to recognize the potential for malpractice issues stemming from not following standards or rights of medication administration, working with broken or wrong medical equipment, not assessing and preventing falls, practicing out of scope of practice, refusal to provide care, failure to deliver a treatment or intervention, as well as documentation errors or deletions (not an all-inclusive list). The legal system has special terms that refer to malpractice issues related to healthcare providers, including:

- **Assault:** Forcing unacceptable touching or violence on a patient
- **Battery:** Aggressive or non-aggressive physical contact with a patient without permission
- **Breach of duty:** Failure to meet standards of care
- **Defamation of character:** False information verbally (slander) or in writing (libel) about another person that can grossly affect their reputation
- **Duty:** Formal relationship between patient and healthcare provider
- **False imprisonment:** The use of unauthorized restraints of patient
- **Invasion of privacy:** HIPAA violations

■ **Negligence:** A deviation from acceptable standard of care that a reasonable person would perform

■ **Proximate cause:** The direct reason for an injury

⬤ ETHICS

Ethics are moral codes that guide all decisions and practices. Ethics is at the foundation of nursing, and it is a nurse's duty to abide by ethical standards to provide the highest quality of care to patients (Barton-Burke, 2019). Nurses utilize ethical principles to aid decision-making by weighing options that are not necessarily easy to make but are morally just and have the patient at the heart of the decisions.

Theories exist to guide human ethical decision-making and devise an ethical framework for assessing behavior choices. There are many different approaches to ethics within healthcare, which nurses may use to guide their own practice. Some focus on the characteristics or actions of the decision-maker, while others focus on the relationship between healthcare provider and patient, and finally others focus on outcomes or past cases:

■ **Utilitarianism** judges an action as ethical when the consequence or outcome of the action causes happiness for the greatest amount of people, and unethical when the outcome of the action causes unhappiness (Flach & Jennings-Dozier, 2000).

■ **Formalism**, or deontology, focuses on obligations and intentions rather than consequences of actions, and applies the universal golden rule prior to deciding rather than after a decision is made (Jenson, 1934).

■ The **principle-based theory**, or principlism, involves assessing how a specific set of principles applies to various situations within nursing (Beauchamp & Childress, 2012):
  ● Non-maleficence: Not harming, preventing harm, or correcting harm for patients
  ● Beneficence: Doing good for patients
  ● Justice: Appropriate and fair distribution of healthcare resources to patients
  ● Autonomy: Respecting patients' decisions about their care and providing enough information for them to make informed decisions
  ● Veracity: Being honest in all interactions with patients

■ **Casuistry** is ability to refer to previous cases that have been addressed to assist in guiding the ethical decision.

■ **Ethics of care theory** encompasses an emotional aspect of caring as well as the technical skills provided to patients and is based upon the relationship developed between a nurse and a patient (Flach & Jennings-Dozier, 2000; Reich, 1995).

■ **Virtue-based ethics** describes the virtuous traits and intentions developed by healthcare providers instead of their actions or the outcome of their decisions (Flach & Jennings-Dozier, 2000; Pellegrino, 1995).

■ **Relational narrative-based ethics** allows nurses to gather the specifics of a patient's story and develop empathy as well as develop a relationship to guide decision-making in the patient's care based upon the ethical values ascertained by understanding the patient's journey (Gadow, 1999).

■ **Rights-based theory** focuses on the individual rather than community and bases ethical and moral decisions on the rights of humans (Arras, Steinbock, & London, 1995).

There is a newer and controversial principle that is not initially focused upon in principlism, addressed as avoidance of killing. Both ANA and ONS's positions note that nurses have the right to refuse to participate in assisted suicide (Haddad, 2016).

▶ ETHICAL DILEMMAS IN CLINICAL PRACTICE

Ethical dilemmas occur within oncology nursing practice when conflict arises between ethical principles, and outcomes that may not be ideal for either party. Dilemmas occur among nurses, between a nurse and another member of the interdisciplinary team or the healthcare organization, and between nurses and patients, or nurses and patients' loved ones (Cohen & Erickson, 2007). Nurses practicing in an oncology setting experience a wide variety of ethical issues, and patients and their families look to the nurses for guidance throughout. Examples of ethical issues that oncology nurses may experience include confidentiality and privacy, cultural, research and clinical trial, and palliative and end-of-life care issues.

Oncology nurses are meant to be **advocates** for patients and their desires or wishes as they relate to their care. The most effective means of advocating for patients include communicating effectively with patients, families, and healthcare providers. To communicate effectively, the nurse needs to have astute listening and assessment skills, paying attention to both the verbal as well as well as nonverbal communication. It is also imperative to show empathy when a patient receives news that will affect them emotionally and physically.

Ensuring **confidentiality** and **privacy** of patients and their personal health information are two key roles of oncology nurses. The Health Insurance Portability and Accountability Act (HIPAA; 1996) requires nurses to protect all personal health information, whether it be electronically in medical records or via email communications, by phone, when written, or even when spoken in conversation with anyone.

The **culture** of patients and their loved ones can cause ethical distress for oncology nurses when advocating for the patient. The oncology nurse's role with cultural diversity includes being able to understand different cultures, engage family members in difficult conversations when culturally appropriate, and employ the aid of language interpreters when necessary and provide educational materials in patients' preferred languages when available.

Balancing obligations to patients with **obligations to research clinical trials** is ethically concerning to oncology nurses or oncology clinical trial nurses (OCTNs; NCI, 2012). Clinical trials gather new evidence to benefit future patient populations with similar diagnoses, so patients participating in the trials may or may not benefit from treatment, which can cause an ethical distress for nurses. The oncology nurse or OCTN's role with clinical trials includes:

- Understanding the risks and the benefits of a clinical trial
- Advocating for the patient and family related and aiding in the enrollment process for the trial
- Ensuring informed consent is signed appropriately and documented in the patient's charts
- Comprehending current education and knowledge regarding the trial
- Assessing and documenting responses of patients to the interventions within the trial
- Providing comprehensive care
- Supporting patients and families with appropriate communication to best identify their needs throughout the trial (Nelson-Marten & Glover, 2016)
- Ensuring knowledge regarding ethical guidelines for human subjects in research from the Belmont Report, which are respect for persons, beneficence, and justice (National Commission for the Protection of Human Subjects of Biomedical and Behavioral Research, 1979)

Palliative and end-of-life care is a difficult topic for many oncology nurses (Barton-Burke, 2015; Beysal, Sari, & Erdem, 2019). The nurse must not allow their own values and beliefs to affect the patient or family and their decisions (Nelson-Marten & Glover, 2016). Utilizing appropriate terminology is necessary when discussing palliative and end-of-life care. *Palliative care* has a primary goal of treating the patient and managing symptoms to improve the quality of life and that of the patient's family, but the intent is not to reverse the disease process, meaning it is not curative. *End-of-life care* most often refers to comfort care and is most appropriate in the hospice setting, whether inpatient or at home. Two other terms that often arise are *ordinary* care and *extraordinary* care for patients in this phase of the care spectrum. Ordinary care is morally appropriate and necessary, while extraordinary care is optional and often based upon the needs of the patient and family on a case-by-case basis (Nelson-Marten & Glover, 2016).

▶ ADVANCE DIRECTIVES

Oncology nurses must be knowledgeable about advance directives that outline patients' wishes for care when they are not able to express their wishes, including:

- **Living will:** Advises the physician on life-prolonging interventions when terminally ill or irreversibly unconscious and allows for pain relief and comfort promoting measures.
- **Medical power of attorney:** A document that allows a person to name another individual capable of making health decisions when the patient is not able to make their own decisions.
- **DNAR (do not attempt resuscitation):** A physician's order to not perform cardiopulmonary resuscitation
- **POLSTs (physicians' orders for patients who have a medical condition):** Can be transported between healthcare settings.

The oncology nurse's role with advance directives includes referring patients to appropriate resources that help write out these advance directives, being aware of state-specific regulations regarding each advance directive, as well as ensuring the healthcare team is aware of them and that they are a part of the patient's medical records.

▶ EXAM TIP

Know the terms related to advance directives.

▶ MECHANISMS TO FACILITATE ETHICAL DECISION-MAKING

The Joint Commission mandates that organizations have processes for evaluating ethical issues. Nurses must have knowledge of the *ethical review board* or *ethics committee* process within their organizations (Beysal, Sari, & Erdem, 2019). Ethics committees are meant to consult on patient cases, to develop policy because of cases, and to provide education to healthcare staff on ethical issues (Nelson-Marten & Glover, 2016).

⬤ EVIDENCE-BASED PRACTICE

Evidence-based practice (EBP) and research are components of one standard of professional performance required of an oncology nurse that guides nursing interventions and improves the quality of cancer care (Wickham, 2016). Oncology nurses apply the best evidence from current research and clinical expertise into everyday practice, along with taking into consideration patient and families' values and wishes when implementing EBP (Jyothi, 2012). This in turn ensures that the patient and family shares decision-making with the clinical care team. EBP is important to nursing practice as it:

- Ensures nursing practices are current by appraising most current research
- Advances nurses' knowledge to best care for their patient populations
- Improves nurses' confidence in skills and decision-making abilities
- Improves quality of care and patient outcomes
- When incorporated into policies and protocols, it supports institutional readiness (Jyothi, 2012)

Following an EBP process is helpful in making EBP a part of everyday practice for oncology nurses. The framework of EBP includes seven essential steps (Melnyk, Fineout-Overholt, Stillwell & Willamson, 2010):

A. **Step 1**: Grow a spirit of inquiry within the immediate practice area as well as across the profession.
B. **Step 2**: Ask relevant clinical questions using the following PICOT format:
    1. P= Patient population of interest
    2. I= Intervention
    3. C= Comparison population group or intervention
    4. O= Outcome
    5. T= Timeframe
C. **Step 3**: Search for the best evidence from relevant and current literature, using nursing and medical literature databases (e.g., Medline, Cumulative Index of Nursing and Allied Health [CINAHL], Cochrane Library).
D. **Step 4**: Critically appraise the evidence found among database searches.
E. **Step 5**: Integrate the evidence using clinical expertise from patient assessments and other patient data and patient/family preferences and values.
F. **Step 6**: Monitor and evaluate the outcomes resulting after the practice change.
G. **Step 7**: Disseminate EBP findings/results.

Several EBP models with systematic frameworks exist that promote sustainability of a practice change and incorporate essential questions. Nurses should consult with their healthcare organization to determine which model(s) are used. Regardless of the EBP model, all ask the same essential questions and series of steps:

- **Ask:** Recognize a clinical problem.
- **Attain:** Examine literature from qualified sources that address the clinical problem.
- **Appraise:** Critique the evidence to ensure applicability to practice and strength of evidence.
- **Apply:** Implement the EBP change into practice.
- **Assess:** Evaluate the outcomes of the EBP change (Wyant, 2017)

RESEARCH

Research is the systematic method of problem solving or answering a clinical question by developing new knowledge on a particular subject (U.S. Department of Health and Human Services, n.d.). Research is broken into two designs:

1. **Quantitative Research:** Study of cause-and-effect relationships or the impact an intervention has on a patient population. Quantitative, empirical studies state the purpose and clinical question upfront, have an outlined study design or methodology, and a specific treatment, generating hard data that are analyzed. The most common types include experimental and quasi-experimental studies.

2. **Qualitative Research:** Selects participants based upon their experience, culture, or behavior, and the design of the research is less structured than quantitative research (Driessnack, Sousa & Mendes, 2007). The most common types in nursing are case studies.

QUALITY OF PRACTICE

Quality in healthcare is the degree to which healthcare programs and patient care reflect the most current and up-to-date evidence from research, and produce preferred patient outcomes (Gilden et al., 2006). The IOM (2001) report, *Crossing the Quality Chasm: A New Health System for the 21st Century*, defined six aims of quality healthcare: safe, effective, patient-centered, timely, efficient, and equitable. Oncology nurses must assess and evaluate these factors across all settings of care (Brant & Wickham, 2013).

▶ SAFETY

Patient care errors, or medical errors, occur in every oncology setting during different phases of patient care. Common types of errors include:

- **Diagnostic:** Error in diagnosis or a delay in the diagnosis, indicated tests not utilized, outdated use of tests or therapies, monitoring patients with tests but not acting upon questionable results
- **Treatment or Medication Administration:** Error in the dose or method of administration; performance error related to a surgery, procedure, or exam; prescribing and administering inappropriate treatment
- **Preventive:** Delaying treatment or not providing prophylactic treatment; not assessing falls and suicide risk
- **Equipment or Process Failures:** Communication breakdown, equipment malfunction

It is a patient's right to have the correct medication and treatment, so patients must be told when errors occur, according to the ethical principles of beneficence, justice, and autonomy (White et al., 2017). The process for reporting an error to a patient includes:

- Accurately state that an error has occurred.
- Explain the type of error and what potential impact it has on the patient clinically.
- Explain how the error happened and how it will be prevented from occurring again.
- Apologize for the error.

▶ QUALITY IMPROVEMENT

The IOM (2013) released a report calling for improvement in quality of care delivered in oncology settings titled *Delivering High-Quality Cancer Care: Charting a New Course for a System in Crisis*. This report has specific indications for oncology nurses and patients' needs that must be met across the trajectory of the cancer care continuum from diagnosis to survivorship or end of life care (Becze, 2014):

- Provide education according to patients' preferences, values, and language needs for them to make well-educated healthcare decisions.
- Provide psychosocial support throughout the cancer continuum from diagnosis to survivorship or end of life.
- Receive education and training for proper communication techniques for end-of-life conversations with patients.
- Advocate and promote palliative treatments that improve quality of life.
- Operate at fullest scope of training and participate in multidisciplinary collaboration of care for patients while initiating referrals to other disciplines and having treatment and continuing care discussions with patients and families.
- Increase number of oncology-certified nurses as certification is essential to the growth of the oncology nursing profession.
- Expand nursing research and clinical trials to include more vulnerable patient populations, especially the geriatric population, including topics such as patient-centered outcomes in more studies due to lack of current research.
- Contribute to the use of health IT in performance and quality measure development.
- Address the financial needs of underserved and underrepresented patient populations.

QUALITY IMPROVEMENT MODELS

There are several common quality improvement (QI) models that oncology nurses may use to improve quality of care. The Model for Quality Improvement (Langley et al., 2009; IHI, 2020) asks three primary questions about what is trying to be accomplished, how to know when change is an improvement, and what change will result in improvement. It implements the Plan-Do-Study-Act (PDSA) cycle that is meant to test the suggested changes:

- **Step 1 Plan:** State the objective, predict what will occur and why, decide what needs to be collected and how
- **Step 2 Do:** Test the intervention, document problems
- **Step 3 Study:** Analyze data, compare data against initial predictions in step 1, summarize and reflect
- **Step 4 Act:** Make modifications based upon what was learned, prepare for the next cycle of PDSA

Other concepts to promote quality include LEAN **Healthcare.** LEAN processes focus on eliminating waste in the clinical area or eliminates processes that add no value. Another tool, which was created by **Six Sigma,** emphasizes the importance of reducing variation in practices among providers to decrease costs and increase the use of EBP (ONS, 2020e).

EDUCATION

Education is a vital aspect of oncology nursing, both personal education and patient/family education. There are several learning theories that can be utilized for personal, professional growth and development of appropriate teaching plans for oncology patients.

▶ NURSE EDUCATION

Oncology nurses must be competent to care for cancer patients. Competencies are a set of qualities that are necessary to perform a specific job requirement. In oncology nursing, competencies are essential for guiding novice nurses with goal setting within 1 to 2 years of fulfilling a particular role within oncology nursing. Oncology Nurse Generalist Competencies provide guidance to nurses starting their careers in any oncology setting. These competencies provide a general overview of ONS recommendations for practice to help nurses new to oncology and guide their learning within the first 1 to 2 years of oncology practice. They are grouped into five categories: teamwork, professional development, clinical care, financial, and quality.

NURSE EDUCATORS AND MENTORS

In-depth oncology education begins at the time of orientation in an oncology nursing role. Nurse educators and mentors are important roles within any oncology setting that guide nurses new to a position, regardless of the level of prior oncology knowledge. **Nurse educators** are important roles within an oncology setting. They provide orientation, function as expert consultants, implement educational programs, lead nursing QI projects, and coordinate nurse skills' competency assessments.

Pairing nurse mentors with newer nurses on an oncology unit is a method of providing education and guidance through the sharing of experiences and difficult moments. Mentors should be experienced oncology nurses who are approachable, accessible, and have the knowledge necessary to build self-esteem and confidence in nurses newer to oncology practice.

▶ PATIENT EDUCATION

The ability to educate the oncology patient is essential, especially newly diagnosed patients. A diagnosis of cancer can be a life-altering event for a patient and family members. Oncology nurses provide a wealth of information to assist patients in their daily living activities and navigate life dealing with the disease, treatments, and side effects. The education delivered to the patient needs to be current, based upon the evidence, and conveyed in a matter in which patients and families can understand. There are several learning theories that can be used to teach patients specific information:

- **Adult Learning Theory:** Describes how adults learn.
- **Behavioral Learning Theory:** Focuses on repeating behaviors that provide a positive response.
- **Cognitive Learning Theory:** Uses critical thinking and "asking questions" to retain, make sense of, and apply information.

- **Humanistic Learning Theory:** Focuses on the learner and their potential rather than the presented material.
- **Motivational Learning Theory:** Uses intrinsic and extrinsic motivators to learn the information.
- **Social-Learning Theory:** Uses observation to learn information.

● ACCREDITATION

Accreditation is a process of approving and officially recognizing healthcare organizations. There are several types of accrediting bodies based on the needs and requirements of an organization, as well as the type of services they provide. For example, a bone marrow transplant program will require a FACT accreditation to prepare, store, and administer cellular products. Common accrediting agencies include The Joint Commission (TJC), ANCC Magnet Recognition Programs, Accreditation Association for Hospitals and Health Systems/Health Facilities Accreditation Program (AAHHS/HFAP), Accreditation Association for Ambulatory Health Care (AAAHC), and the Foundation for the Accreditation of Cellular Therapy (FACT)

● COMMUNICATION

Communication is the exchange of information from a sender to a receiver, and it is delivered in three different modes: verbal, nonverbal, and written. Nonverbal communication includes the body language of both the sender and receiver of information and visual cues. The four standards of effective communication, whether written or verbal, are "clear, concise, brief, and timely" (AHRQ, 2014, "Standards of Effective Communication").

It is the oncology nurse's responsibility to effectively communicate with the interprofessional care team, and effective therapeutic communication with patients and their families or caregivers is an oncology nurse generalist competency (Brant & Rixman, 2013; Gaguski et al., 2017). Effective communication can foster trust and build relationships, improving satisfaction and outcomes; improve adherence; and reduce compassion fatigue and burnout.

Patient-centered communication is an ongoing effort in which patient needs are continuously assessed throughout the care continuum. An oncology nurse must also assess how much a patient and family understand regarding their diagnosis, treatment options, and possible outcomes, and effective communication techniques can aid in this.

▶ EVIDENCE-BASED COMMUNICATION TECHNIQUES

Several evidence-based communication strategies can be used to ensure patient-centered communication as well as team communication to promote safety and quality of care for patients and overcome common barriers to effective communication.

NURSE-TO-PATIENT COMMUNICATION TECHNIQUES

- Sit with patients when discussing information, as it improves patient satisfaction.
- Speak at a timely pace and use language that focuses on basic information, not medical terminology.

- Speak to the patient and provide educational materials to the patient and family in their preferred language, using translation services when necessary.
- Utilize the teach-back method by asking patients and caregivers to repeat in their own words what was just said to them to best gauge how well the patient and/or caregiver absorbed information.
- Ask open-ended questions to assess the emotional status and develop meaningful relationships with patients and caregivers.
- Set goals for discussions with patients and families who are receiving bad news; deliver the news in a quiet and private setting; and utilize evidence-based practice models of communication such as the SPIKES (setting, patient perception, invitation, knowledge, emotions, summary, and strategy) or the Ask-Tell-Ask model where nurses ask patients or families what they understand, then tell or share medical information with them, and then ask about the emotions of the patients and caregivers (Kaplan, 2010; Bumb et al., 2017).

CARE TEAM COMMUNICATION TECHNIQUES

- Role-play delivering bad news to patients including news about recurrence, diagnosis, or end of life care with a small group to provide feedback (Bumb et al., 2017).
- Implement the use of a standardized situational briefing guide such as the SBAR (situation, background, assessment, and recommendation) to relay changes in patients' status.
- Utilize shift or daily team huddles to disseminate patient and staff information.
- Use closed-loop communication such as the check-back method, where a member of the multidisciplinary team confirms the message that was received, and the sender verifies the information is correct.
- Incorporate daily multidisciplinary rounds to discuss clinical, social, and financial aspects of patients' care.

▶ LEADERSHIP

The oncology nurse must be able to demonstrate leadership skills and abilities in both the practice setting and within the entire nursing profession. This is achieved by adapting to the ever-changing needs of patients as well as the care environment. Leading is a process of influencing another nurse or group of nurses and staff to achieve specific goals (Longest & Darr, 2008). Influence is the ability to persuade others to follow advice and suggestions. Common traits of successful nurse leaders include adaptability, diplomacy, dependability, decisiveness, assertiveness, and self-confidence.

There are several common leadership styles that exist to guide healthcare and nursing professionals. In **servant leadership** the leader prioritizes the needs of individuals on a team, focuses on building relationships by developing those on the team, and all team members have input into decision-making. **Transformational leaders** are charismatic and relay their visions and mission through effective communication. **Democratic leadership** build relationships through staff participation and open communication. The **laissez-fair** style uses a hands-off approach and offers little to no direction to staff members. An **autocratic leader** makes all decisions without staff input, which can lead to a culture of blame.

▶ LEADERSHIP COMPETENCIES

To guide oncology nurses through their own professional and personal growth, ONS developed leadership competencies in five categories ("ONS defines nurse," 2012):

1. **Personal mastery:** Consistently evaluating personal leadership skills and striving to close gaps in them
2. **Vision:** Effectively communicating goals to meet and how to meet the goals
3. **Knowledge:** Application of evidence-based information into practice and educating others about up-to-date practices
4. **Interpersonal effectiveness:** Creating and sustaining relationships
5. **Systems thinking:** Comprehending the healthcare relationships needed to drive positive change and outcomes

● COLLABORATION

Collaboration is another essential standard of professional performance for oncology nurses and the oncology specialty. Many different roles are required on the oncology interprofessional team to ensure care provided to patients is centered on their various needs throughout the continuum. The roles include nurses, advanced practice nurses, nurse navigators, physicians, pathologists, pharmacists, physical/occupational therapists, social workers, dieticians, and religious caregivers. Essential elements of collaboration include open communication, valuing the expertise of different roles, and learning to trust team members (Pirschel, 2018a).

Barriers to effective collaboration include a lack of standardized preparation, competency, and experience within the same profession, such as nurses who act within various roles (staff nurse, educator, charge nurse, manager; Chadwick & Clinton, 2016); lack of trust or value in another profession's opinion due to a lack of understanding of scope of practice in each profession; lack of communication or a forum for communicating with different professions; perceived competition and a threat to personal autonomy due to overlapping care from multiple professions; and inadequate support and opportunities from administration and leadership for collaboration (Chadwick & Clinton, 2016).

● PROFESSIONAL PRACTICE EVALUATION

Just as a nurse evaluates how well patients respond to intervention implementation, nurses must evaluate their own professional performance and practice. Nurses must maintain personal accountability and responsibility for learning as the oncology environment changes and assess their current professional abilities to abide by the ethical, legal, and state regulations for practice. This can be done by evaluating performance against institutional, state, and national resources (e.g., scope and standards of practice, rules and regulations, policies and procedures), self-reflection, or a combination of methods.

Personal evaluation should also assess how the nurse personally contributes to the growth of the nursing profession. This may take into consideration involvement in committees and professional organizations, professional publications to spread knowledge, and volunteering opportunities. Nurses must also evaluate participation in committees and boards for policy development on a unit or system-wide level, or on a larger scale with local, regional, state, or national policies.

▶ PEER EVALUATION

Nurses not only evaluate themselves but also identify external sources that can evaluate their professional performance. This is done by seeking feedback from peers, supervisors, and even patients and families that nurses work alongside on a regular basis (Hickey, 2016). Personnel from other disciplines may also be a good source of feedback. Job-specific performance appraisals are conducted annually and include supervisor and peer feedback and should be used to guide growth and development goals for the following year.

Oncology nurses must also provide guidance and feedback to other nurses regarding professional practice to enable improvement and development of the profession (Hickey, 2016). Acting as a resource and mentor to fellow nurses, oncology nurses can provide or suggest overall performance feedback, specific experiences or cases as examples for growth, opportunities for education and development, and constructive feedback. The nurse must always ensure that the message is positive and that suggestions are provided for improvement.

▶ CONTINUING EDUCATION EVALUATION

A nurse is accountable for holding themselves responsible for maintaining knowledge and constantly learning as each clinical setting changes and new treatments become available or best practices for symptom management are unveiled. To renew state nursing licenses and professional certifications, requirements for continuing education hours and topics are mandated, and nurses must be aware of and fulfill requirements, as well as evaluate associated learnings and performance.

▶ DEVELOPMENT PLAN

After a self and peer evaluation of performance and knowledge is completed, areas for growth and development must be identified and a plan outlined. The self-evaluation process should be periodic and systemic, include formal and informal methods of evaluation, and the action plan used to measure success. The action plan should include educational opportunities to continue to grow knowledge base, conferences to attend, organizations to join to advance the profession, and personal goals to improve job performance (Hickey, 2016).

● RESOURCE UTILIZATION

Utilization of only necessary healthcare services aids the healthcare team in providing the most cost-effective, high-quality, and appropriate care and recommendations for patients, while eliminating unnecessary visits and services. Linking patients to appropriate and essential resources is a role of an oncology nurse and another standard of professional performance. Patients experience high out-of-pocket costs related to treatment, diagnostic imaging, surgery, and office visits, and many are not even able to work as a result of their cancer diagnosis. Social determinants of health have a large impact on cancer outcomes, and it is essential for nurses to recognize other costs associated with cancer care including transportation, housing, cost of nutritional aids, and healthy foods (Edward, 2020). Due to the high costs associated with cancer care, compliance can even become a major issue.

Nurses must assess for financial needs and make financial assistance referrals a part of patients' care plans. It is important to understand resources that are available within the organization and local community. Assistance is often available from government agencies, charitable organizations, and pharmaceutical companies to supplement cancer care and help with costs. Patients must be enrolled and eligible to receive funding and assistance. Types of financial assistance include (Edward, 2020):

- Payment plans for those who cannot afford to pay in full
- Help with selecting and applying for the most appropriate insurance according to needs
- Financial counseling regarding expected total out of pocket costs
- Charity care at some hospitals or settings for those who lack health insurance coverage and meet specific income requirements
- Prescription drug discounts and patient assistance programs
- Temporary housing or free programs for those who travel long distances for care

Reducing acute care utilization is essential in reducing overall healthcare costs as well. Most often, these are preventable with proper coordinator of care in the outpatient setting. The three most common acute care utilization measures for patients with cancer are ED visits, admissions or hospitalizations, and re-hospitalization within 30 days of a previous admission. Inpatient admissions are especially linked with higher costs of care. Strategies for reducing ED visits and admissions include:

- Identifying patients who are at high risk for ED visits and unplanned admissions
- Improving access and coordination of care utilizing nurse navigators
- Implementing best practice clinical pathways for symptom management and supportive care
- Implementing symptom management clinics into daily practice to triage urgent needs
- Initiate early referrals to palliative care services

Metastatic cancer is causally related to increased healthcare resource utilization and costs compared to non-metastatic cancer (Tangirala, Appukkuttan & Simmons, 2019). Quick and efficient initiation of treatment is one strategy to delay and even prevent metastases, which in turn can reduce healthcare resource use and costs of care.

Managing healthcare costs and resource utilization is a multidisciplinary effort. Other members of the oncology care team are essential with equitable resource utilization for patients. Physicians have a responsibility to be fiscally responsible by offering treatments with documented outcomes offer the most benefit to patients, and social workers, Oncology Nurse Navigators, and financial counselors are responsible for assessing financial toxicity, identifying and estimating costs, educating patients and caregivers about expected out-of-pocket costs, and locating community and charitable resources.

● CONCLUSION

This chapter has highlighted the most common professional development and performance topics related to nursing and oncology practice. Oncology nurses must understand these concepts to provide high quality, comprehensive, and compassionate care on a daily basis, while maintaining patient safety.

The bibliography and references for this chapter are available on ExamPrepConnect; see inside front cover for access instructions.

1. What are the three types of communication?

   A. Verbal, written, clear and concise
   B. Body language, visual cues, and written
   C. Verbal, nonverbal, and written
   D. Clear, concise, brief, and timely

2. What is the format for asking an appropriate clinical question in the EBP framework?

   A. EBP
   B. PICOT
   C. JHNEBP
   D. QI

3. All of the following are elements of the IOM's Six Aims of Quality Healthcare, except:

   A. Safe and effective
   B. Patient-centered and timely
   C. Safe and rapid
   D. Efficient and equitable

4. Eliminating wasteful processes in healthcare is an example of which of the following QI models?

   A. Model for Quality Improvement
   B. PDSA
   C. Lean
   D. Six Sigma

5. What is the difference between competence and competency?

   A. There is no difference between competence and competency
   B. Competency is the ability to perform to a standard, and competence demonstrates performing the standard
   C. Nurses who are competent also have competency
   D. Competency demonstrates performing the standard of practice, while competence is the ability to perform the practice

1. C) Verbal, nonverbal, and written
The three types of communication are verbal, nonverbal, and written. Body language and visual cues are elements of nonverbal communication. The standards of effective communication are clear, concise, brief, and timely.

2. B) PICOT
The PICOT format is step 2 in the EBP Framework. PICOT stands for **P**atient population, **I**ntervention, **C**omparing intervention, determine the **O**utcome, and **T**ime frame.

3. C) Safe and rapid
The IOM's Six Aims of Quality Healthcare include safe, effective, patient-centered, timely, efficient, and equitable care. Care should not deliver rapidly as it can cause errors.

4. C) Lean
Lean processes are meant to eliminate wasteful processes. Six Sigma emphasizes the importance of reducing variation in practices amongst providers to decrease costs and increased use of EBP. PDSA (Plan-Do-Study-Act) is a cycle used in the Model for Quality Improvement.

5. D) Competency demonstrates performing the standard of practice, while competence is the ability to perform the practice
Competency demonstrates performing the standard of practice for oncology nurses, while competence is the ability iself. Nurses who are competent may not necessarily have competency in one area of practice.

Part VIII

Practice Test

Practice Test

1. The nurse is caring for a patient post thyroid surgery for cancer. The nurse examines the patient and notes blood soaking the gown. The most appropriate INITIAL nursing action is to:

   A. Assess the patient for breath sounds and respiratory effort
   B. Reassure the patient and change the gown
   C. Reinforce the dressing and notify the surgeon
   D. Raise the head of the bed to high Fowler's position

2. A patient is 10 days postoperative from a radical prostatectomy. The patient's chief complaint is "urine leaking out when I cough." The nurse recognizes that the patient is experiencing:

   A. Overflow incontinence
   B. Urge incontinence
   C. Reflex incontinence
   D. Stress incontinence

3. Ixempra (ixabepilone) is used to treat metastatic:

   A. Lung cancer
   B. Prostate cancer
   C. Breast cancer
   D. Colon cancer

4. Asbestos exposure can cause which of the following carcinogenesis mechanisms?

   A. Chromosomal mutation
   B. Chronic inflammation
   C. Apoptosis
   D. Genetic instability

5. All of the following are alternative, non-opioid treatments for cancer pain, EXCEPT:

   A. Biofeedback
   B. Hypnosis
   C. Breathing and relaxation
   D. Yoga

6. Which ethical principle requires that a nurse's actions inflict no harm?

   A. Veracity
   B. Autonomy
   C. Beneficence
   D. Nonmaleficence

7. A patient who has consented to enroll in a clinical trial asks about the timeframe to complete the screening procedures. The nurse knows that the BEST place to find this information is in which of the following sections of the protocol?

   A. Adverse event reporting
   B. Pharmacology and toxicology information
   C. Schedule of assessments
   D. Required monitoring schedule

8. A cancer patient describes to the nurse an episode of breakthrough pain. Which statement by the patient indicates the need for further teaching about the treatment options for breakthrough pain?

   A. "I put one dose of fentanyl in my cheek area as prescribed by my doctor."
   B. "I doubled my dose of MS Contin."
   C. "I listened to a meditation program to help me relax."
   D. "I used a heating pad for my back pain."

9. The nurse is caring for a patient immediately after administration of cisplatin therapy. The nurse's PRIORITY intervention is to monitor:

   A. Vital signs every 2 hours
   B. Urine output hourly
   C. Diet choices daily
   D. Pulmonary function every 4 hours

10. A stem cell transplant patient who had a pheresis catheter placed 8 days ago presents with fever and chills. Which of the following is the MOST accurate statement regarding this patient?

    A. The patient has an infection due to maintenance complications of the catheter
    B. The patient has an infection due to insertion complications of the catheter
    C. The patient has a bladder infection
    D. The patient has a lung infection

11. A leukemia patient is experiencing a severe anaphylactic reaction to the first dose of L-asparaginase. The nurse prepares to administer:

    A. Pseudoephedrine
    B. Phenylephrine
    C. Epinephrine
    D. Ephedrine

12. Which medications can increase risk for blood clots?

    A. Decitabine (Dacogen), doxorubicin (Adriamycin), cyclophosphamide (Cytoxan)

    B. Tamoxifen (Nolvadex), doxorubicin (Adriamycin), etoposide (VP-16)

    C. Lenalidomide (Revlimid), cyclophosphamide (Cytoxan), oxaliplatin (Eloxatin)

    D. Tamoxifen (Nolvadex), Lenalidomide (Revlimid), thalidomide

13. A 42-year-old male is brought to the clinic for bladder incontinence after completion of the first cycle of chemotherapy for small cell lung cancer. The nurse anticipates that the provider will order:

    A. X-ray of the spine

    B. MRI of the spine

    C. Lumbar puncture

    D. Ultrasound

14. A patient is receiving vincristine (Oncovin) as part of maintenance therapy for acute myeloid leukemia (AML). The nurse should reinforce which of the following nursing interventions?

    A. Encourage bowel regimen

    B. Restrict fluid intake

    C. Eat foods low in fiber

    D. Take calcium supplements

15. An ovarian cancer patient receiving chemotherapy and radiation therapy tells the nurse, "The oncologist explained that if the cancer doesn't decrease in size, then the chemotherapy treatment may need to be changed. I don't think I can continue with these treatments. I'm exhausted and have no quality of life. What do you think about a holistic approach, such as a macrobiotic diet?" The nurse's BEST response is:

    A. "Holistic approaches can be beneficial, but I'm not sure about the benefits of macrobiotic diets."

    B. "Tell me what you know about the diet and why you think it might be helpful."

    C. "The macrobiotic diet may cause more side effects than chemotherapy and radiation."

    D. "I recommend that you schedule an appointment with the oncologist to further discuss the diet."

16. A patient who is being treated with chemotherapy for lung cancer presents with decreased appetite and nausea and vomiting. To promote adequate nutrition, the nurse will advise the patient to:

    A. Eat three large meals per day

    B. Eat their favorite foods

    C. Eat small frequent meals throughout the day

    D. Eat only when hungry

17. Which of the following treatments is MOST appropriate for a 24-year male patient with acute myeloid leukemia who just completed induction therapy?

    A. Autologous stem cell transplant
    B. Cord blood transplant
    C. Allogeneic stem cell transplant
    D. Radiation therapy

18. Which of the following medical errors would be considered a preventive error?

    A. Administering the incorrect dose of chemotherapy
    B. Administering chemotherapy that is not indicated for the diagnosis
    C. Not addressing abnormal laboratory results
    D. Not completing a falls risk assessment

19. All of the following are signs and symptoms of leukemia, EXCEPT:

    A. Petechiae
    B. Excessive sweating
    C. Bone pain
    D. Pruritus

20. The nurse is caring for four patients: a patient post stereotactic radiation for lung cancer, a melanoma patient receiving alpha-interferon, a colorectal cancer patient receiving oxaliplatin and 5-fluorouracil, and a patient post ABVD for Hodgkin's lymphoma. The nurse recognizes that all four patients are MOST likely to experience:

    A. Acute shortness of breath
    B. Anemia
    C. Fatigue
    D. Abdominal pain

21. Which of the following medication classes should be administered to a patient who is transitioning to late-stage sepsis?

    A. Antibiotics
    B. Antivirals
    C. Anticoagulants
    D. Vasopressors

22. A cancer patient's WBC is 5.2 K/mcL, neutrophils are 52.2%, and bands are 4%. The patient's absolute neutrophil count is:

    A. 292.2 cells/mcL
    B. 2,922 cells/mcL
    C. 3,782 cells/mcL
    D. 378.2 cells/mcL

23. An 89-year-old prostate cancer patient has been given a prognosis of <6 months due to failure to thrive, severe bone pain, and two vertebral fractures. The patient has no children and one elderly sister. The nurse recognizes that the BEST end-of-life care option for this patient is a referral to:

    A. A rehabilitation facility
    B. Home hospice
    C. An acute care facility
    D. An inpatient hospice facility

24. A patient newly diagnosed with acute myeloid leukemia is admitted for emergent induction therapy. The nurse anticipates that which of the following interventions will be prescribed?

    A. Cytarabine only
    B. Radiation only
    C. Cytarabine and an anthracycline
    D. Stem cell transplant

25. Photodynamic therapy is used to treat:

    A. Melanoma
    B. Melanoma and squamous cell cancers
    C. Squamous cell cancer and basal cell cancers
    D. Melanoma and basal cell cancers

26. A site participating in a multicenter treatment trial reports a serious adverse event to the sponsor within 24 hours of occurrence. The sponsor must report the serious adverse event to the FDA within:

    A. 24 hours of notification
    B. 10 days of notification
    C. 5 days of notification
    D. 15 days of notification

27. Which of the following is the MOST accurate statement regarding nadir?

    A. Nadir occurs 7 to 12 days post chemotherapy treatment when white blood cell counts are at their highest level
    B. Nadir occurs 3 to 5 days post chemotherapy treatment when white blood cell counts are at their highest level
    C. Nadir occurs 7 to 12 days post chemotherapy treatment when white blood cell counts are at their lowest level
    D. Nadir occurs 3 to 5 days post chemotherapy treatment when white blood cell counts are at their lowest level

28. The nurse is preparing to administer rituximab (Rituxan) to a patient. The nurse will wear which of the following personal protective equipment?

    A. Mask, gown, and gloves
    B. Mask and chemotherapy-designated gloves and gown
    C. Mask only
    D. Gloves only

29. Which of the following meals is least likely to cause nausea in an oncology patient?

    A. Salad with fried chicken
    B. Bacon and eggs
    C. Grilled chicken with rice
    D. Vegetable curry

30. A patient finishing the third course of chemotherapy tells the nurse that they have a dental cleaning appointment in 2 days. The patient states, "I need to keep my teeth clean, and it's hard to schedule these appointments." The nurse will advise the patient to:

    A. Reschedule the appointment for 10 days post chemo treatment
    B. Keep the appointment; it is important to keep teeth in optimal health during chemotherapy
    C. Speak to the oncologist prior to scheduling any dental/medical appointments or procedures
    D. Reschedule the appointment for the day before the next appointment

31. The nurse is teaching a newly diagnosed breast cancer patient about foods that help to prevent nausea and vomiting. The nurse will recommend:

    A. Turkey chili and lemonade
    B. Cheeseburger and cola
    C. Dry crackers and ginger ale
    D. Bland fish and cola

32. The nurse is caring for a patient receiving furosemide (Lasix) for a pleural effusion secondary to metastatic colon cancer. The nurse will:

    A. Instruct the patient to avoid sun exposure
    B. Advise the patient to change positions slowly
    C. Instruct the patient to take the medication at night
    D. Advise patient to restrict fluid intake

33. A patient completed a cycle of chemotherapy 7 days ago, and their labs are: white blood cell count 2 K/mcL; absolute neutrophil count 1,000 cells/mm^3; hemoglobin 8.2 g/dL; and platelets 125 K/mcL. The nurse understands that:

    A. Nadir occurs 7 to 10 days after chemotherapy
    B. The lab results are expected due to the chemotherapy patient received last week
    C. The cancer is not responding to chemotherapy
    D. Nadir occurs 7 to 10 days after chemotherapy, and the lab results are expected due to the chemotherapy patient received last week

34. A patient with lung cancer presents in the emergency department with shortness of breath, tachycardia, chest pain, low blood pressure, muffled heart sounds, and enlarged, bulging neck veins. The nurse suspects that the patient is experiencing:

A. Bronchial pneumonia

B. Cardiac tamponade

C. Acute myocardial infarction

D. Pulmonary embolism

35. The MOST significant risk factor for melanoma is:

A. Family history of basal and squamous cell cancers

B. Personal history of actinic keratosis

C. Family history of sunburns

D. Personal history of atypical nevus syndrome

36. The treatment plan for a 62-year-old patient newly diagnosed with non-Hodgkin's lymphoma includes bone marrow biopsy followed by chemotherapy. The nurse anticipates that which of the following chemotherapy regimens will be prescribed?

A. A/C (adriamycin/cytoxan)

B. FOLFOX (5FU, oxaliplatin, leucovorin)

C. R-CHOP (rituxan, cytoxan, vincristine, prednisone)

D. BEAM (carmustine, etoposide, cytarabine, melphalan)

37. Which of the following patients has the highest risk of developing an alteration in ventilation?

A. A 63-year-old male patient with lung cancer and a history of radiation therapy

B. A 30-year-old female with breast cancer in remission

C. A 54-year-old male patient with non-Hodgkin's lymphoma who recently quit smoking

D. A 50-year-old female patient with colorectal cancer and asthma

38. Which statement by the oncology patient indicates that further education about measures to prevent nausea is required?

A. "I should eat small meals throughout the day."

B. "Yogurt and protein shakes are good to eat because they have a lot of calories."

C. "I should take my nausea medication as soon as I feel nauseous."

D. "Drinking milk will help to relieve my nausea."

39. The nurse will include all of the following measures in the care plan for a patient who is receiving bleomycin, EXCEPT:

A. Assess PFT results

B. Calculate dose to date

C. Assess MUGA scan results

D. Review test-dose orders

40. A patient with colon cancer visits the clinic for a 3-month follow-up appointment. On initial assessment, the nurse notes that the patient has sclera jaundice. The nurse anticipates that the provider will order:

    A. A complete blood count

    B. A complete blood count with differential

    C. BUN and creatinine levels

    D. ALT, AST, and LD levels

41. Which of the following is the MOST accurate statement regarding cytokines?

    A. Cytokines are created in the laboratory

    B. Cytokines attack foreign agents in the body

    C. Cytokines act at the extracellular level

    D. Cytokines act as messengers for the immune system

42. During a follow-up visit, a 65-year-old male patient with prostate cancer notes that he is having difficulty obtaining an erection. The nurse's BEST response is:

    A. Tell the patient to discuss his concerns with the provider

    B. Refer the patient to a sex therapist

    C. Recommend a drug to treat the erectile dysfunction

    D. Ask the patient for permission to further explore his concerns and issues

43. All of the following cancers have screening tests and early-detection measures, EXCEPT:

    A. Ovarian cancer

    B. Colorectal cancer

    C. Prostate cancer

    D. Breast cancer

44. All of the following are late signs or symptoms of lung cancer, EXCEPT:

    A. Headache

    B. Hypertension

    C. Bone pain

    D. Blood clots

45. A cold cap can be used to prevent alopecia in patients with:

    A. Acute myeloid leukemia

    B. Diffuse B-cell lymphoma

    C. Prostate cancer

    D. Breast cancer

46. A screening test with a specificity of 90% indicates that:

    A. 90% of those who *do not have* the disease will test *negative*

    B. 90% of those who *do have* the disease will test *positive*

    C. 10% of those who *do not have* the disease will test *negative*

    D. 10% of those who *do have* the disease will test *positive*

47. Which of the following agents require a 0.22-micron filter during administration?

    A. Cisplatin (Platinol)
    B. Gemcitabine (Gemzar)
    C. Nivolumab (OPDIVO)
    D. Rituximab (Rituxan)

48. All of the following nursing interventions would be included in the care plan for a patient who is experiencing severe anxiety related to the new diagnosis of stage III T-cell lymphoma, EXCEPT:

    A. Administer antianxiety medications every 4 to 6 hours
    B. Discuss the care plan with the patient's family
    C. Refer patient to a social worker
    D. Encourage the patient to verbalize concerns

49. Which of the following treatment options will the nurse expect to be prescribed to a patient newly diagnosed with metastatic melanoma?

    A. Nivolumab and ipilimumab
    B. Rituxan and nivolumab
    C. Nivolumab and paclitaxel
    D. Ipilimumab and paclitaxel

50. A patient who has been prescribed filgrastim (Neupogen) after receiving the first cycle of ABVD (adriamycin, bleomycin, vincristine, and dacarbazine) tells the nurse that they cannot afford the $1,000 copayment for the drug. The nurse's BEST action is to:

    A. Suggest a different medication that is more affordable
    B. Look into obtaining the medication from a specialty pharmacy
    C. Tell the patient that the medication is not essential
    D. Ask the manufacturer if samples are available

51. Which of the following is the MOST accurate statement?

    A. Morphine is more addictive than hydromorphone
    B. Morphine can be used as a cough suppressant
    C. Hydromorphone is 2 to 8 times more potent than morphine
    D. Hydromorphone can be used as a cough suppressant

52. The nurse is preparing to administer vinorelbine IVP to a patient with small cell lung cancer. The nurse will advise the patient that during the infusion they will likely feel:

    A. Pain or burning
    B. Nothing
    C. Nausea
    D. The urge to void

53. Chemotherapy-induced alopecia typically occurs:

    A. Immediately after the start of chemotherapy

    B. 30 to 45 days after exposure to chemotherapy

    C. 3 to 5 days after exposure to chemotherapy

    D. 7 to 10 days after exposure to chemotherapy

54. All of the following nursing interventions should be performed for a patient with left-sided lymphedema from metastatic breast cancer, EXCEPT:

    A. Taking blood pressure on the right arm

    B. Perform blood draws on the left arm

    C. Elevate left arm with pillow when patient is sitting or lying in bed

    D. Apply compression sleeve to the left arm

55. A health assessment technique used to assess for melanoma is:

    A. Rule of nines

    B. TNM system

    C. Ann Arbor system

    D. ABCDE rule

56. The nurse is concerned that a patient may experience a hypersensitivity reaction related to their cancer treatment. The patient is likely being treated with:

    A. Nivolumab

    B. Rituximab

    C. Ipilimumab

    D. Pertuzumab

57. High-fat diets, family history, and genetic malformations are risk factors for:

    A. Colorectal cancer

    B. Mesothelioma of the lung

    C. Adenocarcinoma of the stomach

    D. Pancreatic cancer

58. The nurse will recommend that a patient avoid which foods to manage their constipation?

    A. Fruits and vegetables

    B. Whole grains and nuts

    C. Fish and meat

    D. Rice and pasta

59. Which classification of laxatives can increase fluid in the bowel and peristalsis in patients experiencing chemotherapy-related constipation?

    A. Osmotic

    B. Bulk-forming

    C. Saline

    D. Stimulant

60. All of the following are physiologic changes that occur during the dying process, EXCEPT:

A. Increased confusion
B. Decreased urination
C. Hyperthermia
D. Increased pain

61. Which of the following statements made by a patient indicates that further teaching on alopecia is required?

A. "I need to wear a hat when I'm in the sun."
B. "It's ok to not wear a hat when it's cold; the cold will help regulate my body temperature."
C. "If I lose my eyebrows and eyelashes, I must wear sunglasses when I'm outside."
D. "I should try to limit washing my hair to twice a week."

62. A breast cancer patient is receiving external beam radiation to the left axilla for positive lymph nodes. The nurse will instruct the patient to:

A. Apply cold compresses to the left axilla
B. Apply moisturizer to the radiation field daily
C. Apply deodorant only to the right axilla
D. Apply hot compresses to the left axilla

63. A 65-year-old patient with colorectal cancer has lost 30 pounds in 3 months after starting on 5-fluorouracil, leucovorin, and Avastin therapy. Which laboratory values should be reported to the provider?

A. BUN 21
B. WBC 5.3
C. Albumin 2.3
D. Hemoglobin 11. 6

64. A stem cell transplant donor is preparing for mobilization of cells and is experiencing fever, fatigue, and severe bone pain. The nurse recognizes that these symptoms are MOST likely related to:

A. A *Staphylococcus* infection
B. An acute allergic reaction
C. Colony-stimulating factors
D. A viral infection

65. Which of the following is the MOST appropriate nursing intervention for a patient receiving hospice care?

A. Regularly monitor vital signs
B. Administer medications to manage chronic symptoms
C. Ensure adequate nutrition
D. Provide pain control

66. The nurse will recommend all of the following interventions to a breast cancer patient reporting a sore throat 2 days post chemotherapy, EXCEPT:

    A. Rinse mouth with baking soda twice daily
    B. Avoid acidic/spicy foods and alcohol
    C. Chew on ice chips during the next treatment
    D. Use preferred mouthwash to rinse and freshen dry tissues

67. Two pairs of hazardous drug–approved gloves are required when doing all of the following, EXCEPT:

    A. Emptying the urinal of a patient receiving chemotherapy
    B. Disconnecting chemotherapy
    C. Unpacking hazardous drugs from boxes prior to putting them away or compounding
    D. Handling oral chemotherapy that is intact

68. The "N" in the TNM staging classification represents:

    A. Tumor size and location
    B. No growth beyond the primary site
    C. Metastasis status
    D. Lymph node involvement

69. A patient is enrolled in a phase 3 double-blinded randomized control trial (RCT). The study design involves standard therapy + placebo versus standard therapy + study drug. The nurse's MOST accurate statement to the patient is:

    A. "Even though this trial involves a placebo, I can assure you that you will receive the study drug."
    B. "Although this study involves placebo, you will not be treated with anything less than the standard approved therapy. At this point in time, it is not known which treatment combination is the best."
    C. "The study is double-blinded, which means that your primary oncologist is the only person who will know which treatment you are receiving."
    D. "There are specific side effects related to the study drug. Even though this is double-blinded, you will be told which medications you received."

70. When should a nurse first assess a patient for resource needs and financial toxicity?

    A. Prior to the initiation of treatment
    B. When the patient or family expresses financial toxicity
    C. When the first treatment bills are received
    D. When changes to the treatment plan are made

71. A patient who is enrolled in a clinical trial has questions regarding reimbursement for charges that the insurance company did not cover for the first cycle of treatment. The nurse's BEST response is:

A. "I'm sorry, some items are more expensive because you are enrolled in a clinical trial."

B. "I apologize for the oversight. Since you are enrolled in the clinical trial, the pharmaceutical company will pay for all procedures, tests, lab work, and copayments."

C. "I'm sorry for the inconvenience. I will need to review the clinical trial budget to determine what is covered, as well as review your insurance information."

D. "I should have informed you before that if your insurance will not cover these items, you are not required to participate in them, which will save you money."

72. What is the difference in taste alterations associated with chemotherapy administered every 3 weeks versus weekly?

A. Taste alteration are the same, regardless of whether the chemotherapy is administered weekly or every 3 weeks

B. Taste alterations are more pronounced with chemotherapy administered every 3 weeks

C. Taste alterations are more pronounced with chemotherapy administered weekly

D. Taste alterations are related to the drug(s), not the timeframe in which they are administered

73. A patient informs the nurse that they plan to use herbal supplements before stem cell transplant. The nurse's BEST response is to:

A. Encourage the patient to use the herbal supplements

B. Recommend that the patient not use the supplements

C. Ask the patient for further details about the supplements and inform the provider

D. Encourage the patient to use alternative remedies such as acupuncture instead of herbal supplements

74. Which of the following is a sign or symptom of both hypocalcemia and hypomagnesemia?

A. Seizures

B. Excessive thirst

C. Abdominal pain

D. Hypertension

75. The nurse is caring for a patient with stage IV breast cancer. The patient expresses fear that her two adolescent daughters are predisposed to the same diagnosis. The nurse's BEST response is to:

A. Provide the patient information about genetic testing and counseling

B. Assure the patient that her daughters are not at increased risk of cancer

C. Inform the patient that stress may hinder treatment progress

D. Ask the chaplain to visit with the family

76. An oncology patient complains of fatigue, weakness, and loss of appetite for several days. The nurse anticipates that the patient's laboratory results will include:

    A. Decreased potassium levels
    B. Abnormal white blood cell count
    C. Decreased BUN and creatinine
    D. Elevated specific gravity in the urine

77. Which medication can cause hyperglycemia in the oncology patient?

    A. Mycophenolate mofetil (CellCept)
    B. Dexamethasone (Decadron)
    C. Tamoxifen (Nolvadex)
    D. Ondansetron (Zofran)

78. A 70-year-old patient is being treated with pembrolizumab for stage IV melanoma. Which of the following laboratory values should be assessed prior to administration of the agent?

    A. Magnesium
    B. Cholesterol
    C. Uric acid
    D. T3, T4, and TSH

79. While walking to the bathroom, a patient's chest tube becomes dislodged. The nurse's INITIAL intervention is to:

    A. Call the provider immediately
    B. Apply a sterile gauze and dressing at the insertion site
    C. Reinsert the chest tube
    D. Apply a wet-to-dry dressing

80. Which chemotherapy agent requires monitoring of drug blood levels?

    A. Bleomycin
    B. Doxorubicin
    C. Methotrexate
    D. Cisplatin

81. Which diet is associated with increased risk of colorectal cancer?

    A. High-fat and high-sugar diet
    B. Low-fat and low-sugar diet
    C. High-protein and high-sugar diet
    D. High-protein and low-sugar diet

82. A patient who recently completed 6 weeks of external beam radiation to the axilla related to breast cancer presents with skin irritation. The nurse will instruct the patient to:

    A. Shower weekly to keep the skin dry
    B. Avoid shaving the area and use of scented deodorant
    C. Use cool packs to soothe the skin
    D. Apply a heating pad to the affected area

83. Risk factors for leukemia include all the following, EXCEPT:

    A. Previous cancer treatment
    B. Genetic disorders
    C. Exposure to certain chemicals
    D. History of diabetes

84. The term *comedocarcinoma* is used to describe:

    A. Higher grade ductal carcinoma in situ of the breast
    B. Inflammatory breast cancer
    C. Stage I breast cancer
    D. Stage IV breast cancer

85. Which nurse is the MOST appropriate mentor for a newly graduated nurse who just started on the inpatient solid tumor oncology floor?

    A. A nurse navigator from the bone marrow transplant floor
    B. An oncology certified nurse who has worked in both hematology and solid tumor oncology for 10 years
    C. A nurse who has worked on the solid tumor oncology floor for 5 years
    D. A charge nurse from the radiation oncology center

86. Which of the following patients has the greatest risk of experiencing fear of cancer recurrence?

    A. An 84-year-old retired female with a past medical history of hypertension, diabetes, and depression who was treated for breast cancer at age 50
    B. A 54-year-old male construction worker who refused treatment for small cell lung cancer
    C. A 22-year-old female college student with history of generalized anxiety disorder who is newly diagnosed with diffuse large cell lymphoma
    D. A 62-year-old male with a history of Lynch syndrome who was recently diagnosed with colorectal cancer

87. The nurse is caring for a cancer patient who was prescribed opioids for pain control. What other medication would the nurse expect to be prescribed to control opioid-related side effects?

    A. Zolpidem (Ambien)
    B. Carbamazepine (Tegretol)
    C. Docusate (Colace)
    D. Diazepam (Valium)

88. Which opioid is the MOST appropriate pain medication for a patient with stage IV lung cancer with uncontrolled cough?

    A. Morphine
    B. Hydromorphone
    C. Methadone
    D. Codeine

89. A 74-year-old male patient diagnosed with mantle cell lymphoma is receiving EPOCH therapy (96-hour continuous infusion of etoposide, doxorubicin, and vincristine, prednisone, and cyclophosphamide). The patient refuses to work with the physical therapist. The nurse recognizes that the patient:

    A. May be experiencing neuropathy, which is contributing to the unwillingness to participate in physical therapy
    B. Should be left alone if they do not want to participate in therapy
    C. Is showing signs of depression and "giving up" on treatment
    D. Does not believe physical therapy is a priority

90. All of the following recommendations are included in The Institute of Medicine's *Long-Term Survivorship after Care Treatment*, EXCEPT:

    A. A schedule for recommended screening and tests
    B. Provider referrals for follow-up care
    C. Supplements to promote a healthy lifestyle
    D. Information on the psychosocial effects of cancer and survivorship

91. Which of the following assessment findings is MOST likely to be related to alterations in taste post chemotherapy?

    A. Weight gain of 10 lbs in 3 weeks
    B. Anhedonia
    C. Diarrhea
    D. Mouth sores

92. A patient receiving paclitaxel (Taxol) for newly diagnosed breast cancer complains of shortness of breath 30 minutes into the IV infusion. The nurse's INITIAL action is to:

    A. Continue with the infusion and call the provider
    B. Stop the infusion and call the provider
    C. Obtain an EKG
    D. Prepare to administer antihistamine and steroid

93. A lymphoma patient is returning to the oncology infusion clinic for the third consecutive day of chemotherapy. Which of the following assessment findings is most concerning to the nurse?

    A. Nausea and vomiting
    B. Temperature of 98.9°F
    C. Weight gain of 10 lbs
    D. Dry mouth

94. Which of the following patients is at the greatest risk for recurrence of cancer?

    A. A 45-year-old female patient with breast cancer who is being treated with chemotherapy and surgery
    B. A 42-year-old male patient with a glioblastoma who had a partial craniotomy
    C. An 89-year-old male patient with prostate cancer who was treated with radiation therapy
    D. A 59-year-old male patient with pancreatic cancer who had a Whipple procedure

95. Which of the following is NOT a risk factor for ovarian cancer?

    A. Older age
    B. Family history
    C. Use of oral contraceptives
    D. Early pregnancies

96. A patient newly diagnosed with head and neck cancer is scheduled to begin chemotherapy and radiation therapy. The nurse will educate the patient about all of the following potential adverse effects, EXCEPT:

    A. Febrile neutropenia
    B. Tumor lysis syndrome
    C. Nausea
    D. Dysphagia

97. All of the following findings would lead the nurse to anticipate a modification or discontinuation of anthracycline therapy, EXCEPT:

    A. Decrease in left ventricular ejection fraction >20% from baseline
    B. Decrease in left ventricular ejection fraction <50% during treatment
    C. Symptoms of heart failure
    D. Pleural effusion

98. A patient's neutrophil count is less than 1,000/mm 10 days post Taxol and carboplatin administration for ovarian cancer. The nurse will implement all of the following interventions, EXCEPT:

    A. Encourage daily showering
    B. Instruct patient to limit visitors
    C. Wear personal protective equipment when entering room
    D. Administer filgrastim (Neupogen) daily

99. Li-Fraumeni syndrome is MOST commonly associated with which of the following cancers?

    A. Renal cell, colon, and breast cancer
    B. Breast cancer, leukemia, and adrenal tumors
    C. Glioblastoma, leukemia, and renal cancer
    D. Multiple myeloma, lymphoma, and leukemia

100. Which of the following integumentary side effects is not related to radiation therapy?

    A. Erythema

    B. Acneiform rash

    C. Dry desquamation

    D. Moist desquamation

101. Which of the following medications reduces the risk of tumor lysis syndrome?

    A. Rasburicase

    B. Allopurinol

    C. Dexamethasone

    D. Furosemide

102. A patient presents at the clinic with a crusted and oozing facial wound that will not heal and continues to bleed every morning. The nurse suspects that the patient has:

    A. Squamous cell carcinoma

    B. Basal cell carcinoma

    C. Acneiform rash

    D. Actinic keratosis

103. The oncology nurse recognizes that a patient requires additional education when they say:

    A. "If it is okay with my doctor, I will contact my insurance company to see if any of my medications can be switched to biosimilar medications to reduce my out-of-pocket cost."

    B. "I'm going to ask the oncology nurse navigator if I'm eligible for any patient assistance programs."

    C. "I will call my insurance company before scheduling my PET scan to see if I need a prior authorization."

    D. "I will start filling all my prescriptions at the specialty pharmacy to save money."

104. Which of the following fluids would be ordered for initial fluid resuscitation in a patient with sepsis?

    A. Albumin

    B. Hetastarch

    C. Crystalloids

    D. Packed red blood cells

105. The nurse is caring for a patient with multiple myeloma who was admitted for increased shortness of breath. The patient was treated with an autologous transplant and is day +34. The nurse recognizes that the patient's shortness of breath is MOST likely caused by:

    A. Carmustine

    B. Etoposide

    C. Cytarabine

    D. Melphalan

106. Which of the following oncologic diseases causes the highest risk for deep vein thrombosis?

    A. Breast cancer

    B. Uterine cancer

    C. Bone cancer

    D. Colon cancer

107. Which of the following symptoms is indicative of metastases to the brain?

    A. Chronic back pain

    B. Respiratory depression

    C. Presence of S3 heart sound

    D. Personality changes

108. A patient is being discharged after receiving gemcitabine (Gemzar), and the nurse has finished educating the patient about side effects related to the chemotherapy agent. Which statement by the patient confirms that the education was understood?

    A. "I can use my straight-edged razor."

    B. "I should file my cuticles instead of cutting them."

    C. "I'm glad I'm being discharged today. I am getting my molar pulled tomorrow."

    D. "When I sneeze, I should keep my mouth closed."

109. Hair loss can be distressing to patients as they undergo chemotherapy or radiation. The nurse should do all of the following, EXCEPT:

    A. Prepare patients by providing education on what they can expect

    B. Explore the meaning and significance of hair loss to each patient

    C. Help patients plan for the hair loss prior to it starting

    D. Help patients purchase appropriate head coverings

110. The nurse is assessing a patient who finished cycle 2 of doxorubicin (Adriamycin) and cyclophosphamide (Cytoxan) 10 days ago. Which assessment findings indicate that the patient is experiencing an expected side effect of this therapy?

    A. Decreased white blood cell and platelet counts

    B. Decreased white blood cell count and hemoglobin

    C. Increased white blood cell and platelet counts

    D. Increased white blood cell count and hemoglobin

111. A breast cancer patient presents in the clinic with shortness of breath, temperature of 101.3°F, nausea, and fatigue. The nurse will review the patient's CBC, chem-screen, and:

    A. Lactic acid levels

    B. Troponin levels

    C. CA 27–29 levels

    D. Cholesterol levels

112. A patient is prescribed morphine sulfate extended-release for pain. The initiating dose is MS Contin 15 mg PO every 12 hours. The nurse anticipates that the patient will exhibit all of the following symptoms, EXCEPT:

    A. Hypotension
    B. Drowsiness
    C. Polyuria
    D. Constipation

113. All of the following are common signs and symptoms of pancreatic cancer, EXCEPT:

    A. Unintended weight gain
    B. Nausea
    C. Jaundice
    D. Dark urine

114. The nurse manager of an oncology infusion unit announces that a nutritionist will be joining the multidisciplinary team and that all nutrition queries should be directed to this individual. Some of the infusion nurses are hesitant to contact the nutritionist as they believe it will impede their patient education efforts. What barrier to collaboration is demonstrated in this scenario?

    A. A lack of standardized preparation, competency, and experience within the same profession
    B. A lack of trust or value in another profession's opinion related to a lack of understanding of scope of practice in each profession
    C. A lack of communication or a forum for communicating with different professions
    D. Perceived competition and a threat to personal autonomy as a result of overlapping care from multiple professions

115. All of the following foods are recommended for a patient with diarrhea, EXCEPT:

    A. Rice
    B. Cooked vegetables
    C. Apple sauce
    D. Salad

116. Which of the following treatment options for prostate cancer poses the greatest risk for the development of erectile dysfunction?

    A. Watchful waiting
    B. External beam radiation therapy
    C. Retopuberant prostatectomy
    D. Anti-androgen medications

117. The BEST treatment option for gemcitabine-induced thrombotic microangiopathy is:

    A. Plasmapheresis
    B. Administration of eculizumab
    C. Discontinuation of gemcitabine and supportive care
    D. Dialysis

118. All of the following treatment-related side effects can lead to anorexia if left untreated, EXCEPT:

    A. Mucositis
    B. Depression
    C. Extravasation
    D. Constipation

119. A patient diagnosed with lung cancer is receiving pemetrexed and cisplatin chemotherapy. The nurse recognizes that the patient will require supplementation of:

    A. Potassium
    B. Magnesium
    C. Calcium
    D. Folic acid

120. The nurse is providing discharge education to a patient who had a bilateral mastectomy with lymph node removal. Which statement by the patient indicates understanding about how to prevent lymphedema?

    A. "I should try to lift heavy things to promote circulation."
    B. "I can take hot, steamy showers to reduce swelling."
    C. "I need to buy an electric razor."
    D. "The only thing I have to do is watch for swelling."

121. All of the following drugs can be prescribed to decrease the effects of myelosuppression, EXCEPT:

    A. Epoetin alfa (Procrit)
    B. Filgrastim (Neupogen)
    C. Warfarin (Coumadin)
    D. Sargramostim (Leukine)

122. Which strains of the HPV virus are targeted with the HPV vaccine?

    A. HPV 3–6
    B. HPV 14–16
    C. HPV 16–18
    D. HPV 16–22

123. At a 3-month follow-up visit post chemotherapy, a colon cancer patient in remission complains of fatigue and inability to concentrate on their work as an accountant. The patient is MOST likely experiencing:

    A. A recurrence of cancer
    B. Dehydration
    C. Anemia
    D. Depression

124. After completion of treatment with an anthracycline, a patient presents with complaints of heart palpitations and shortness of breath when performing activities of daily living. Upon auscultation, the nurse hears an S3 heart sound. The nurse suspects that the patient is experiencing:

A. Pulmonary hypertension
B. Myocardial infarction
C. Cardiomyopathy
D. Septal wall defect

125. All of the following are common symptoms of tumor lysis syndrome, EXCEPT:

A. Dyspnea
B. Decreased urination
C. Muscle cramps
D. Nausea

126. The oncologist prescribes TENS therapy for a patient. The nurse explains to the patient that TENS therapy is:

A. Physical therapy to improve gait function and decrease pain
B. A mild electrical current that is applied to the skin at the site of pain
C. Nutrition supplements to improve appetite
D. Compression stockings to reduce swelling from lymphedema

127. Which of the following is the MOST accurate statement regarding community-based resources:

A. They are effective in improving quality of life and anxiety for survivors and their families because it is helpful to spend time with others who have had similar experiences
B. They must be individually tailored to meet the preferences and comfort level of the survivor and the family members
C. They are not effective as the survivor should be the primary focus
D. Always take place in large groups

128. The nurse is assessing a 75-year-old patient who has developed congestive heart failure after four cycles of doxorubicin (Adriamycin) and cyclophosphamide (Cytoxan). Which findings indicate that the patient's condition is worsening?

A. Increased shortness of breath and tachycardia
B. Productive cough and weight loss
C. Wheezing and bradycardia
D. Increased blood sugar and lethargy

129. Ascites is most commonly associated with what type of cancer?

A. Hepatocellular carcinoma
B. Breast cancer
C. Lymphoma
D. Osteosarcoma

130. When caring for a patient with possible cord compression, the nurse's PRIORITY intervention is to:

   A. Perform cardiac and lung assessments every 4 hours
   B. Perform neurologic assessment every 4 hours
   C. Perform gastrointestinal assessment every 8 hours
   D. Perform blood glucose checks before each meal and before bedtime

131. Which of the following is a common barrier for patients to participate in phase 1 clinical trials?

   A. Efficacy data are difficult to obtain due to the cohort design
   B. Patients are hesitant to participate due to lack of institutional review board (IRB) approval
   C. Patients have been heavily pretreated and are susceptible to adverse events that must be reviewed to study drug relationship
   D. Each cohort requires 15 participants before safety data can be reviewed to move on to the next drug dose level

132. A non-Hodgkin's lymphoma patient is receiving a chemotherapy regimen that includes a corticosteroid. The nurse explains that this medication is often added to the treatment regimen for all the following reasons, EXCEPT:

   A. Steroids reduce inflammation
   B. Steroids reduce nausea
   C. Steroids prevent urinary retention
   D. Steroids have cancer-fighting properties

133. Which drug classification has the highest risk for reactivation of hepatitis B virus?

   A. Taxanes
   B. Immunotherapy agents
   C. Monoclonal antibodies
   D. Vinca alkaloids

134. An astrocytoma typically affects which part of the brain?

   A. Medulla
   B. Cerebellum
   C. Cerebrum
   D. Frontal lobe

135. A nurse who has worked in an outpatient hematology/oncology clinic for a little over 2 years is interested in advancing professionally. The nurse asks her manager if she meets the requirements for the OCN certification. The manager responds that she must meet all of the following requirements, EXCEPT:

    A. Minimum of 2 years of experience as a RN within the previous 4-year period
    B. Minimum of 2,000 hours of practice within oncology either in a clinical, administrative, educational, research, or consultative settings within the previous 4-year period
    C. Minimum of 10 contact hours of nursing continuing education hours in oncology within 3 years from the time of application
    D. Minimum of 5 of the 10 contact hours in oncology must be continuing medical education (CME)

136. A patient who is enrolled in a clinical trial has neutropenia, which is considered an adverse event. To determine appropriate management, the nurse will review the:

    A. Protocol
    B. Institutional review board (IRB) approval letter
    C. Press release about the trial
    D. Clinicaltrials.gov website

137. Which of the following patients should be assigned to an inpatient private room?

    A. A 35-year-old female with copious, intractable diarrhea and vomiting
    B. A 70-year-old female with colon cancer receiving chemotherapy and radiation
    C. A 43-year-old male admitted for observation after experiencing a reaction to rituximab (Rituxan)
    D. A 24-year-old female admitted for induction therapy for acute myeloid leukemia

138. A patient with head and neck cancer who is receiving external beam radiation has been diagnosed with esophagitis. The patient likely exhibited which of the following symptoms?

    A. Nausea and vomiting
    B. Chest pain
    C. Painful ulcers in mouth
    D. Indigestion

139. Which of the following tumor markers aids in the diagnosis of testicular cancer?

    A. CA 19–9
    B. AFP
    C. CA 125
    D. CEA

140. Which of the following statements BEST describes adaptive immunity?

    A. Adaptive immunity occurs after an exposure to an antigen from a vaccine

    B. Adaptive immunity provides short-term immune protection

    C. Adaptive immunity involves the basophils and eosinophils

    D. Adaptive immunity has no genetic connections

141. Which of the following statements made by the patient indicates that further education regarding infection prevention is required?

    A. "My granddaughter just got the MMR vaccine, so I should wait until next month to see her."

    B. "My husband needs to change the cat litter box."

    C. "I should wear gloves when I'm gardening."

    D. "I should call my provider if I have a temperature higher than 101.0°F."

142. A nurse is orienting a new graduate to the inpatient oncology unit. When educating the graduate about safe administration of chemotherapy and biotherapy, the nurse will include all of the following teaching points, EXCEPT:

    A. Review the patient's BSA

    B. Wear chemotherapy gloves and lab coat when preparing chemotherapy agents

    C. Dispose of antineoplastic waste in hazardous waste containers

    D. Review the CBC and chem-screen prior to preparing chemotherapy agents

143. Discharge education post colostomy should include the following, EXCEPT:

    A. Avoid contact sports

    B. Resume sexual activity

    C. Avoid dining out

    D. Monitor stoma for skin breakdown

144. Which of the following transplants is used to treat aggressive multiple myeloma?

    A. Cord blood transplant

    B. Allogeneic stem cell transplant

    C. Autologous stem cell transplant

    D. Synergistic transplant

145. While assessing a patient who is receiving treatment with cytarabine, the provider asks the patient to sign their name on a piece of paper. The nurse recognizes that the provider is assessing for:

    A. Cerebellar toxicity

    B. Cranial nerve toxicity

    C. Cardiac toxicity

    D. Liver toxicity

146. All of the following nursing interventions help to prevent infection in oncology patients, EXCEPT:

    A. Maintain sterile technique when accessing PAC
    B. Administer antiemetics
    C. Provide perineal care to indwelling bladder catheter
    D. Educate patient to avoid eating raw fish

147. Which metabolic state is NOT expected with tumor lysis syndrome?

    A. Hyperkalemia
    B. Hypercalcemia
    C. Hyperphosphatemia
    D. Hyperuricemia

148. A 62-year-old female patient complains of severe abdominal pain, gross hematuria, and a palpable abdominal mass. The nurse anticipates that which of the following diagnostic tests will be ordered?

    A. MRI of the abdomen
    B. CT of the abdomen and pelvis
    C. CA-125 level
    D. CA 19–9 level

149. The nurse is caring for a patient who has a chest tube with a closed drainage system after a lobectomy. Nursing care interventions include:

    A. Monitor chest tube output every 2 hours initially, then 4 or 8 hours per protocol
    B. Notify the physician if chest tube output exceeds 125 mL/hr
    C. Position patient with chest tubes and surgical side up
    D. Position patient on the affected side (surgical side down, good lung up)

150. A patient with metastatic bone cancer who is moaning, grimacing, and acting restless is prescribed additional pain medication. The family at the bedside is concerned because the patient has past addictive behavior. The nurse's BEST action is to:

    A. Educate the family about ethical responsibility in regard to pain management, give the prescribed pain medication, and evaluate the patient in 30 minutes
    B. Withhold the prescribed pain medication, educate the family about ethical responsibility in regard to pain management, and call the physician
    C. Ask the family to go to the waiting room, give the prescribed pain medication, and call the healthcare provider
    D. Withhold the prescribed pain medication, ask the family to go to the waiting room, and evaluate the patient in 30 minutes

151. A clinical trial site participating in a large multicenter trial has decided to use both a local and central institutional review board (IRB). The MOST accurate statement regarding the rationale for involving both IRBs is:

  A. Operating costs are high for local IRBs; therefore, the use of a local and central IRB will offset the costs
  B. The local IRB has members who know the patients personally and will ensure their safety
  C. The central IRB does not have enough members to oversee the trial
  D. The use of both IRBs will increase patient protection and safety

152. All of the following gram-negative bacteria are common causes of sepsis, EXCEPT:

  A. *Klebsiella*
  B. *Streptococcus pyogenes*
  C. *Staphylococcus aureus*
  D. *Clostridioides difficile*

153. A patient who was receiving a 3-day course of ifosfamide presents with acute hematuria and pain and burning on urination. The nurse suspects that the patient is experiencing:

  A. Neutropenia
  B. Thrombocytopenia
  C. Tumor lysis syndrome
  D. Hemorrhagic cystitis

154. Which of the following is the MOST accurate statement regarding informed consent for a patient newly diagnosed with cancer who speaks only Spanish?

  A. The consent must be translated into the patient's preferred language
  B. It is not necessary for the provider to speak with the patient; instead, the patient can be provided with reading materials in Spanish
  C. Proceeding with English is acceptable as the patient requires urgent treatment
  D. A translator is not needed if the provider speaks Spanish

155. Peutz-Jegher syndrome is associated with which types of cancer?

  A. Renal and breast
  B. Colorectal and breast
  C. Leukemias and lymphomas
  D. Prostate and breast

156. Which of the following lab values would require immediate attention in a patient who is being treated for multiple myeloma?

  A. Potassium 3.4 mmol/L
  B. Creatinine 4.5 mg/dL
  C. Sodium level 139 mEq/L
  D. Magnesium 1.5 mg/dL

157. The nurse is reviewing the chart of a colon cancer patient who has been complaining of vaginal discharge. The provider prescribed fluconazole 400 mg PO in an initial dose, followed by 100 mg PO for 2 days. The nurse recognizes that the patient is being treated for:

A. Aspergillosis
B. Vaginal candidiasis
C. Bacterial vaginosis
D. Rectal abscess

158. A patient who has breast cancer and is taking tamoxifen has expressed concerns that it is interfering with her sexual relationship with her husband. The nurse has provided several suggestions over the last month, but the patient explains that there has been no change in her sexual relationship. The nurse understands that:

A. This is a normal side effect of hormone therapy that the patient will have to learn to tolerate if she wants to continue treatment
B. This is treatment-related toxicity, and the hormone therapy will need to be discontinued
C. The patient needs additional education to effectively implement the suggestions the nurse discussed during their previous visit
D. The patient may need to be referred to a trained specialist since previous sexual counseling by the nurse was ineffective in resolving her issues

159. During the patient education process for a patient receiving doxorubicin and cyclophosphamide, the patient asks, "Why do I have to worry about mouth sores when I have breast cancer?" The nurse's BEST response is:

A. "Chemotherapy affects rapidly growing cells, such as the cells in your mouth, leading to mouth sores."
B. "Chemotherapy causes white blood cells to increase, which causes mouth sores."
C. "Mouth sores can occur at any time for patients receiving chemotherapy."
D. "Only patients receiving radiation will experience mouth sores."

160. A patient being treated with radiation therapy for stomach cancer suddenly develops severe right flank pain that radiates to the groin. The patient is nauseous and afebrile. Urinalysis shows marked hematuria and no casts. The most appropriate INITIAL nursing intervention is to:

A. Administer narcotic analgesia
B. Call the provider and request a CT scan of the abdomen
C. Prepare the patient for a lithotripsy procedure
D. Provide the patient with a strainer

161. A patient who was just transferred from another hospital asks the nurse if the form they completed at the other hospital with all of their end-of-life wishes was entered into the computer system. The nurse recognizes that the patient is referring to a:

   A. Palliative care order form
   B. POLST form
   C. DNR order
   D. Hospice form

162. The nurse is preparing to review the side effects of interferon with a patient newly diagnosed with melanoma. The nurse will include which of the following teaching points?

   A. The drug can cause flu-like symptoms and depression
   B. Avoid drinking grapefruit juice during treatment
   C. The drug can cause severe nausea and vomiting
   D. Avoid using salt substitutes and high-potassium foods

163. All of the following contributing factors are related to poor survival rates in under-served populations, EXCEPT:

   A. Decreased access to preventive care
   B. Decreased compliance with treatment
   C. Increased risk of genetic mutations
   D. Increased risk of diagnosis at advanced stages of disease

164. A patient expresses financial distress to the nurse during an assessment of the patient's income and insurance. The patient's insurance will cover all medications and treatment; however, the co-pays will be high, and the patient is not currently able to work. The patient cannot afford their own apartment right now, so they live with a sibling. The nurse will recommend all of the following financial assistance, EXCEPT:

   A. Temporary housing program for patients receiving cancer treatment
   B. Payment plan with hospital billing department
   C. Financial counseling regarding expected out-of-pocket costs
   D. Prescription drug discount programs

165. Which of the following is the BEST nursing recommendation for a patient with grade 2 mucositis?

   A. Restrict fluid intake
   B. Avoid spicy foods
   C. Brush teeth four times a day
   D. Use alcohol-based mouth rinse four times a day

Practice Test: Answers with Rationales

1. A) Assess the patient for breath sounds and respiratory effort
A soaked gown indicates that the incision is bleeding excessively. This could indicate edema and pressure in the surgical site that can affect the patient's breathing, and blood could be compromising the airway. Assessing the patient for breath sounds and respiratory effort is the priority action. Reassuring the patient and changing the gown can be done after the airway is secured. Reinforcing the dressing and calling the surgeon should be completed after the airway is secured. Raising the head of the bed is dependent on the airway assessment.

2. D) Stress incontinence
The patient is experiencing stress incontinence, which is urine leakage that occurs as a result of activity such as coughing, sneezing, running, or laughing. Stress incontinence can occur in patients postoperative from radical prostatectomy. Overflow incontinence occurs when the bladder does not completely empty after urinations. Urge incontinence, also known as overactive bladder, happens when one feels the urgency to urinate. Reflex incontinence primarily occurs in disease states with serious neurological impairment.

3. C) Breast cancer
Ixempra (Ixabepilone) is a chemotherapy agent used to treat metastatic breast cancer.

4. B) Chronic inflammation
Asbestos can cause chronic inflammation, which is a mechanism for carcinogenesis. Asbestos does not cause chromosomal mutations, apoptosis, or genetic instability.

5. D) Yoga
Providers may recommend nonpharmacologic treatments for managing cancer pain in addition to pain medication. Options include biofeedback, breathing and relaxation exercises, distraction, heat or cold, hypnosis, imagery, massage, pressure and/or vibration, and transcutaneous electrical nerve stimulation (TENS). While yoga can be beneficial to patients, it is not effective at reducing cancer pain.

6. D) Nonmaleficence
The ethical principle that requires that the nurse's actions inflict no harm is nonmaleficence. The nurse also has a duty, to tell the truth, which is called veracity. Autonomy stipulates that patients have the right to determine their own care and the right to refuse treatment. Beneficence refers to the nurse's responsibility to maximize the benefit to the patient.

7. C) Schedule of assessments

The schedule of assessments provides a timeline of the events that occur during the clinical trial. Screening period, treatment assessments, and post follow-up periods are time points that appear on the schedule of assessments. The adverse event reporting, pharmacology/toxicology information, and monitoring schedule do not provide any information on treatment procedure completion timelines.

8. B) "I doubled my dose of MS Contin."

Breakthrough pain is a transient exacerbation of pain that occurs either spontaneously or in relation to a specific predictable or unpredictable trigger, despite relatively stable and adequately controlled background pain. Treatment includes taking a rapid-onset dose of pain medication (e.g., one dose of fentanyl), in addition to the prescribed dosage of long-term pain medication and employing nonpharmacologic pain relief techniques such as meditation and heating pads. The patient should not increase the dose of long-acting pain medications without first consulting with their physician.

9. B) Urine output hourly

Monitor urine output hourly. Cisplatin can cause severe nephrotoxicity; therefore, it is imperative to monitor urine output hourly so that replacement fluids can be promptly administered if necessary. It is also important to monitor vital signs; however, urine output is the priority intervention. Pulmonary function should be assessed once per shift. It is not necessary to monitor the patient's diet choices.

10. B) The patient has an infection due to insertion complications of the catheter

Fever and chills that present within 7 to 10 days of insertion of a catheter are signs of an infection due to insertion complications. Symptoms that present more than 10 days after insertion are generally related to issues with care and maintenance of the catheter.

11. C) Epinephrine

The patient would prepare to administer epinephrine to a patient who is experiencing an acute anaphylactic reaction to L-asparaginase. Epinephrine is the drug of choice for acute anaphylactic reactions. Pseudoephedrine and phenylephrine are decongestants, and ephedrine can be used to treat hypotension during spinal anesthesia.

12. D) Tamoxifen (Nolvadex), lenalidomide (Revlimid), thalidomide

Tamoxifen (Nolvadex), lenalidomide (Revlimid), and thalidomide can increase risk for blood clots. Decitabine (Dacogen), doxorubicin (Adriamycin), cyclophosphamide (Cytoxan), etoposide (VP-16), and oxaliplatin (Eloxatin) do not increase risk for blood clots.

13. B) MRI of the spine

A patient with small cell lung cancer who presents with bladder incontinence should be evaluated for a possible spinal cord tumor. The provider would likely order an MRI of the spine to determine if there is a spinal cord tumor. X-ray, lumbar puncture, and ultrasound would not be used to diagnose a spinal tumor.

14. A) Encourage bowel regimen

Patients receiving treatment with vincristine should be encouraged to follow a bowel regimen as vincristine causes severe constipation. The bowel regimen should include a high-fiber diet with fruits and vegetables, 8 to 10 glasses of fluids/day, and regular physical activity. A stool softener once or twice a day can also help to prevent constipation. Calcium supplements should be directed by the provider and avoided, if possible, as they can cause constipation.

15. B) "Tell me what you know about the diet and why you think it might be helpful."

In addition to asking about a potential holistic approach to treatment, the patient is expressing many concerns to the nurse, including concern that the existing treatment may not be effective, anxiety about a potential change in treatment, despair about the impact treatment is having on their quality of life, and extreme fatigue that could be both a side effect of the treatment and/or a sign of depression. It is essential that the nurse encourage open communication so that the patient feels comfortable talking more deeply about their concerns so that they can be addressed. The nurse can best accomplish this by reframing the question and asking the patient why they think the diet may be helpful. The other options do not represent therapeutic communication.

16. C) Eat small frequent meals throughout the day

Side effects of chemotherapy are nausea/vomiting and decreased appetite. To promote adequate nutrition, the nurse will advise the patient to eat small frequent meals throughout the day to ensure adequate intake of calories and promote balanced nutrition. The patient can eat their favorite foods, provided that they align with their nutrition needs and do not exacerbate their nausea/vomiting.

17. C) Allogeneic stem cell transplant

Allogeneic stem cell transplant (donor cells) is the most appropriate treatment for a 24-year-old patient with acute myeloid leukemia who just completed induction therapy. Autologous stem cell transplant (patient cells) is used for multiple myeloma, not leukemias. Cord blood (cells from umbilical cord) is used for patients who do not have a matched donor. A 24-year-old male patient is unlikely to have poor donor options.

18. D) Not completing a falls risk assessment

Not completing a falls risk assessment is an example of a preventive error. Administering the incorrect dose of chemotherapy or chemotherapy that is not indicated for the diagnosis are medication administration errors. Failing to address abnormal laboratory results is a diagnostic error.

19. D) Pruritus

Leukemia symptoms vary based on the type of leukemia. Common leukemia signs and symptoms include fever and/or chills, persistent fatigue and weakness, frequent or severe infections, unintentional weight loss, swollen lymph nodes, enlarged liver or spleen, easy bleeding or bruising, recurrent nosebleeds, petechiae (tiny red spots on the skin), excessive sweating (especially at night), and bone pain or tenderness. Pruritus can be a sign of pancreatic cancer, not leukemia.

20. C) Fatigue
All four patients are likely to experience fatigue, which is a common side effect of treatment with stereotactic radiation, alpha interferon, receiving oxaliplatin and 5-fluorouracil, and ABVD (adriamycin, bleomycin, vinblastine, dacarbazine). Acute shortness of breath would indicate a hypersensitivity reaction. Anemia is a potential side effect of all treatments except stereotactic radiation. Only the colorectal cancer patient would be expected to experience abdominal pain.

21. D) Vasopressors
Vasopressors are administered to patients in late-stage sepsis to increase blood pressure. Antibiotics and antivirals are used to treat early sepsis, and anticoagulants are used to treat disseminated intravascular coagulation (DIC).

22. B) 2,922 cells/mcL
Absolute neutrophil count is calculated as follows:
ANC = WBC (cells/mcL) × [percent (PMNs + bands) ÷ 100]
ANC = 5,200 cells/mcL × [(52.2%+4%) ÷ 100]
ANC = 2,922 cells/mcL

23. D) An inpatient hospice facility
This patient has a terminal illness and is likely a candidate for hospice given their prognosis of <6 months. Provided that the patient meets all of the criteria for hospice, the best option would be an inpatient hospice facility since the patient has limited family support. A rehabilitation or acute care facility is not an appropriate option for this patient.

24. C) Cytarabine and an anthracycline
Cytarabine and anthracycline will most likely be prescribed for a patient with acute myeloid leukemia admitted for emergent induction therapy. Radiation would not be used as single agent, nor would cytarabine. A stem cell transplant may be recommended but not for induction therapy.

25. C) Squamous cell cancer and basal cell cancers
Photodynamic therapy is used to treat squamous and basal cell cancers. Melanoma is treated with surgery and biotherapy agents.

26. D) 15 days of notification
The clinical trial sponsor is required to report the event to the FDA on a MedWatch 3500A Form within 15 days of notification of the adverse event.

27. C) Nadir occurs 7 to 12 days post chemotherapy treatment when white blood cell counts are at their lowest level
Nadir occurs when white blood cell counts are at their lowest level, which is typically 7 to 12 days after chemotherapy treatment.

28. B) Mask and chemotherapy-designated gloves and gown
When administered chemotherapy and biotherapy agents such as rituximab (Rituxan), personal protective equipment (PPE) requirements include mask and chemotherapy-designated gloves and gown.

29. C) Grilled chicken with rice
Oncology patients often experience nausea and vomiting as a result of their cancer and treatment. They should eat foods that are bland, low in fat, and include carbohydrates like rice to fill the stomach and reduce gastric acids. High-fat, fried, and spicy foods can cause nausea.

30. C) Speak to the oncologist prior to scheduling any dental/medical appointments or procedures
Chemotherapy weakens the immune system, so patients may be more susceptible to bacterial infections, particularly endocarditis. Because of this, many doctors recommend having a dental check-up, cleanings, and/or dental treatment before chemotherapy starts. Since treatment has already started, the patient should clear any necessary dental/medical appointments with the oncologist prior to scheduling them.

31. C) Dry crackers and ginger ale
To help a patient prevent and deal with nausea and vomiting, the nurse should recommend carbohydrates such as dry crackers and ginger ale. Carbohydrates keep the stomach full, which helps to avoid the effects of gastric acids, and the carbonation and ginger in ginger ale help to settle the stomach. Heavy or spicy foods, such as cheeseburgers and turkey chili, should be avoided, as should sugary drinks (e.g., lemonade and cola). While bland foods are recommended, fish is light and will not help to keep the stomach full.

32. B) Advise the patient to change positions slowly
Furosemide (Lasix), a loop diuretic, can cause changes in blood pressure, so the nurse should advise the patient to move and change positions slowly. Furosemide is not affected by sun exposure and should be taken in the morning, not at night. The patient should be advised to drink normal amounts of fluid while on a diuretic, otherwise there is risk for acute dehydration.

33. D) Nadir occurs 7 to 10 days after chemotherapy, and the lab results are expected due to the chemotherapy patient received last week
After chemotherapy administration, blood cell counts begin to drop. Nadir occurs approximately 7 to 10 days after the treatment. The lab results are expected due to the chemotherapy patient received last week. They are not a sign that cancer is not responding to chemotherapy.

34. B) Cardiac tamponade
Cardiac tamponade typically presents with three classic signs called *Beck's triad*: low pressure in the arteries (hypotension), bulging and distended neck veins, and muffled heart sounds. In addition, patients can present with shortness of breath, tachycardia, and chest pain. Bronchial pneumonia commonly presents with fever, productive cough, shortness of breath, tachycardia, and chest pain. Acute myocardial infarction commonly presents with pressure, tightness, pain, or a squeezing or aching sensation in the chest and/or arms that may spread to the neck, jaw, and back. Patients may also have shortness of breath, nausea, and indigestion. Pulmonary embolism commonly presents with sudden-onset shortness of breath, chest pain, and cough with blood-tinged sputum.

35. D) Personal history of atypical nevus syndrome
The most significant risk factor for melanoma is personal history of atypical nevus syndrome. Other risk factors for melanoma include family history of basal and squamous cell cancers and personal history of actinic keratosis. Personal history of sunburn is a risk factor for melanoma, not family history of sunburn.

36. C) R-CHOP (rituxan, cytoxan, vincristine, prednisone)
Non-Hodgkin's lymphoma is commonly treated with rituxan, followed by CHOP (cytoxan, vincristine, prednisone). A/C (adriamycin/cytoxan) is used to treat breast cancer, FOLFOX (5FU, oxaliplatin, leucovorin) is used to treat colorectal cancer, and BEAM (carmustine, etoposide, cytarabine, melphalan) is used prior to stem cell transplantation.

37. A) A 63-year-old male patient with lung cancer and a history of radiation therapy
A lung cancer patient is at highest risk for respiratory comprise and alteration in ventilation. While the female patient with colorectal cancer and asthma and the male patient with non-Hodgkin's lymphoma who recently quit smoking may be at risk for respiratory compromise, the patient with lung cancer has the greatest risk. A breast cancer patient in remission is not at increased risk for respiratory compromise.

38. D) "Drinking milk will help to relieve my nausea."
Milk and milk products will not help to relieve nausea; in fact, they may increase nausea, as will fatty, fried, spicy, and overly sweet foods. Patients should be encouraged to eat small meals throughout the day and eat yogurt and protein shakes to promote adequate calorie intake. In addition, patients should take nausea medication as soon as they feel nauseous.

39. C) Assess MUGA scan results
Pulmonary function tests (PFTs) should be assessed prior to administration of bleomycin as it can cause pulmonary fibrosis. In addition, the nurse should calculate dose to date because bleomycin has a lifetime max of 400 units per m^2. Bleomycin also requires a test dose. MUGA (multigated acquisition) scan results would be reviewed prior to administration of doxorubicin, not bleomycin.

40. D) ALT, AST, and LD levels
Alanine aminotransferase (ALT), aspartate transaminase (AST), and lactate dehydrogenase (LD) levels are used to measure liver functions. They should be evaluated when a patient presents with sclera jaundice. BUN and creatinine levels are used to assess kidney function. CBC is used to measure bone marrow blood counts.

41. D) Cytokines act as messengers for the immune system
Cytokines are proteins that act as the messengers of the immune system, helping to control the activity of other immune system cells and blood cells. They do not directly attack foreign agents in the body. They increase anticancer activity by sending signs to promote abnormal cell death. Cytokines act at the intracellular level. They are not created in the laboratory.

42. D) Ask the patient for permission to further explore his concerns and issues

Ask the patient for permission to ask further questions about his concerns. Healthcare providers should try to normalize conversations about the sexual concerns of cancer patients and survivors and encourage open communication. Using the PLISSIT model (Permission, Limited Information, Specific Suggestions, Intensive Therapy) as a conversation guide, the nurse should first ask permission to discuss the patient's concerns related to sexuality to ensure the patient is comfortable with the discussion. Once the patient's concerns are understood, the nurse would provide limited information about what may be causing the issue and provide specific suggestions about what might be done to resolve the issue. If the issue continues, the nurse would refer the patient to a sex therapist or specially trained counselor for intensive therapy.

43. A) Ovarian cancer

There are screening tests and early-detection measures for colorectal cancer (e.g., colonoscopies), prostate cancer (e.g., digital rectal exam, prostate-specific antigen [PSA] levels), and breast cancer (e.g., mammography, genetic testing). There are no screening tests or early-detection measures for ovarian cancer.

44. B) Hypertension

Late signs and symptoms of lung cancer include weight loss, loss of appetite, headaches, bone pain or fractures, and blood clots. Early symptoms include cough, hoarseness, constant chest pain, shortness of breath or wheezing, frequent lung infections (e.g., bronchitis or pneumonia), and coughing up blood. Hypertension is not a late or early sign of lung cancer.

45. D) Breast cancer

Cold caps, or scalp cooling systems, are tightly fitting caps filled with a cold gel that constricts the blood vessels in the scalp, reducing the amount of chemotherapy that reaches the hair follicle. They can be used to prevent scalp alopecia in breast cancer patients. Cold caps are not recommended for liquid tumors. Prostate cancer patients usually do not have chemotherapy as first-line treatment; therefore, cold caps are not required or recommended.

46. A) 90% of those who *do not have* the disease will test *negative*

Specificity is the ability of a test to correctly identify people without the disease. Essentially, it is the percentage of true negatives. A specificity of 90% indicates that 90% of those who *do not have* the disease will test *negative*. *Sensitivity* is the ability of a test to correctly identify people with the disease—percentage of true positives. A sensitivity of 90% indicates that 90% of those who *do have* the disease will test *positive*.

47. C) Nivolumab (OPDIVO)

Nivolumab (OPDIVO) is a immunotherapy agent in the monoclonal antibody class used to treat a wide range of cancers. A 0.22-micron filter is used with the IV administration of OPDIVO to filter out particulate matter, bacteria, and air emboli to protect the patient. Micron filters are not required for the administration of cisplatin (Platinol), gemcitabine (Gemzar), and rituximab (Rituxan).

48. B) Discuss the care plan with the patient's family
Patients with new cancer diagnoses often experience severe anxiety, particularly those who have a history of anxiety or depression. Appropriate nursing interventions include the administration of prescribed antianxiety medications every 4 to 6 hours, referral to a social worker, and encouraging the patient to verbalize their concerns. While families can be encouraged to support the patient, they are not included in the development of a care plan.

49. A) Nivolumab and ipilimumab
Nivolumab and ipilimumab, which are monoclonal antibodies, is a combination immunotherapy used to treat metastatic melanoma. Chemotherapy is not effective for treating melanoma, so paclitaxel should not be used. Rituxan, which is also a monoclonal antibody, is used to treat lymphoma and autoimmune disorders.

50. B) Look into obtaining the medication from a specialty pharmacy
Drugs used to treat cancer are highly specialized and can be very costly for pharmacies to dispense. Specialty pharmacies that focus on high-cost, high-touch medication therapy for complex disease states such as oncology may be able to provide drugs such as filgrastim at a lower cost. Because cancer drugs are so specialized, alternate lower-cost options are often not available. The nurse should not tell the patient that the drug is not necessary. While the manufacturer may be able to provide a sample, it will not help the patient in the long term.

51. C) Hydromorphone is 2 to 8 times more potent than morphine
Hydromorphone is 2 to 8 more times potent than morphine, so it has the potential to be more addictive than morphine. Neither hydromorphone nor morphine can be used as a cough suppressant.

52. B) Nothing
During an IVP (intravenous push) infusion of a vesicant such as vinorelbine, the patient should feel nothing. Pain or burning and redness at the injection site are indications of extravasation. Vinorelbine does not typically cause acute-onset nausea. Urge to void can occur with IV contrast, not IVP infusions.

53. D) 7 to 10 days after exposure to chemotherapy
Chemotherapy-induced alopecia typically occurs 7 to 10 days after exposure to chemotherapy. Hair will usually fall out unevenly and in clumps, which can be exceedingly difficult for many patients.

54. B) Perform blood draws on the left arm
Blood draws and blood pressure should be performed on the unaffected (right) arm. It is imperative to elevate the left arm when patient is sitting or lying in bed to assist with drainage. Compression sleeves should be worn whenever possible.

55. D) ABCDE rule
The ABCDE rule is used to assess melanoma. A is for Asymmetry, B is for Border, C is for Color, D is for diameter, and E is for evolving. The Rule of Nines is to determine total body surface area for burns. TNM (tumor, node, metastasis) is a solid tumor staging system, and the Ann Arbor system is a system previously used to stage lymphoma.

56. B) Rituximab

The patient is likely being treated with rituximab, which increases the risk for hypersensitivity reactions due to the chimeric component of the drug. Nivolumab and ipilimumab increase the risk for inflammatory processes such as colitis and thyroiditis. Pertuzumab increases the risk for hypertension.

57. A) Colorectal cancer

High-fat diets, family history, and genetic malformations are risk factors for colorectal cancer. Mesothelioma has been associated with asbestos, smoking, and exposure to other chemical irritants. Pancreatic cancer and adenocarcinoma of the stomach can be caused by smoking, exposure to chemicals, and obesity.

58. D) Rice and pasta

Rice and pasta can compound constipation; therefore, patients with constipation should avoid those food items. Fruits, vegetables, whole grains, and nuts are high in fiber and can assist with peristalsis, so they should be encouraged. Consumption of fish and meat does not significantly impact bowel function.

59. A) Osmotic

Constipation is a side effect of many chemotherapy agents. Bulk-forming laxatives increase fluid in the bowel and stool bulk, aiding peristalsis. Saline laxatives increase water absorption into the bowel and intestinal transit time. Stimulant laxatives increase GI motility.

60. C) Hyperthermia

When a patient is dying, they will experience increased confusion and pain, decreased urination and appetite, and hypothermia (not hyperthermia).

61. B) "It's ok to not wear a hat when it's cold; the cold will help regulate my body temperature."

During treatment, hair becomes fragile and breaks easily; therefore, patients should limit the number of times they wash their hair to twice a week with a mild shampoo. Eyebrows protect against rain and sweat, eyelashes protect against foreign bodies and dust, and hair protects against sun and cold. If the patient loses their eyebrows and eyelashes, they must wear sunglasses when they are outside. If they lose their hair, they must wear a hat outside.

62. C) Apply deodorant only to the right axilla

Deodorant should be applied only to the axilla that is not being radiated to prevent skin irritation. Other preventive measures include avoiding hot or cold compresses and moisturizers during radiation therapy.

63. C) Albumin 2.3

The patient's albumin level is low, which is a sign of anorexia and poor nutritional status. BUN, WBC, and hemoglobin levels are within the normal range for a patient receiving this therapy.

64. C) Colony-stimulating factors

When a donor is preparing for mobilization of cells, colony-stimulating factors are administered, which can cause severe bone pain, fever, chills, and fatigue. It is unlikely that this patient's symptoms are caused by a *Staphylococcus* or viral infection or an acute allergic reaction.

65. D) Provide pain control

Patients receiving hospice care have a prognosis of <6 months. The focus is on comfort care, not curative care. Providing pain control is a priority intervention. The monitoring of vital signs is often discontinued to minimize interventions, as are medications for chronic symptom management. In the final stages of life, patients often begin to refuse intake. Nutrition and hydration should be provided as comfort measures per the preference of the patient. It is not necessary that the nurse ensure adequate nutrition.

66. E) Use preferred mouthwash to rinse and freshen dry tissues

Dry, sore, and/or raw mouth/throat tissues are a side effect of chemotherapy and radiation treatments. Patient education should include avoiding acidic, spicy foods (can irritate sensitive oral tissues) and alcohol (can cause dryness). Many OTC types of mouthwash contain alcohol, which may dry and further irritate tissues, so the patient should not be instructed to use their preferred mouthwash. Instead, they should rinse their mouth with a salt–water solution to soothe sore tissues. To lessen symptoms in the future, the patient should chew on ice chips during upcoming treatments.

67. D) Handling oral chemotherapy that is intact

Two pairs of hazardous drug (HD)-tested and approved gloves are required when receiving and unpacking HDs, compounding HDs, administering and disconnecting HDs, and disposing of, cleaning, and handling of patient excreta within 48 hours of receiving HDs. Only one pair of HD-approved gloves is necessary when dispensing intact oral chemotherapy.

68. D) Lymph node involvement

Tumor staging is used to determine the spread of solid malignancies. The TNM classification system is used to determine the cancer stage for many solid malignancies. Each letter in the TNM classification stands for a staging protocol: T—tumor size and location, N—regional lymph node involvement, M—metastasis status (cancer spread to other organs).

69. B) "Although this study involves placebo, you will not be treated with anything less than the standard approved therapy. At this point in time, it is not known which treatment combination is the best."

The oncology nurse is incorrect in telling the patient that the investigational + standard therapy is superior as the phase 3 trial is directly comparing these arms and results are not available. Patients feel uncertain when they see the use of a placebo and need to be reassured that even if they are going to potentially receive a placebo, they will not receive it without at least the best currently approved therapy. It is unethical to provide a placebo to a patient who requires treatment. A double-blind study means that the research staff and patient will not be aware of which combination the patient will be taking. In an emergency, the patient can be unblinded if there are concerns that threaten the health or well-being of the patient. The potential adverse events related to study drugs are not conclusive to inform the patient or research team which combination the patient is assigned.

70. A) Prior to the initiation of treatment
Nurses should assess for social determinants and financial distress or toxicity as soon after diagnosis as possible and prior to the initiation of treatment so that any potential issues with insurance coverage can be addressed and assistance programs applied for prior to incurring any bills. The nurse should not wait until the patient or family expresses financial toxicity or asks for assistance as many people are uncomfortable discussing financial issues.

71. C) "I'm sorry for the inconvenience. I will need to review the clinical trial budget to determine what is covered, as well as review your insurance information."
The clinical trial sponsor, sometimes a pharmaceutical company, provides a budget to the study site that covers tests, medications, and procedures that are required outside of the usual insurance coverage for patients receiving oncology treatment. The budget may also provide funds for travel and accommodations reimbursement. Participating in a clinical trial does require additional visits and/or phone calls in which the patient must participate. The sponsor may not pay for all of the protocol-required items, as many are covered by the patient's insurance. Tests and procedures are not more expensive because the patient is enrolled in a clinical trial. If the budget and the patient's insurance do not cover a specific item, additional resources should be explored to prevent financial hardship and prevent trial withdrawal.

72. B) Taste alterations are more pronounced with chemotherapy administered every 3 weeks
Taste cells regenerate approximately every 20 days. Patients who receive chemotherapy every 21 days start to recover their taste cells by the time they start the next cycle, so the fluctuations in taste changes can be more noticeable and distressing. The taste cells in patients receiving weekly chemo do not have time to recover, so the taste alternation is more consistent with no fluctuation, making it less pronounced.

73. C) Ask the patient for further details about the supplements and inform the provider
Some herbal supplements can cause severe liver and kidney toxicity and interact with the chemotherapy and biotherapy agents. The nurse should ask the patient for further details about the supplements and inform the provider to ensure that they are safe for use prior to encourage or discouraging use. While acupuncture may be an appropriate alternative therapy for this patient, the nurse should address the supplement issue before discussing other options.

74. A) Seizures
Seizures are a sign of both hypocalcemia and hypomagnesemia. Excessive thirst, abdominal pain, and hypertension are signs of hypercalcemia and hypermagnesemia.

75. A) Provide the patient information about genetic testing and counseling
The nurse's role as a patient advocate is crucial, and providing the patient with information on genetic counseling may put the patient's mind at ease and reduce their stress levels. Inaccurate reassurance or avoidance does not respect patient concerns. Informing the patient that stress may worsen their treatment progress is not a therapeutic response. While the nurse can suggest that a chaplain visit the family (if it aligns with their spiritual beliefs), the nurse should address the patient's concerns before doing so.

76. D) Elevated specific gravity in the urine
The patient is exhibiting signs and symptoms of dehydration, including fatigue, weakness, dark urine, and decreased appetite. The nurse should anticipate elevated specific gravity in the urine, as well as increased BUN, creatinine, and potassium levels.

77. B) Dexamethasone (Decadron)
Steroids such as dexamethasone (Decadron) can cause hyperglycemia in the oncology patient. Hyperglycemia is not a side effect of mycophenolate mofetil (CellCept), tamoxifen (Nolvadex), or ondansetron (Zofran).

78. D) T3, T4, and TSH
Thyroid function should be evaluated prior to administration of pembrolizumab due to the risk of thyroiditis complications. It is not necessary to monitor magnesium, cholesterol, and uric acid levels prior to administration of pembrolizumab.

79. B) Apply a sterile gauze and dressing at the insertion site
When a patient's chest tube becomes dislodged, the nurse should first apply sterile gauze and dressing at the insertion site and then call the provider. The nurse should not attempt to reinsert the chest tube as it may cause harm to the patient. A wet-to-dry dressing may also cause harm to the patient.

80. C) Methotrexate
Leucovorin is administered with methotrexate to reduce the risk of renal side effects. Drug blood levels must be monitored properly to dose leucovorin. Drug levels do not need to be monitored with bleomycin, doxorubicin, and cisplatin therapy.

81. A) High-fat and high-sugar diet
Diets high in fat and sugar place individuals at greater risk for developing colorectal cancer.

82. B) Avoid shaving the area and use of scented deodorant
The entrance and exit skin may become irritated after radiation therapy. Patients with skin irritation should be advised to clean the area daily with mild soap, apply moisturizer daily, and avoid shaving, the use of scented deodorant, thermal irritants such as heat or cool packs, and sun exposure to the affected area for life.

83. D) History of diabetes
Risk factors for leukemia include previous cancer treatment, genetic disorders (e.g., Down syndrome), exposure to certain chemicals (e.g., benzene), smoking, and family history of leukemia. History of diabetes is not a risk factor for leukemia.

84. A) Higher grade ductal carcinoma in situ of the breast
Comedocarcinoma is a term used to describe higher grade ductal carcinoma in situ (DCIS) of the breast and DSCIS with significant necrosis. It is not used to describe stage I or IV of breast cancer.

85. B) An oncology certified nurse who has worked in both hematology and solid tumor oncology for 10 years

The nurse who has worked in both hematology and solid tumor oncology for 10 years would be the most appropriate mentor given their length of direct experience in the area in which the new nurse will be working. While the nurse who has worked on the solid tumor oncology floor for 5 years would also be a good mentor, and perhaps could more easily relate to the challenges a new nurse may encounter, a nurse who is certified and has worked in the area for more years will have greater insight to share with the trainee. When possible, mentors should also be certified in their areas of expertise. A nurse navigator from the bone transplant floor and a charge nurse in radiology have different job roles and areas of expertise, so they would not appropriate selections.

86. C) A 22-year-old female college student with history of generalized anxiety disorder who is newly diagnosed with diffuse large cell lymphoma

Risk factors for fear of cancer recurrence (FCR) include existing psychological disorders such as anxiety and depression, new diagnosis, and younger age. A 22-year-old female with a history of generalized anxiety disorder with a new diagnosis is most at risk for FCR.

87. C) Docusate (Colace)

A common side effect of opioid medications is constipation. Docusate is indicated to treat/prevent constipation. Zolpidem is used to treat sleeping disorders, carbamazepine is indicated for seizures, and diazepam is indicated for anxiety. These medications should be avoided in patients taking opioids due to potential drug interactions.

88. D) Codeine

In addition to reducing pain, codeine also has antitussive properties, so it is the most appropriate pain medication for a patient with stage IV lung cancer with uncontrolled cough. Morphine, hydromorphone, and methadone should be avoided as they will decrease the respiratory rate of the patient.

89. A) May be experiencing neuropathy, which is contributing to the unwillingness to participate in physical therapy

The patient may be experiencing peripheral neuropathy, a treatment-related side effect of vincristine, which is making it difficult for him to participate in physical therapy. It does not indicate that the patient has depression and is giving up on treatment or does not believe physical therapy is a priority. The nurse should assess for potential reasons the patient is unwilling to participate and treat the underlying causes.

90. C) Supplements to promote a healthy lifestyle

The Institute of Medicine's *Long-Term Survivorship after Care Treatment* includes recommendations that address the unique needs of cancer survivors, including recommended screening and tests, key referrals for follow-up care, and information on the psychosocial effects of cancer and survivorship. It does not provide recommendations for supplements to promote a healthy lifestyle.

91. B) Anhedonia
Taste cells are affected by chemotherapy, which can cause significant alterations in taste and lead to depression, anhedonia, weight loss (not gain), and constipation (not diarrhea). Some patients may even avoid social gatherings because of the inability to enjoy eating. While chemotherapy can cause mouth sores, and mouth sores can cause pain and related difficulty eating, they do not alter taste.

92. B) Stop the infusion and call the provider
Shortness of breath is a sign of a possible anaphylactic reaction to treatment. The nurse should immediately stop the infusion and call the provider. The provider may order an EKG, antihistamines, and steroids.

93. C) Weight gain of 10 lbs
A 10-pound weight gain is significant and indicates that the patient is retaining fluids, which can be related to cardiac or renal dysfunction. A temperature of 98.9°F is considered normal, and nausea and vomiting and dry mouth are expected side effects of chemotherapy.

94. B) A 42-year-old male patient with a glioblastoma who had a partial craniotomy
Data show nearly 100% of patients with a glioblastoma will experience disease recurrence, regardless of treatment.

95. C) Use of oral contraceptives
Risk factors for ovarian cancer include older age, family history, and early pregnancies. Use of oral contraceptives is not a risk factor for ovarian cancer; however, it is a risk factor for breast and cervical cancers.

96. B) Tumor lysis syndrome
Combination therapy with chemotherapy and radiation increases a patient's risk for neutropenia. Patients receiving this therapy are also likely to experience nausea and dysphagia. Tumor lysis syndrome is not a risk for patients with head and neck cancers. It is a risk for patients with lymphomas.

97. D) Pleural effusion
Anthracycline therapy can cause cardiotoxicity leading to cardiomyopathy. The nurse would anticipate a change or discontinuation of anthracycline therapy in a patient with a decrease in left ventricular ejection fraction (LVEF) >20% from baseline or <50% during treatment or symptoms of heart failure. Pleural effusion would likely not lead to modification or discontinuation of treatment.

98. C) Wear personal protective equipment when entering room
The patient's neutrophil count indicates that the patient has neutropenia and is at risk of infection. The nurse should encourage the patient to shower daily to avoid self-infection and limit visitors due to the high risk for infection. Filgrastim (Neupogen) stimulates the growth of the white blood cells, making patients less vulnerable to infections, so it should be administered daily. Personal protective equipment (PPE) is worn when administering chemotherapy; it is not necessary for neutropenia.

99. B) Breast cancer, leukemia, and adrenal tumors

Li-Fraumeni syndrome is an inherited disorder caused by mutations in the *TP53* gene. This genetic mutation is associated with breast cancer, leukemia, and adrenal tumors, as well as brain cancer and osteosarcoma.

100. B) Acneiform rash

Skin reactions to radiation include erythema and dry and moist desquamation. Acneiform rash is not a side effect of radiation therapy; however, it can be caused by epidermal growth factor receptor (EGFR) inhibitors.

101. B) Allopurinol

Allopurinol is a prophylactic medication administered to reduce risk of tumor lysis syndrome (TLS). It reduces the conversion of nucleic acid byproducts to uric acid, preventing urate nephropathy and oliguric renal failure. Rasburicase is used to treat acute TLS. Dexamethasone is a steroid used to reduce inflammation and suppress the immune response. Furosemide is a loop diuretic.

102. B) Basal cell carcinoma

Basal cell cancer is characterized by wounds that do not heal and continue to bleed for an extended period. The wounds may be crusting and oozing and are often found on the face and back. Squamous cell carcinoma is characterized by red, rough, scaly patches that can bleed and become crusty. Acneiform rash can be caused by cancer drugs and is characterized by small, raised, acne-type bumps on the face, scalp, chest, and upper back. They can be filled with pus and crust over; however, they do not bleed. Actinic keratosis are precancerous rough, scaly patches that develop from prolonged sun exposure. They are commonly found on the face, lips, and ears.

103. D) "I will start filling all my prescriptions at the specialty pharmacy to save money."

Specialty pharmacies dispense only select medications that are typically associated with complex management and administration guidelines, so they are often able to offer lower costs. Specialty pharmacies do not typically fill all prescriptions for all patient medications. With the provider's consent, the patient can discuss lower cost treatment options with the insurance company. They should also contact the insurance company to inquire about prior authorization before scheduling any diagnostics. The oncology nurse navigator can identify any potential patient assistance programs for the patient.

104. C) Crystalloids

The initial fluid resuscitation recommendation for sepsis is crystalloids. If the patient requires substantial amounts of fluids to meet the goal of volume resuscitation, then albumin can be added. Blood is a colloid, not a crystalloid. Hetastarch is not recommended for sepsis due to the worsening effect it has on the kidneys.

105. D) Melphalan

Melphalan is a chemotherapy agent that is commonly given as the conditioning regimen for patients with multiple myeloma prior to autologous stem cell transplant. Melphalan causes respiratory complications such as shortness of breath. Carmustine, etoposide, and cytarabine are not used in the conditioning regimen.

106. B) Uterine cancer
Although all cancers can cause blood clots and resulting deep vein thrombosis, the highest risk cancers include brain, liver, kidney, lung, ovarian, pancreatic, and uterine, as well as lymphomas, leukemias, and multiple myeloma.

107. D) Personality changes
Brain metastases can present with personality changes. Patients with brain metastases will have pain in the head or headaches, not back pain. Respiratory depression and the presence of S3 heart sound do not present initially with brain metastases.

108. B) "I should file my cuticles instead of cutting them."
The nurse should teach patients to avoid any injury or trauma and discourage any activities that would pose a risk for injury. Maintaining skin integrity is important, so patients should use an electric razor for shaving and an Emery board for nail care. They should also avoid restrictive clothing, minimize invasive procedures (e.g., dental procedures), and sneeze and blow their nose gently with mouth open to prevent increased intracranial pressure.

109. D) Help patients purchase appropriate head coverings
The nurse can best assist the patients with their hair loss by preparing them for what they can expect, exploring the meaning and significance of hair loss, and helping patients plan for hair loss before it starts. Helping patients purchase appropriate head coverings is beyond the oncology scope of practice.

110. A) Decreased white blood cell and platelet counts
Doxorubicin (Adriamycin) and cyclophosphamide (Cytoxan) can cause myelosuppression 10 to 14 days post infusion. A patient with myelosuppression will have decreased white blood cell and platelet counts.

111. A) Lactic acid levels
A breast cancer patient who presents with shortness of breath, temperature of 101.3°F, nausea, and fatigue may be neutropenic or have an infection or anemia. To determine the cause, the nurse should review the patient's complete blood count (CBC); chem screen to monitor kidney, liver, and electrolytes; and lactic acid levels to identify an infection process. CA 27–29 levels are used to monitor response to breast cancer treatment and risk of recurrence. It is not necessary to monitor those levels at this time or cholesterol levels.

112. C) Polyuria
Morphine may cause serious side effects, including hypotension, slow and shallow breathing, shortness of breath, drowsiness, apnea, circulatory depression, weakness, constipation, tachycardia, sweating, anxiety, and increased thirst. Morphine does not cause polyuria.

113. A) Unintended weight gain
Common signs and symptoms of pancreatic cancer include jaundice (yellowing of eyes/skin), dark urine, light-colored/greasy stools, itchy skin, belly or back pain, weight loss (not weight gain), decreased appetite, nausea and vomiting, gallbladder or liver enlargement, blood clots, and (infrequently) diabetes.

114. D) Perceived competition and a threat to personal autonomy as a result of overlapping care from multiple professions

Some of the infusion nurses may see the new nutritionist as a threat to their ability to conduct their jobs comprehensively, or their autonomy, and the overlap in care will create a problem. This will lead to a barrier of collaboration with the nutritionist. To overcome this barrier, the nurse manager should meet with the infusion nurses to fully discuss their concerns and develop a plan to resolve the issues and enable productive collaboration.

115. D) Salad

Patients with diarrhea should consume a diet that is low in insoluble fiber, high in soluble fiber, and low in fat and lactulose. Rice, cooked vegetables, and apple cause are recommended foods. Patients should avoid eating raw vegetables (e.g., salad) as they can be harder to digest and, in some cases, exacerbate diarrhea.

116. C) Retopuberant prostatectomy

The majority of men will experience erectile dysfunction following radical retropuberant prostatectomy. It may be temporary or permanent due to nerve damage during surgery. External beam radiation can also cause erectile dysfunction, but surgery poses the greatest risk. Watchful waiting and anti-androgen medications do not directly cause erectile dysfunction.

117. C) Discontinuation of gemcitabine and supportive care

Gemcitabine is a chemotherapy agent that can cause thrombotic microangiopathy, which is a group of disorders defined by the presence of hemolytic anemia, low platelet count, and organ damage resulting from the formation of microscopic blood clots in capillaries and small arteries. While both plasmapheresis and eculizumab can be used in the treatment of gemcitabine-induced thrombotic microangiopathy, there is little evidence that outcomes of these treatments are superior to discontinuation and supportive care alone.

118. C) Extravasation

If left untreated, mucositis, depression, and constipation can lead to anorexia. Mucositis is the inflammation and ulceration of the membranes that line the digestive tract and mouth, which can make eating very painful. Depression can cause loss of appetite, and constipation can cause abdominal pain and bloating, which can contribute to anorexia. Extravasation, which causes skin breakdown, is not associated with anorexia.

119. D) Folic acid

Pemetrexed is a multitargeted antifolate drug used to treat lung cancer. Patients treated with pemetrexed require folic acid and vitamin B12 supplementation to reduce hematologic and gastrointestinal side effects. Potassium, magnesium, and calcium are not required.

120. C) "I need to buy an electric razor."

Patients who receive a bilateral mastectomy with lymph node removal should take all measures to avoid a cut in the axillary area, which can lead to infection and lymphedema. If shaving is necessary, the patient should use an electric razor. The patient should not lift heavy things or take hot showers to reduce swelling.

121. C) Warfarin (Coumadin)
The following medications may be given after each cycle of chemotherapy to prevent myelosuppression: epoetin alfa (Procrit), filgrastim (Neupogen), sargramostim (Leukine), and pegfilgrastim (Neulasta). Warfarin (Coumadin) is not prescribed to decrease the effects of myelosuppression.

122. C) HPV 16–18
The HPV vaccine targets the HPV strains 16–18. It is not effective at preventing strains 3–6, 14–16, or 16–22.

123. C) Anemia
The patient is likely experiencing anemia post chemotherapy. Anemia is caused by a reduction in red blood cells. Red blood cells can continue to be affected by chemotherapy, even 3 months after the last treatment. Anemia can present as fatigue and an inability to focus or concentrate. The patient's scenario is not indicative of a recurrence of cancer or depression. While fatigue is a symptom of dehydration, the patient would likely also complain of thirst, less frequent urination, and dark-colored urine.

124. C) Cardiomyopathy
Anthracycline-induced cardiotoxicity can lead to cardiomyopathy. Signs of cardiomyopathy include weakness, fatigue, dizziness, hypertension, tachycardia, palpitations, irregular heartbeat, S3 hearts sound, orthopnea, dyspnea on exertion, and chest pressure. While pulmonary hypertension can cause similar symptoms, the nurse should suspect cardiopathy due to the increased cardiotoxicity with anthracycline therapy. A patient with myocardial infarction would present with pain, pressure, or tightness in the chest, back, or jaw, as well as pain that radiates down the arm, shortness of breath, nausea, sweating, and anxiety. Septal wall defect is a congenital condition; it is not caused by anthracycline treatment.

125. A) Dyspnea
Tumor lysis syndrome (TLS) is a condition that occurs when a large number of cancer cells die within a short period, releasing their contents into the blood. It can occur after chemotherapy treatment for large, bulky, or fast-growing tumors such as lymphoma. Symptoms of TLS include nausea, vomiting, diarrhea, muscle cramps or twitches, weakness, numbness or tingling, fatigue, decreased urination, irregular heart rate, confusion, restlessness, irritability, delirium, hallucinations, and seizures. Other clinical manifestations of tumor lysis syndrome include syncopal attack, lethargy, pitting edema, facial edema, abdominal distention, and other sign of fluid overload. Dyspnea is not a common symptom of TLS.

126. B) A mild electrical current that is applied to the skin at the site of pain
TENS is the acronym for transcutaneous electrical nerve stimulation. This therapy involves a mild electrical current applied to the skin at the site of pain.

127. B) Must be individually tailored to meet the preferences and comfort level of the survivor and the family members
While community-based interventions can be a valuable resource to reduce anxiety and improve the quality of life for survivors and their families, it is important for the oncology nurse to recognize that preferences on environment and method of support can vary among participants. Community-based resources can include a wide range of activities, not just large-group activities.

128. A) Increased shortness of breath and tachycardia

Increased shortness of breath and tachycardia are signs of worsening congestive heart failure (CHF). Patients with CHF will have weight gain (due to fluid retention), not weight loss. While patients with CHF may have wheezing and lethargy, they will not have bradycardia. Blood glucose levels are related to diabetes, not CHF.

129. A) Hepatocellular carcinoma

Ascites, the accumulation of fluid in the peritoneal cavity, is most commonly associated with hepatocellular carcinoma, as well as ovarian, pancreatic, liver, and colon cancers. Ascites is not commonly associated with breast cancer, lymphoma, osteosarcoma.

130. B) Perform neurologic assessment every 4 hours

Performing neurologic assessments every 4 hours is vital to determine the status of cord compression. Cardiac and lung assessments would be performed every 4 hours for a patient with cardiac tamponade or pleural effusion. Gastrointestinal assessment would be performed every 8 hours for patients with colon cancer. Blood glucose levels would be checked before each meal and before bedtime for diabetic patients and patients on high-dose steroids.

131. C) Patients have been heavily pretreated and are susceptible to adverse events that must be reviewed to study drug relationship

Efficacy data are not an endpoint for phase 1 clinical trials; safety and drug dosing/administration are central endpoints. Efficacy is associated with phase 2 clinical trials. Patients are not eligible to participate in clinical trials that have not been IRB approved. Cohort designs are specific to each trial, although 3+3 is a common cohort design; fifteen participants per cohort is not a standard requirement. Phase 1 trial participants are usually pretreated, relapsed, and do not have sound standard or phase 2-4 options for treatment. Participants can have treatment or disease-related toxicities that prevent them from continuing study participation due to adverse events (related or unrelated to the investigational agent).

132. C) Steroids prevent urinary retention

Inflammation is the body's natural response to an event, whether it is trying to heal a wound or fight an infection. Both of those are good things, but they can sometimes cause pain. Steroids can help bring down inflammation and in turn can help manage pain. Steroids can play multiple roles in cancer treatment. First, they can be part of the cancer treatment itself, such as with some lymphomas and multiple myeloma. Second, they can be highly effective at reducing nausea and vomiting related to chemotherapy. Steroids do not prevent urinary retention.

133. B) Immunotherapy agents

Immunotherapy agents have the highest risk for reactivation of hepatitis B infections in a patient with previous exposure.

134. C) Cerebrum

An astrocytoma is a glioma that develops from the astrocytes that support nerve cells. Astrocytomas typically affect the cerebrum portion of the brain.

135. D) Minimum of 5 of the 10 contact hours in oncology must be continuing medical education (CME)

To be eligible for initial OCN certification, a nurse must have a current, active, unencumbered license as a registered nurse in the United States, its territories, or Canada at the time of application and examination; a minimum of 2 years of experience as a RN within the previous 4-year period; a minimum of 2,000 hours of practice within oncology either in clinical, administrative, educational, research, or consultative settings within the previous 4-year period; and a minimum of 10 contact hours of nursing continuing education hours in oncology within 3 years from the time of application. A maximum (not minimum) of 5 of the 10 contact hours in oncology can be continuing medical education (CME).

136. A) Protocol

The protocol and the investigator's brochure (IB) have the most updated information regarding guidelines for adverse event management and potential relationship to investigational agents. The protocol includes guidelines for drug delay, dose reduction, drug interactions, permitted concomitant medications, and drug resumption. The institutional review board (IRB) approval letter, press releases, and clinicaltrials.gov will not list side effects of the drug.

137. A) A 35-year-old female with copious, intractable diarrhea and vomiting

Patients with cancer are at increased risk for infection due to their immunocompromised status. A cancer patient with copious, intractable diarrhea and vomiting should be evaluated to rule out *Clostridioides difficile*, a gram-positive bacteria. Patients with suspected *C. diff* should be placed in private rooms to prevent spread to other patients. In addition, healthcare providers should wear gloves and a gown when entering the patient's room. Private rooms are not required for patients who are receiving chemotherapy and radiation, experienced a reaction to rituximab (Rituxan), or are receiving induction therapy for acute myeloid leukemia.

138. B) Chest pain

Radiation-induced esophagitis, an inflammation of the esophagus, is a side effect of radiation therapy for head and neck cancers. Patients with esophagitis will likely present with dysphagia and chest pain. Nausea and vomiting, painful ulcers in mouth, and indigestion are not symptoms of esophagitis.

139. B) AFP

AFP can be detected in non-seminoma testicular cancer. CA 19–9 is a tumor marker for both pancreatic and ovarian cancers and ovarian cancer. CA 125 is a marker for ovarian cancer, and CEA is a marker for colon cancer.

140. A) Adaptive immunity occurs after an exposure to an antigen from a vaccine

Adaptive immunity occurs after exposure to an antigen from a vaccine. It provides long-term protection, involves the T and B lymphocytes, and can be related to genetics.

141. D) "I should call my provider if I have a temperature higher than 101.0°F."

Patients should be taught to call their provider if their temperature is ≥100.4°F or if they have pain, respiratory issues, chills, or dysuria. They should also maintain skin integrity by protecting themselves from cuts and burns and avoid contact with people who have received any live vaccine, such as the MMR, within the past 30 days. Patients should wear gloves when gardening to prevent cuts and scrapes and avoid contact with bacteria in the soil. They should also avoid changing cat litter boxes.

142. B) Wear chemotherapy gloves and lab coat when preparing chemotherapy agents

Safe administration of chemotherapy and biotherapy begins with a review of patient's CBC, chem-screen, and body surface area (BSA) prior to preparing chemotherapy agents. These elements will help to determine proper dosing. Thorough hand washing is essential before administration. Personal protective equipment (PPE) includes chemotherapy gown, gloves, and mask. A lab coat does not provide enough protection. Antineoplastic waste should be disposed of in hazardous waste containers.

143. C) Avoid dining out

Patients post colostomy should be encouraged to resume their activities of daily living, including sexual activity and dining out. They should avoid contact sports and monitor the stoma for skin breakdown.

144. C) Autologous stem cell transplant

Autologous stem cell transplant is used to treat multiple myeloma, lymphoma, and auto-immune disorders. In autologous stem cell transplantation, the donor cells come from the patient. In allogeneic stem cell transplantation, the donor cells come from a person other than the patient, such as a related or unrelated donor. Allogeneic transplants are used to treat leukemias. Cord blood transplantation uses cord blood collected from the umbilical cord and placenta of healthy newborns. It is used to treat some leukemias and lymphomas. A syngeneic transplant is an allogeneic transplant in which the donor cells are provided by an identical twin.

145. A) Cerebellar toxicity

Cerebellar toxicity is a dose-dependent adverse effect of cytarabine therapy, which is a drug that is used to treat certain kinds of leukemia and lymphoma. Patients receiving cytarabine should be monitored for signs of cerebellar toxicity, including ataxia, dysarthria, unsteady gait, confusion, memory loss, and cognitive dysfunction. Patients should be asked to sign their names on a piece of paper so that it can be compared to the signature on the informed consent to determine if the patient is experiencing any cognitive or motor changes.

146. B) Administer antiemetics

To prevent infection in oncology patients, it is essential to maintain sterile technique when accessing the Port-A-Cath (PAC), provide perineal care to indwelling bladder catheter, and advise the patient to avoid eating raw fish and meat. Antiemetics are administered to prevent nausea and vomiting, not prevent infection.

147. B) Hypercalcemia

The metabolic derangement associated with tumor lysis syndrome includes hyperkalemia, hypocalcemia (not hypercalcemia), hyperphosphatemia, and hyperuricemia.

148. B) CT of the abdomen and pelvis

A CT scan (not MRI) would be the first imaging test ordered for a patient with complaints of severe abdominal pain, gross hematuria, and a palpable abdominal mass. A CA-125 (cancer antigen-125) level is most commonly used to monitor treatment for endometrial, peritoneal or fallopian tube cancer; check for cancer recurrence; and screen patients at high risk for ovarian cancer. A CA 19–9 (cancer antigen 19–9) level is most commonly used to monitor treatment for pancreatic cancer and check for cancer recurrence.

149. C) Position patient with chest tubes and surgical side up

The nurse should monitor chest tube output every hour initially, then every 2 to 4 or 8 hours as indicated. The nurse should notify the provider if chest tube output exceeds 70 mL/hour and/or is bright red, warm, and free flowing. Increased amounts of warm, free-flowing blood indicate intrathoracic hemorrhage that may necessitate surgical intervention. Maintaining a patent, intact chest drainage system is vital to reestablish negative pressure within the chest cavity and expansion of the lungs. The patient should be positioned with chest tubes and surgical side up.

150. A) Educate the family about ethical responsibility in regard to pain management, give the prescribed pain medication, and evaluate the patient in 30 minutes

Many families fear that end-of-life pain control will cause a resurgence of an addiction in a patient. It is the nurse's ethical responsibility to provide adequate pain management without bias. Withholding pain medication would not be ethical. The nurse should provide the family with appropriate education.

151. D) The use of both IRBs will increase patient protection and safety

Utilization of local and central institutional review boards (IRBs) provides additional review with committees who are not working in tandem to ensure human subject clinical trial participants are safe and research is being performed per guidelines from regulatory authorities. The local IRB, although affiliated with the institution performing the research, is not privy to information about the participants as they are still protected by HIPAA. When local and central IRBs review a project, they do not approve individual pieces of the clinical trial as they require all the information to make an informed decision.

152. D) *Clostridioides difficile*

Klebsiella, Streptococcus pyogenes, and *Staphylococcus aureus* are gram-negative bacteria that commonly cause sepsis. *Clostridioides difficile* is gram-positive bacteria.

153. D) Hemorrhagic cystitis

Ifosfamide can cause hemorrhagic cystitis, which is a diffuse inflammatory condition of the bladder resulting in bleeding from the bladder mucosa. Symptoms include the sudden onset of gross hematuria and pain in urination. Prophylactic treatment with Mesna is recommended to protect the lining of the bladder against damage from ifosfamide and reduce the risk of hemorrhagic cystitis. Neutropenia and thrombocytopenia can be related to the use of ifosfamide, but they would not present with acute hematuria and pain and burning on urination. Tumor lysis syndrome is not related to use of ifosfamide.

154. A) The consent must be translated into the patient's preferred language

The consent must be translated into the patient's preferred language by a certified medical. It is imperative that the healthcare provider speaks with the patient about all of the elements of informed consent according to FDA requirements. The patient's family cannot serve as the translator, nor can the healthcare provider translate for themselves.

155. B) Colorectal and breast

Peutz-Jegher syndrome is an inherited condition that increases risk of developing hamartomatous polyps in the digestive tract. Individuals with Peutz-Jeghers syndrome are at a greater risk of developing colorectal, breast, cervical, uterine, ovarian, pancreatic, and lung cancers. Peutz-Jeghers syndrome does not increase risk for renal or prostate cancers, leukemias, or lymphomas.

156. B) Creatinine 4.5 mg/dL

Patients with multiple myeloma are at risk of acute kidney failure. Creatinine measures how well the kidneys are filtering waste from the blood. Elevated creatinine levels indicate abnormal kidney function and require immediate attention. Often patients will require dialysis until the disease is under control.

157. B) Vaginal candidiasis

Vaginal candidiasis is a fungal infection caused by *Candida,* a yeast. Vaginal candidiasis is commonly called a "vaginal yeast infection." Symptoms include vaginal discharge, vaginal itching/soreness, and pain during urination or sexual intercourse. Patients who are receiving chemotherapy or steroids are at an increased risk for developing vaginal candidiasis. It is treated with antifungal medications such as fluconazole. Aspergillosis is a fungal infection that typically affects the respiratory system. Bacterial vaginosis (BV) is a bacterial infection that also causes discharge, but it tends to be white/gray and thin, compared to the white, thick, clumpy discharge seen in candidiasis. BV is also characterized by a fishy odor. It is treated with antibiotics, not antifungals. A patient with rectal abscess would not present with vaginal discharge.

158. D) The patient may need to be referred to a trained specialist since previous sexual counseling by the nurse was ineffective in resolving her issues

Using the PLISSIT Model of Addressing Sexual Functioning, the nurse would first give the patient Permission to raise sexual issues, then give them Limited Information about sexual side effects of treatment, make Specific Suggestions based on evaluation of the presenting problem, and then refer for Intensive Therapy if the patient's issues are not resolving. Since the first three levels were ineffective, the nurse understands that the patient may need the assistance of a trained specialist.

159. A) "Chemotherapy affects rapidly growing cells, such as the cells in your mouth, leading to mouth sores."

Doxorubicin and cyclophosphamide treatment is chemotherapy, not radiation. Chemotherapy affects any cells in the body that rapidly grow and divide. Cells in the mucosal lining along the GI tract, hair cells, and stem cells are all rapidly growing and dividing cells that are affected during chemotherapy.

160. A) Administer narcotic analgesia

The symptoms suggest that an obstruction of the urinary tract is present, which can be caused by scar tissues from radiation therapy. The pain of an obstruction can be excruciating; therefore, the administration of a narcotic analgesia is the most appropriate first response. A CT scan of the abdomen can be helpful in diagnosing the problem, particularly high-speed or dual-energy CT, which may reveal scar tissues. Simple abdominal X-rays are used less frequently because this kind of imaging test can miss scar tissue or small stones. Lithotripsy may be ordered if there is a conclusive diagnosis of stones, but this would not be indicated in patients with scar tissue. Providing the patient with a strainer to catch passed stones will not treat the pain being experienced by the patient, nor will it identify any other cause of pain.

161. B) POLST form

POLST is an order from a provider that specifies the medical care and end-of-life wishes of a person with a serious illness. A Do Not Resuscitate (DNR) form also includes similar details; however, a DNR cannot be transferred between hospitals in many states. The POLST form is more likely to be transferred with a patient. Palliative care and hospice forms are not official documents.

162. A) The drug can cause flu-like symptoms and depression

Interferon is an immunotherapy agent used to treat certain kinds of cancers. The nurse should advise the patient that it can cause flu-like symptoms and depression. It does not generally cause severe nausea and vomiting. Grapefruit juice does not interfere with the mechanism of action of interferon, so the patient does not have to avoid grapefruit juice during treatment. The patient can continue to use salt substitutes and eat high-potassium foods.

163. C) Increased risk of genetic mutations

Due to a number of socioeconomic factors, underserved populations have decreased access to preventive care, decreased compliance with treatment, and increased risk of diagnosis at advanced stages of the disease. Genetic mutations are related to specific ethnic groups and are correlated with poor survival rates in underserved populations.

164. A) Temporary housing program for patients receiving cancer treatment

The patient may benefit from financial counseling regarding all expected out-of-pocket costs, a payment plan with the hospital billing department, drug discount programs, and other Patient Assistance Programs (PAPs). Although the patient cannot currently afford to live on their own, a temporary housing program is not required, as the patient is able to live with a sibling.

165. B) Avoid spicy foods

A patient with grade 2 mucositis will have erythema and ulcers with moderate pain. It should not interfere with oral intake; however, the patient should be instructed to avoid foods that are spicy, acidic, salty, coarse, or dry. They should keep their mouth moist by sucking on ice chips and taking frequent sips of water. While they should keep their mouths clean, brushing teeth four times a time may further irritate the ulcers. Mouth rinse may be used, but it should be a non-alcohol-based solution as alcohol can dry the mouth.

Index

NOTE: Page numbers followed by "f" and "t" refer to figures and tables, respectively.